• • • • • • •
The Cognitive Neuroscience of Memory

THE

COGNITIVE

NEUROSCIENCE

OF MEMORY

an introduction

• • • • • • • • • • • • •

Howard Eichenbaum

Laboratory of Cognitive Neurobiology
Boston University
Boston, Massachusetts

OXFORD
UNIVERSITY PRESS

2002

OXFORD
UNIVERSITY PRESS

Oxford   New York
Athens   Auckland   Bangkok   Bogotá   Buenos Aires   Cape Town
Chennai   Dar es Salaam   Delhi   Florence   Hong Kong   Istanbul   Karachi
Kolkata   Kuala Lumpur   Madrid   Melbourne   Mexico City   Mumbai   Nairobi
Paris   São Paulo   Shanghai   Singapore   Taipei   Tokyo   Toronto   Warsaw

and associated companies in
Berlin   Ibadan

Published by Oxford University Press, Inc.
198 Madison Avenue, New York, New York 10016
http://www.oup-usa.org
1-800-334-4249

Oxford is a registered trademark of Oxford University Press.

Library of Congress Cataloging-in-Publication Data
Eichenbaum, Howard.
The cognitive neuroscience of memory : an introduction/
Howard Eichenbaum.
p.;cm   Includes bibliographical references and index.
ISBN 0-19-514174-1 (cloth)—ISBN 0-19-514175-X (pbk.)
1. Memory. I. Title
[DNLM: 1. Memory—physiology. 2. Brain—physiology.
3. Cognition—physiology.
WL   102 E338c 2002]   QP406 .E334 2002   612.89—dc21   2001036607

1 3 5 7 9 8 6 4 2
Printed in the United States of America
on acid-free paper.

• • • • • •
Preface

This book is written for undergraduate students and others who seek an overview of progress in understanding how the brain accomplishes one of its most marvelous acts, memory. At the outset I review the history of thinking and research on the biological bases of memory, and highlight discoveries made in a "Golden Era" that spanned from the late nineteenth century into the twentieth century. During this period major breakthroughs were made, revealing secrets about the fundamental elements of the brain and how they work. Although these discoveries were about brain function in general, many of the researchers were interested in the applicability of their findings to the phenomenon of memory. Also, during the Golden Era four main themes in memory research were initiated. In my introduction, I attempt to give the reader an appreciation for how those themes emerged from the discoveries made in that period.

Those four themes provide the framework for the remainder of the book. The first theme is "connection," and it considers how memory is fundamentally based on alterations in the connectivity of neurons. This section of the book covers the most well-studied models of cellular mechanisms of neural plasticity that may underlie memory. The second theme is "cognition," which involves fundamental issues in the psychological structure of memory. This section of the book considers the competition among views on the nature of cognitive processes that underlie memory, and tells how the controversy was eventually resolved. The third theme is "compartmentalization," which is akin to the classic problem of memory localization. However, unlike localization, the notion of "compartments" is intended to avoid the notion that particular memories are pigeonholed into specific loci, and instead emphasize that different forms of memory are accomplished by distinct modules or brain systems. This section of the book surveys the evidence for multiple memory systems, and outlines how they are mediated by different brain structures and systems. The fourth and final theme is "consolidation," the process by which memories are transformed from a labile trace into a permanent store. In this section of the book, I summarize our current understanding of two distinct stages in memory consolidation. One stage involves molecular and cellular mechanisms that underlie a fixation of changes in the connection strengths introduced earlier. The other stage of consolidation occurs at the level of brain systems and involves a reorganization and restructuring of the circuits that store and retrieve memories. For heuristic purposes I attempt to deal with these two stages separately, although they are highly interrelated by the brain mechanisms involved.

I hope the book will be of use to cognitive scientists, biologists, and psychologists who seek an introduction to biological investigations of memory, and to undergraduate students seeking an expanded coverage of the neurobiology of memory for courses in learning and memory or behavioral and cognitive neuroscience. Readers will benefit from a solid background in basic molecular biology and neurobiology. However, a brief overview of the necessary biological background is included.

It bears mentioning that substantial portions of the material presented in this book are derived from another recent book, *From Conditioning to Conscious Recollection: Multiple Memory Systems of the Brain* (Oxford University Press), coauthored by myself and Neal Cohen. Although there is overlap in the materials of the two books, they differ substantially in two ways. First, the earlier book has a much more limited scope. It is a comprehensive presentation and synthesis, as well as an attempt at reconciliation of current controversies, on the specific topic of multiple memory systems. Its aim is focused on a thorough analysis of one of the central themes of the present book, the theme of "compartmentalization." By contrast, the scope of the present book is much broader. It provides a general introduction to the history of brain and memory research, and is constructed as a comprehensive survey of topics in memory research, including the molecular and cellular bases of memory in cells, invertebrate model systems, and vertebrate systems, the psychological foundations of learning theory, and the phenomena of memory consolidation, as well as the topic of multiple memory systems. Second, the earlier book is constructed for an advanced readership, primarily scientific colleagues and graduate students with considerable previous background in relevant areas of neuroscience and the neurobiology of memory. By contrast, the treatment of topics in the present book is introductory. This book intentionally makes no effort at being detailed or thorough in the described experiments in any research area. Rather, it is aimed to show how we address central questions in brain mechanisms of memory, and seeks to provide a basic understanding of each of several central issues through a presentation of a selected set of classic and recent exemplary experiments.

In addition, for students and instructors who plan to use this book as a text, I have included a set of heuristic aids. First, I emphasize a historical perspective at the outset, with a review of memory research from its very beginnings. Second, the book is divided into four sections, each of which distinguishes a fundamental theme in memory research. Each section is introduced with a theoretical and historical overview. Third, each chapter begins with a set of "Study Questions" aimed to guide the student toward the central issues in that chapter. I encourage students to think about these questions as they read the text, and then write out detailed answers in preparation for exams. Fourth, each chapter ends with a "Summing Up" section that recaps the major take home points in that chapter and attempts to synthesize the several issues that arose. Fifth, I have included a Glossary that contains definitions of frequently used and important terms. In addition, it may be useful to have a basic neuroscience text available as an adjunct reference for the course. Such a text will help orient students to anatomical terms and provide supplementary information about the anatomy and physiology of brain structures described here. It is hoped that these aids will help students in formulating their "schemas" for the topics in this book and permit them to take more away from the information in it.

Considerable appreciation goes to Michelle Barbera who created the illustrations for this book, and to Fiona Stevens of Oxford University Press for her counsel on its organization and content. Thanks also to Neal Cohen, my long time collaborator in thinking and writing about memory, including the related co-authored book described above. More generally, I am indebted to the many students whom I have had the pleasure of teaching over the last couple of decades; they have contributed by asking the hard questions and demanding clear explanations, some of which I hope are conveyed in this text. Finally, I owe a fundamental debt to Edith Eichenbaum, a professional teacher like me, who has provided generous encouragement and guidance throughout my scholarly life.

• • • • • •
Contents

Part IV Consolidation:
The Fixation and Reorganization of Memories, 283

●●●●●●
The Cognitive Neuroscience of Memory

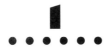

Introduction:
Four Themes in Research on
the Neurobiology of Memory

STUDY QUESTIONS

What is the neurobiology of memory?

What major questions about memory are pursued with a neurobiological approach, and how are these questions addressed in experimental analyses?

What are meant by "connection," "cognition," "compartmentalization," and "consolidation"?

Our memories reflect the accumulation of a lifetime of experience and, in this sense, our memories are who we are. Surely the background of our makeup is determined largely by our genes; genetics sets the range of what we can aspire to be. However, by contrast to generality of genetic limitations, the specifics are a matter of *memory*. We learn to walk, to dance, to drive a car, to throw a ball, and to play a video game—a myriad of acquired skills we come to take for granted. We learn to fear dangerous situations, to appreciate particular types of music and styles of art—a broad range of aversions and enjoyments we have assumed as elements of our preferences and personality. We learn to speak, and to speak and understand our particular language. We learn world history, and we learn our own family tree and personal autobiography—all of these, and much, much more, compose the vast contents and intricate, complex organization of memories that make each of us a unique human being. So, the analysis of memory is a search for self-understanding, an adventure that promises to reveal the inner secrets of how we came to be who we are.

The nature of memory—its basic biological structure, its psychological character and organization, and its longevity—has been the subject of investigations by philosophers, writers, and scientists for hundreds of years, and each approach offers its own distinct avenue for understanding memory. Recently, with the rise of modern methods of cognitive science and neuroscience, and their combination, many new and deep insights about the mechanisms of memory have emerged. These observations have also led us to a greater general understanding about the mind and about brain functions that mediate cognition, emotion, behavior, and consciousness. The aim of this book is to explore memory from the perspective of cognitive neuroscience, offering a historical and a current overview of how brain functions in memory have been studied and what we have learned about memory as an encompassing aspect of the mind.

The present chapter introduces some of the philosophical and historical underpinnings of research on the biological bases of memory. I begin by presenting four central themes that have guided memory research for over a hundred years. Substantial preliminary evidence regarding each of these themes emerged during a "Golden Era" for neuroscience in the latter half of the nineteenth century and the beginning of the twentieth century. A brief introduction to some of these accomplishments provides the background for a subsequent, more detailed summary of progress on each of the four central themes in the remainder of the book.

The four "C's"

At the outset of systematic investigations of the nervous system four major themes dominated considerations of brain function of relevance to memory. In part to facilitate your memory for them, I refer to these themes as the four "C's": *connection*, *cognition*, *compartmentalization*, and *consolidation*.

√ The first theme—*connection*—concerns the most basic level of analysis of memory function, the basic nature of the circuitry of the brain including the elements of information processing and how they communicate with one another in the service of memory. The emphasis on "connection" here reflects the major conclusion that has emerged in this research—that memory is encoded within the dynamics, that is, the changeability or plasticity, of connections between nerve cells. More specifically, the consensual view from the perspective of memory as a phenomenon of brain cells is that memories are instantiated by alterations of the strength

or reliability of communication between cells via their synaptic connections. Efforts to understand the nature of the storage mechanism are aimed
at identifying the biological materials, the cellular "switch," from which
memories are made. Accordingly, cellular and molecular analyses of memory have been focused on characterizing the modifiability or plasticity of
neural connections that underlie memory performance. Experimental research in this area seeks to discover specific molecular events that form
the basis of a memory, and subcellular structures that support neural connections that accomplish memory. This research also asks how the basic
memory storage mechanism can be modulated by natural neurochemical
events and manipulated by genetic and pharmacological interventions.

√ The second theme—*cognition*—refers to the nature of memories at the
highest level of analysis, the psychological level. Consider the following
unusual instance of memory. You walk into a new room, an odd colored
light fills the room, then a loud and frightening rattling noise goes off and
persists—you exit with haste. Subsequently, you happen to enter that room
again, and again the odd light comes on. You immediately leave. Is the
memory for that event represented in terms of a new association between
particular novel sensory stimulus, the odd light, and the escape behavior
you executed in response to it, what psychologists call a "stimulus–
response association"? Or is the fundamental association between the light
and the consequent irritation the loud sound evoked in you, what psychologists call a "stimulus–reinforcer association"? Or are the concepts of
stimulus–response and stimulus–reinforcer associations altogether too sim-
plistic a view of how your memory is stored? Does your memory representation contain a record of the entire series of relevant and peripheral
events that constituted the learning episode? Is that memory isolated among
a large and loose *collection* of episodic memories? Or is that memory contained within a systematic *organization* of other experiences in the same
building that form a network of knowledge about your experiences there?

Questions about the nature of memory representations have been at
the center of debates about whether the complexity of memory can or cannot be reduced to a set of simple associative principles. During the Golden
Era there were divergent and strong views espousing either that memory
can be simplified to a set of principles about stimulus–response and stimulus–reinforcer associations or that memory involves complex networks
that can be understood only in terms of cognitive operations that are not
reducible to simple associative mechanisms. The understanding that has
emerged from this area of research is that there are mechanisms that guide
behavior from stimulus–response and from stimulus–reinforcer associations, and there is a "cognitive" form of memory that is distinguished in

both its psychological mechanisms and anatomical pathways from the other forms of memory.

The third theme—*compartmentalization*—addresses the question of memory localization. This question appeared early on in debates about whether memory can be localized to a particular area of the brain, especially the cerebral cortex, or whether it is distributed throughout the cortex, or indeed the entire brain. The major conclusion that has emerged on this theme is that memory as a whole is distributed widely in the brain. But, at the same time, different kinds of memory are accomplished by specific brain modules, circuits, pathways, or systems. That is, memory is *compartmentalized*. The compartmentalization occurs at two levels. First, the cerebral cortex is composed of many anatomically circumscribed "modules," each of which makes a correspondingly specific contribution to memory function. Second, there are multiple memory systems in the brain, all of which involve the cerebral cortex but they diverge in pathways leading from the cortex to other structures that lie beneath the cortex (subcortical structures), and the systems formed by these cortical–subcortical pathways accomplish different kinds of memory. This research area also considers the relationship between memory and other cognitive processes, including consciousness, coordinated movement, and emotion. The major aim of research on brain modules and systems is to identify and distinguish the different roles of specific brain structures and pathways, usually by contrasting the effects of selective damage to specific brain areas. Another major strategy in attacking this issue focuses on localizing brain areas that are activated, that is, whose neurons are "turned on" during particular aspects of memory processing. Some of these studies use new functional imaging techniques to view activation of brain areas in humans performing memory tests. Another approach seeks to characterize the "code" for memory within the activity patterns of single nerve cells in animals, by asking how information is represented by the activity patterns within the circuits of different structures in the relevant brain systems.

The fourth theme—*consolidation*—concerns when and how memories become permanent. It is well known that some experiences are rapidly forgotten, whereas others are remembered for a lifetime. And there have been many anecdotal and clinical reports that various forms of interference or head or brain injury can "wipe out" memories that were recently acquired but have less effect on memories acquired remotely before the interfering event or injury. These observations suggest that memories are initially labile and later become resistant to loss, suggesting a process of consolidation during which memories take on a permanent form. Modern research has shown that there are two general kinds of consolidation. One of these—which I call "fixation"—involves a cascade of molecular and cellular events during which the changes in connections between cells become permanent in several minutes to hours after a memory is formed. This process can be influenced by many factors, including among them a specific brain system for modulation of memory fixation. The other kind of consolidation process is called "reorganization" because this process involves a prolonged period during which distinct brain structures interact with one another, and the outcome is that newly acquired information is integrated into one's previously existing body of knowledge. This reorganizational process therefore involves an entire brain system, and discovering how it works involves a consideration of both the individual contributions of particular parts of the brain system and the nature of interactions among the parts.

The Golden Era

The aim of this chapter is to set the stage for the succeeding sections that will review our understanding of each of the four major themes in memory research, and in doing so provide a framework for understanding the neurobiological bases of memory. I pursue an historical approach, elaborating on each of the four "Cs," beginning with a summary of discoveries made at the threshold of modern neuroscience research on memory in the latter half of the 1800s.

Before that period, some of the critical background had already long been established. In 1664 the early anatomist Willis published the first description of the anatomy of the brain and had suggested that different brain areas controlled distinct functions. Simplified views of the brain and its main components are provided in Figures 1–1 and 1–2. Also, in 1791 Galvani introduced the notion that electricity is the mechanism of nervous conduction. But around the turn of the twentieth century several additional major discoveries formed the full beginning of a scientific analysis of the brain, a Golden Era in which several key findings led toward real progress in understanding brain function and memory. Some of these contributions represented major advances to the field of neuroscience in general, and others pertained to memory research in particular. Here I highlight a few of the major insights of that period that have had lasting impact. Put together, these observations should give the reader a sense of the field of neuroscience, and especially about the neurobiology of memory, upon which all subsequent progress is based.

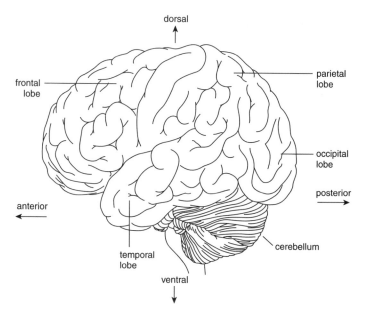

Figure 1–1. Side view of the human brain, showing the major subdivisions of the cerebral cortex, the cerebellum, and terminology used to describe relative locations in the brain.

Connection: Cellular substrates of brain communication and memory

One main set of advances that laid the foundation for memory research involved discoveries about the basic building blocks of brain circuits. These discoveries identified the fundamental elements of the brain, characterized

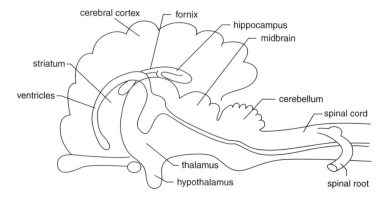

Figure 1–2. Cut-away side view schematic of a generic mammalian brain and spinal cord, showing locations of major subcortical brain structures and the system of ventricles (a hollow circulatory system running throughout).

how they are assembled into simple functional circuits, and demonstrated that they can be modified during learning.

The neuron doctrine

One major area of discovery about the brain that contributed directly to our understanding of the cellular and molecular substrates of memory was the development of the "neuron doctrine" by the Spanish anatomist Santiago Ramon y Cajal. The neuron doctrine is the notion that the brain is composed of discrete nerve cells, and that these cells are the essential units of information processing, connected to one another so as to transfer and integrate information in large-scale networks. At the time of Cajal, this view was not entirely new, but it was also not widely accepted. Rather, Cajal's work addressed a major controversy about the nature of connections between neurons. In the debate, one camp, called the "reticularists," argued that the brain is a single unified interconnected network of fibers in which all the cells were fused to one another. By contrast, the other camp, called the "antireticularists," suspected that the brain was composed of independent nerve cells as units, but they had no definitive evidence. Before Cajal, the strongest argument for independent cells came from the observation that small lesions in one area resulted in sharply defined areas of degeneration, not what one would expect of a fused network.

Cajal's success was based on his adoption of a new staining method that was developed by another anatomist named Camillo Golgi in 1873. The method involved a "black reaction," a new silver stain that had the remarkable quality of darkening the entire cell membrane of a neuron. At the same time, the staining was selective to only a small fraction of the neuron population in an area of brain tissue. Thick sections of the brain stained this way provided a full view of individual cells standing out clearly against the background of many other surrounding pale cells. Using this method Cajal was able to provide the most striking confirmation of the already existing identification of the major elements of nerve cells. As shown in Figure 1–3, these include the cell body, the multiple fine processes that extended from one end of the cell body called dendrites, and the single larger process extending from the other end of the cell body called the axon. Also, he noted the specialization of the axon as it contacted the dendrites of other cells; this specialization would later be called the synapse (see next section).

Cajal attempted many variations of the procedure. He found that tissue with less myelin, the insulation layer of axons, produced the clearest images of neuronal processes, and the best cases were found in young brains and in birds. He also found that thicker sections allowed one to examine all of the extensions of the cell membrane that connect with other

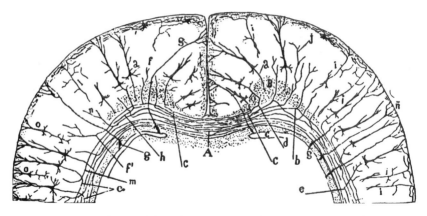

Figure 1–3. Drawing by Cajal based on a section through the cortex of a 20-day-old mouse. Note the different types of cells, all oriented vertically from the superficial layer at the top to the corpus callosum (indicated by the letter A) at the bottom, where the axons of the cortex bundle (from DeFelipe and Jones, 1988).

cells. In each of several different preparations he found elaborate endings of axons in nests or baskets of axonal "arborization"—a treelike branching—of the axon connecting it to multiple parts of another cell or multiple cells. In no case did he observe the stain continuing into the next cell, as would be expected if there was a fusion of the axonal ending with dendrites of another cell. Cajal concluded that there must be some method of communication between cells that did not involve a joining of their membranes. Cajal's preparations and the evidence they provided were elegant, and convinced other anatomists and physiologists that each cell was contained within a membrane and was separate although in contact with other cells. These observations won him the Nobel Prize in 1906.

Cajal was also able to make key conclusions about the function of neurons from his observations on their anatomy. As said previously, he confirmed the existence of all of the major components of the nerve cell. Moreover, in his studies on visual and olfactory sensory structures, Cajal noted that the dendrites pointed toward the outside world and that the axon pointed toward the brain. From these observations he deduced that nerve cells were functionally polarized, such that information flows from the dendrites to the axon and is subsequently conveyed by the specialized connection to the dendrites of another nerve cell.

These conclusions established the essential view that the integration of information occurred by the summation of signals converging from the axons of several neurons onto the dendrites of cells receiving those inputs. In addition, Cajal developed some important and prescient ideas directly relevant to the basic memory mechanism. He studied the brains of several species and observed that the vertebrates higher in the phylogenetic scale had a greater number of connections between nerve cells. He concluded that the increase in connectivity could be the basis of greater intellectual power of the higher species. He suggested that mental exercise could facilitate increased connectivity through a greater number and intensity of the connections, and that these changes in connectivity could coincide with the acquisition of skills such as playing a musical instrument. Cajal's insights have become key axioms for the study of neuronal function and communication. Moreover, his suggestion that "plasticity" in number and strength of neuronal connections underlies learning guides the search for molecular and cellular substrates of memory.

The reflex arc

In the same period other major advances were made from studies on the physiology of the nervous system. Perhaps most important among these were Charles Sherrington's observations on the nature of reflexes in the spinal cord. Before Sherrington the existence of involuntary muscle actions was already well recognized, including the basic observation that specific sensory stimulation could be "reflected," as if by a mirror, to generate muscle movements—hence the "reflex arc" (Fig. 1–4). In addition it was known that complex reflexes, such as those mediating jumping in frogs or coordinated flying movements in birds, could be elicited even following decapitation, suggesting control of complex coordination could happen at a level below the brain—at the level of the spinal cord. And it was clear that reflex arcs accomplished within the spinal cord could be inhibited by higher level control. However, there was very little understanding of the underlying circuitry that accomplished either simple or complex reflexes.

Sherrington made many contributions that provided the foundations for our understanding of neural circuitry that are as relevant today as they were when he made his discoveries. Even before Cajal's convincing anatomical evidence was provided, Sherrington had reached the conclusion that neurons must be independent elements. Part of the evidence came from his studies on neural degeneration, showing that cortical lesions, damage induced by heat or cutting, resulted in restricted, not diffuse patterns of degeneration. He also realized that the neuron doctrine, and the detailed evidence showing the connection was from axons to dendrites, could explain why neural transmission was one-way. And the discontiguity between cells provided a mechanism for why there was a time lag in reflexes such that they were much slower than predicted from the speed of conduction of the neural impulse—the loss of time in long-range conduction had to involve the extra time re-

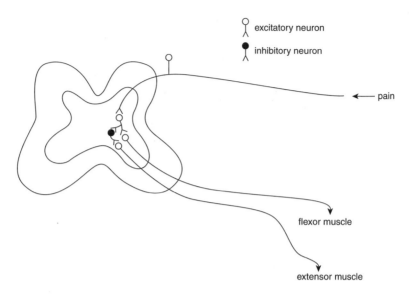

Figure 1–4. A schematic diagram of some components of the pain withdrawal reflex arc. Pain to the skin activates a sensory neuron whose cell body is just outside the spinal cord. The axon synapses with an interneuron within the spinal cord, which excites a motor neuron that causes contraction of the relevant flexor muscle, and excites an inhibitory interneuron that decreases activity in motor neurons that activate the extensor muscles in the same limb.

quired for an impulse to jump a "gap" between the neural elements. Sherrington is credited for inventing the term *synapse* to describe the hypothetical junction between neurons where transmission occurs.

In his classic studies on the "knee jerk" reflex, Sherrington demonstrated the details of his model reflex arc, wherein specific sensory information is gathered at the input end of the arc and then relayed to turn specific muscles on and off at the output end. He provided critical evidence for the existence of the "sixth sense"—specialized sensory receptors in the muscle that monitor muscle length and tension, and showed that these sensory elements send nerves into the spinal cord. He also contributed to the characterization of the maps of sensory inputs from the skin surface into the spinal cord, the so-called dermatomes. By isolating and stimulating sensory roots he could determine which regions of the skin evoked reflexive movements. Conversely, to map the output pattern, he stimulated individual spinal cord motor roots and characterized which muscles were activated.

Important as these discoveries were, perhaps Sherrington's most outstanding contribution was elucidating some of the complexities of the circuitry that underlie reflexes. He concluded that, even at the level of the spinal cord, reflex arcs are not entirely separate or independent. In these circuits the initial sensory neurons in the spinal cord receive dedicated inputs, but the output neurons of even the simplest reflexes received information from many of those input cells (Fig. 1–4). Thus, consistent with Cajal's observations on the anatomy of nerve cells, there was a summation or integration of both inputs into a common path that could guide complex behavioral actions. And there were two major kinds of inputs that combined in this integration. There were excitatory inputs by which an impulse from the input cell increased the likelihood of impulse generation in the next cell. And there were inhibitory inputs by which an impulse in the input cell decreased the likelihood of impulse generation in the next cell. He also made major discoveries about the phenomenon of reciprocal innervation, the basic mechanism by which excitatory and inhibitory influences are coordinated to mediate movement. Within this scheme every action by one muscle is coordinated with an opposing action of complementary muscles. For example, the simple act of walking involves the coordinated actions of flexing one group of muscles during the extension of others, followed by the opposite complementary actions in executing the next step in walking.

In addition, Sherrington employed the technique of decerebration, cutting the spinal cord just behind the brain, to show that complex coordinated actions existed even without higher level cerebral control. He showed, for example, in a decerebrate cat, when a forelimb was excited to move forward, the hindlimb on the same side moved back and the two legs on the other side of the body exhibited the opposing movements, producing the pattern seen in normal walking, but without conscious cerebral control. In studies on the "scratch reflex" he showed the specificity of arm movements for scratching evoked in response to small areas of skin stimulation. Furthermore, in extensions of these studies he revealed that coordinated and directed scratching movement patterns could be played out over time, with alternating extension and flexion of muscles at different levels of the limb to produce repeated scratching movements, plus postural adjustments in the other limbs to support standing without the use of the scratching limb.

Sherrington envisioned all of this as accomplished within the spinal cord, by a "chaining" of reflexes wherein successive coordinated movements are elicited by their predecessors. These elements provided the outline for his formulation on the integrative action of the nervous system. In this prototype for modern views, Sherrington proposed a hierarchy of coordinated control wherein the cerebral cortex is acknowledged as the newest and most complicated switchboard of reflexes, and successively lower centers in the brain stem and spinal cord to mediate more and more specific, yet still complex and coordinated actions.

The conditioned reflex

Initially unrelated to this course of research, the Russian physiologist Ivan Pavlov was making landmark discoveries about the nervous control of digestion. He discovered that the release of digestive fluids was controlled by the nervous system, contrary to the prevailing view that digestive fluids were released as a consequence of mechanical stimulation by food directly onto the stomach wall. To test his hypothesis that the nervous system was involved, Pavlov developed a surgical procedure in which he severed the gullet and attached both open ends to the skin of the neck. This allowed him to either introduce food into the mouth and upper gullet and then retrieve it without going to the stomach, or introduce food directly into the stomach. He found that food stimulation associated with ingestion caused the release of gastric fluids in the stomach, even when the food never reached its normal target. He concluded that food excites the gustatory sensory apparatus in the mouth and gullet, transmitting signals into the brain stem, which, via the vagus nerve, controls the release of gastric fluids. From a neurophysiological perspective, one can say that Pavlov identified a reflex arc for digestion, and for this he received the Nobel Prize in 1904.

But by the time he received the prize, Pavlov had already turned his interest to an intriguing report that gastric juices of a horse could begin to flow not only with a direct application of gustatory stimuli but also even when the animal only caught sight of hay. Pavlov replicated the phenomenon of "psychic secretion" using dogs and measured the generation of fluids from the salivary glands. He found that the sight of a piece of beef indeed caused salivation, but he also found that the phenomenon was unreliable. The salivation tended to decrease following repeated presentations of the sight of beef. Conversely, sometimes salivation was initiated by events that preceded the sight of beef, for example, when the person who regularly provided the food merely appeared in the testing room.

Pavlov set out to meticulously control the stimuli available to the animal, and he tried out many arbitrary stimuli—including the famous bell rung prior to the presentation of food. Based on the results from a broad range of experimental manipulations, Pavlov concluded there were two kinds of reflexes. One kind of reflex is "unconditioned," identical with the innate and stable reflexes of Sherrington. The unconditioned reflex is composed of a particular unconditioned stimulus (US) that inevitably elicits its characteristic unconditioned response (UR). The other kind of reflex is "conditioned," that is, acquired through experience. This kind of reflex is the unstable one, and is composed of an arbitrary conditioned stimulus (CS) that when paired with a US comes to elicit a conditioned response (CR) similar in form to the UR. Pavlov identified the critical importance of two parameters in establishing and maintaining the conditioned reflex: the close temporal contiguity of the CR and US—the CS must lead the US by a particular time interval, and the CS must consistently predict the US.

Combined, the contributions of Cajal, Sherrington, and Pavlov, as well as many others, laid the basic framework for succeeding views of brain circuitry and function, as well as its role in memory. They showed that the basic elements of the circuits are independent neurons that communicate across synapses, that these elements are integrated within complex patterns of circuitry for coordinated action built up from simple reflex arcs, and that these circuits can be modified to support learned reflexes. These insights set the stage for future investigations on the mechanisms of how connections between neurons are modified during learning, and guided the development of views on the organization of memory for both simple and complex behaviors.

Cognition and memory

During the same period, distinct developments were made toward characterizing the nature of memory from a purely psychological perspective. Two main and competing lines of theorizing developed. One school, called "behaviorism," developed out of a desire to provide a rigorous science of memory consistent with the findings on the neurophysiology of conditioned reflexes, and attempted to explain all of learned behavior on the basis of elements of association and conditioned responses. The other school, called "cognitivism," emphasized the complexity of learned behavior, and its promoters could not be persuaded that all aspects of cognition, insight, and planning could be captured in an elaborate account of associations or reflex chains and instead required a more elaborate conception and, correspondingly, a more complex neural instantiation.

Behaviorism

The tradition of rigorous methodology in memory research began with Herman Ebbinghaus, who admired the mathematical analyses that had been brought to the psychophysics of perception, and he sought to develop similarly precise and quantitative methods for the study of memory. Basing his work on a large number of pioneering studies, in 1885 Ebbinghaus published a monograph that set a new standard for the systematic study of memory. Ebbinghaus rejected the use of introspection as a methodology that was prominent in previous conceptual schemes about memory. In its place he developed several key new techniques that would control the nature of the material to be learned and provide quantitative objective assessments of memory performance. To create learning materials that were both simple and homogeneous in content Ebbinghaus invented the "nonsense syllable," a meaningless letter string composed of two consonants with a vowel between (e.g., "ket," "poc." "baf"). With this invention he avoided the confounding influences of what he called "interest," "beauty," and other features that he felt might affect the memorability of real words. In addition, the nonsense syllable simultaneously equalized the length and meaningfulness of the items, albeit by minimizing the former and eliminating the latter. Furthermore, to measure memory Ebbinghaus invented the use of "savings" scores that measured retention in terms of the reduction in trials required to relearn material. In addition, he was the first to employ mathematical–statistical analyses to test the reliability of his findings.

It was also in this period that systematic studies on animal learning and memory had their beginnings. In 1901 Small introduced the maze to studies of animal learning, inspired by the famous garden maze at Hampton Court in London (Fig. 1–5). He began what would become an industry of systematic and quantitative studies to identify the minute details of how rats acquired specific responses in repetitions of turns taken in the maze. But he observed that within a trial or two rats prefer a shortcut over the response route that had been reinforced on many previous trials, leading Small to conclude that future experiments should investigate the natural biological character of the animal if one is to be able to interpret the findings. These initial observations set forth a major controversy in the field of animal learning. Can learning be reduced to a set of arbitrary associations between external stimuli and behavioral responses, or must one consider issues such as cognition, insight, and motive?

At the turn of the century, Edward Thorndike had invented a "puzzle box" in which he observed cats learning to manipulate a door latch to allow escape from a holding chamber. Based on his observations he proposed the "law of effect," which stated that rewards reinforced repetitions of the specific behaviors that preceded them. (This simple law would be reinvented and extensively elaborated by B.F. Skinner in the 1950s to explain all of learned behavior.) In the same period John Watson published his accounts on maze learning by rats. In one of his most famous experi-

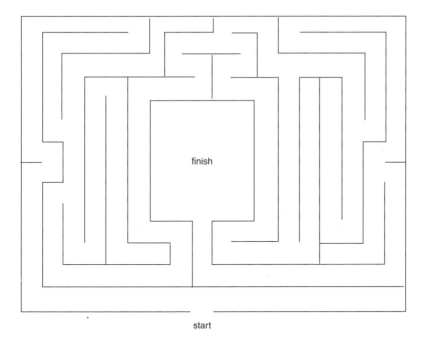

Figure 1–5. Small's maze, based on the maze at Hampton Court. The animal entered at the bottom of the maze and had to find its way to the central open area.

ments, Watson trained rats to run a maze and then searched for the un-derlying stimulus control by eliminating one sense after another. He found the rats could still run the maze with only the kinesthetic (muscle) sense remaining, leading him to conclude that the learning must be mediated by a chain of reflexes, consistent with the evidence from physiology. By 1913 he had accumulated sufficiently compelling evidence for the reductionist strategy that he wrote a "behaviorist manifesto," formalizing the view that learning could be understood in terms of simple stimulus and response as-sociations without resorting to considerations of vague concepts such as consciousness.

Cognitivism

William James captured prevalent views of the time on the origins of both the behaviorist and cognitivist perspectives in his classic *The Principles of Psychology*. Within this treatise, James considered reflex mechanisms and pathways as the essential building blocks of memory, and he called these the mechanisms for the formation of a "habit." James viewed habits as built upon a very primitive mechanism that is common among biological systems and due to an inherent plasticity of organic materials. Within the nervous system he viewed the mechanism of habit in terms of its known electrical activity, and suggested that electrical currents should more readily traverse paths previously taken. Thus, James felt that a simple habit was nothing more than the discharge of a well-worn reflex path, entirely consistent with the views of emerging behaviorism. Furthermore, James expanded on this notion, attributing great importance to habits as the building blocks of more complicated behavioral repertoires. He suggested that well-practiced behaviors and skills, including walking, writing, fencing, and singing, are mediated by concatenated discharges in connected reflex paths, organized to awaken each other in succession to mediate the serial production of learned movement sequences.

However, while acknowledging the importance of habits as the fundamental mechanism that underlies memory, James recognized real "memory" as something altogether different from habit. James argued that there were two forms of memory, differentiated by their timing and by their role. He suggested that initially there is a *primary memory*, what we today call short-term or working memory, a short-lived state where new information has achieved consciousness and belongs to our stream of thought. Primary memory also serves as the gateway by which material would enter *secondary memory*, what we now call long-term memory. James emphasized that secondary memory involves both the intellectual content of information we have learned and the additional consciousness of the experience during learning.

In addition to the feature of personal consciousness, the full characterization of memory was framed in terms of its structure as an elaborate network of associations. James argued that, while memory is based on the habit mechanism, it is vastly elaborated such that the formation of associations among habits supports the richness of our experience of a memory. Thus, the underlying foundation of recall involves a complex, yet systematic set of associations between any particular item and many other co-occurring items during one's experiences.

It is of interest that James also offered speculations that touched on the biological basis of memory. He suggested that memory depends on two aspects of the habit mechanism. First, how good a memory is depends on the strength or persistence of the pathway—this aspect James suggested was innate. Second, he suggested that memory depends on the number of pathways through which an item is associated. He emphasized the latter as more malleable, and argued that the key to a good memory is to build diverse and multiple associations with one's experiences, weaving information and experiences into systematic relations with each other. The capacity to search through one's network associations was held to be the basis of conscious recollection, and could lead to creative use of memory to address new problems. Conversely, James admonished his students not to simply rehearse learned materials. This, he argued, could lead only to the concatenation of habit pathways that could only be expressed by repetition.

James never contrasted "habit" and "memory" as distinct forms of memory. A more direct recognition of two forms of memory can be attributed to the philosopher Henri Bergson, who in 1911 explicitly proposed that representations of the past survive under two distinct forms, one in the ability to facilitate repetition of specific actions, and the other in independent recollections. The suggestion that habits and memories might both have a common cellular basis, and at the same time exist as distinct forms of memory, would ultimately resolve the controversy between the behaviorist and cognitivist schools. In addition, the notion of different forms of memory would reappear in the solution to the controversy about the compartmentalization of memory discussed next.

Compartmentalization of cortical function and memory

In this same period as advances were made in characterizing reflex circuitry, and the controversy about the nature of memory was brewing, a separate battle was engaged over another critical puzzle about the brain and memory. This controversy focused on the organization of the cerebral cortex. There was already scattered evidence from studies of patients with circumscribed brain damage that the anterior (front) and posterior (back) regions of the cerebral cortex played different functional roles. But no clear functional specifications arose from the early observations. Two dramatically different views emerged during the nineteenth century.

"Organology"

The earliest specific and systematic formulation on cortical localization came in the early 1800s from the German physician Franz Joseph Gall. Following a trend early in the eighteenth century in which scientists were attempting to associate body features with aspects of personality, Gall sought to determine whether there existed variation in structure and function of the brain. He developed a theory of cortical localization, which he called organology, in which each of many independent psychological faculties is mediated by a specialized organ in the brain. The central axiom of this theory was that individual differences in specific faculties were reflected in greater development of the mediating brain organ and, correspondingly, the size of the overlying skull area. The theory was developed using a combination of observations on individual variation in specific psychological faculties and skull areas in humans and on comparisons between the abilities and skulls of animals versus humans. Gall's detailed investigations on humans included a variety of individuals that represented extreme variations in behavioral capacities. He sought out people with a special talent, such as writers, statesmen, and musical and mathematical prodigies, or with a behavioral abnormality, such as lunatics, the feebleminded, and criminals. For each he would interview the person extensively to characterize their unusual behavioral qualities and carefully examine the head for irregularities. Based on his insights about the functional aspects of their abilities and on discovery of unusual skull features, he envisioned a tight correlation between the skull and brain anatomy and a direct link to the unusual aspect of behavior. For example, among his earliest findings on humans was the observation that some people who were outstanding in memorizing verbal material had bulging eyes, suggesting to Gall an enhanced development of an organ in the frontal lobes specialized for verbal memory.

In addition, Gall collected hundreds of skulls from animals and made detailed comparisons between the anatomical features of those skulls and those of humans. The same sort of loose correlation was applied, in this case comparing the psychological abilities of animals both between different species and with humans. From a combination of all this material he devised a system of faculties, some shared by humans and animals and some exclusively human (Fig. 1–6). An example of his reasoning comes

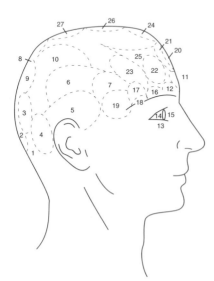

Figure 1–6. Gall's organology scheme. The assignments were: 1. Instinct for reproduction. 2. Love of offspring. 3. Affection. 4. Instinct of self-defense. 5. Carnivorous instinct, tendency to murder. 6. Guile. 7. The feeling of property, theft, hoarding. 8. Pride. 9. Vanity, ambition. 10. Forethought. 11. Educability. 12. Places. 13. Memory of people. 14. Words. 15. Language and speech. 16. Colors. 17. Sounds, music. 18. Sense of connections between numbers. 19. Mechanics of construction. 20. Wisdom. 21. Metaphysics. 22. Satire. 23. Poetry. 24. Kindness. 25. Ability to imitate. 26. Religion. 27. Perseverance.

from his deductions about the faculty of "destructiveness, carnivorous instinct, or tendency to murder," localized to an area above the ears. This designation was strongly based on a combination of observations on animals and humans. That area was larger in carnivores than in grass-eating animals. And the area was overly large in a successful businessman who gave up his profession to become a butcher, in a student who was fond of torturing animals and became a surgeon, and in a pharmacist who became an executioner.

Gall's early attempts to make functional assignments of cortical areas were considerably off-base, due to two major flaws in his methodology. First, Gall's methods were based on individual cases, each of which was subject to considerable interpretation about the nature of the basis of their unusual abilities. Second, Gall simply assumed a close correlation between skull and brain anatomy, and had little interest in examining brain directly. Gall's assumptions led him in the wrong direction in almost every case. Later clinical and experimental studies consistently failed to confirm Gall's specific functional assignments. However, these later studies would demonstrate localization of cortical functions, albeit with different functional designations. Thus, quite rightfully Gall is given considerable credit for the basic insight that the cortex is composed of multiple, functionally distinct areas.

Case studies of human patients with localized cortical damage

More compelling evidence for specific functional designations within the cerebral cortex came from observations of neurological case studies of patients with selective brain damage, and from parallel physiological studies. Among the most important of the case studies on brain pathology was one made by the French physician Paul Broca in 1861. The study involved a 51-year-old man named Lebourgne who had suffered from epilepsy since birth and had later lost the power to speak and developed a right side paralysis and loss of sensitivity. This patient came to Broca's attention when he was admitted to Broca's surgical ward at the hospital for an unrelated disorder, and died within a week. The autopsy revealed a circumscribed area of damage in the third convolution of the frontal lobe on the left side of the cerebral cortex. The patient's disorder was also well circumscribed. He was virtually unable to speak—indeed, he acquired the nickname "Tan" from the only sound he made—but his mouth was not paralyzed and he retained the capacity to hear and understand speech. This case provided a compelling demonstration of a highly severe and selective behavioral disorder related to a specific cortical zone. The argument for localization of higher functions was made all the more compelling with the description of a complementary case by Carl Wernike in 1894. In this case the patient was severely impaired in speech comprehension, without hearing loss or a disorder of speech production, and the damage was circumscribed to a zone within the left temporal cortex.

Experimental neurology and neurophysiology

The evidence from neurological cases was strongly supported by concurrent findings from experimental work on animals. The earliest studies on animals, specifically aimed to test Gall's theory, were reported in 1824 by Flourens. He failed to find localization of sensory and motor functions following cortical damage in birds. These findings and other studies that could not demonstrate selective losses in mammals became the strongest evidence against localization of cortical function. However, the use of birds and other animals with relatively less differentiated cortical areas turned out to be a poor choice for an experimental model in analyses of cortical function. The case for localization was eventually made, from studies using brain stimulation in dogs, by Gustav Fritsch and Eduard Hitzig published in 1870, and with the careful work of David Ferrier using brain lesions in monkeys, presented in 1874.

Based on earlier work showing that stimulation of the head or cortex could produce twitching movements of the musculature, Fritsch and Hitzig employed minimal levels of electrical stimulation to map the cortex of dogs. They found that stimulation of a zone within the frontal cortex resulted in specific muscle movements. Moreover, they discovered that minimal stimulation of one cortical area more anterior and dorsal produced selective movements of the forepaw on the contralateral side of the body, whereas nearby regions of stimulation resulted in muscle movements in adjacent body areas. Low-level stimulation of other cortical areas did not produce movements in any part of the body, indicating that they had isolated a specialized motor area of the cortex and that area was organized as a kind of mapping of the musculature of the body.

Based on the physiological findings of Fritsch and Hitzig, Ferrier was convinced there had to be separate cortical areas that mediated specific sensory functions, such as vision, hearing, smell, and touch, and other areas that controlled movement. He suspected that previous studies had failed to find selective behavioral–anatomical correlations because the lesions were too small or the animals selected did not have sufficiently differentiated cortical areas. He prepared two monkeys, and in each showed a selective disorder associated with a specific area of cortical damage. One monkey had a severe paralysis on the right side of the body associated with a circumscribed lesion within the left frontal area. The other monkey was completely deaf following a bilateral removal of the temporal lobe. Ferrier's evidence held up to close scrutiny by his colleagues and provided the most compelling initial evidence of distinct sensory and motor functional areas in the cerebral cortex.

This combination of studies settled the debate on localization, making it clear that the cerebral cortex does not operate as a unitary organ, but rather is composed of many functionally distinct compartments. Subsequently, the localization controversy would arise again, this time about the locus of memory traces *per se*, as distinct from the more general issue of functional localization. This time, the strong localizationist view would not hold, at least with regard to the cortex. However, a new perspective, based on anatomical considerations beyond the cortex, would show that memory is subdivided according to larger pathways or compartments that involve connections between the cortex and other brain regions.

Consolidation

A major topic in research of the Golden Era directly associated with the phenomenon of memory involved studies on memory performance in neurological patients with memory disorders, as well as in normal human subjects. Two phenomena of amnesia following brain damage were prominent. First, patients with memory deficits could acquire new information and remember it briefly, but showed an abnormally rapid amount and rate of forgetfulness. This phenomenon in amnesia, called anterograde amnesia, was intimately tied to the diagnosis of memory impairment, in that the disorder of memory could be contrasted with intact perception and comprehension, as well as a spared ability to hold information long enough to demonstrate the latter capacities. Second, and even more impressive, was the observation of retrograde amnesia, the loss of memories acquired before the brain trauma. Both phenomena of memory loss were systematically studied first in the Golden Era.

The neuropathology of memory

In 1882, the French philosopher and psychologist Theodore Ribot reviewed a large number of cases of retrograde amnesia associated with brain damage and head trauma. He observed that in those cases where memory impairment is the major consequence, memories acquired remotely before the insult were relatively preserved compared to those acquired recently just before. His formulation, which came to be known as Ribot's law, was stated as a "law of regression" by which the loss of memory is inversely related to the time elapsed between the event to be remembered and the injury. Ribot thus concluded that memories required a certain amount of time to be organized and fixed.

Further early systematic characterizations of memory disorders, and the incumbent insights they provide about normal memory, began with the descriptions of two forms of dementia in which memory loss plays a prominent role. In 1906, Alois Alzheimer reported on an institutionalized female patient with progressive dementia. Her first symptoms involved personality changes, but soon after she exhibited a profound memory impairment. After being shown objects and recognizing them, she immediately forgot them and the circumstances in which she had learned about them. Patients with Alzheimer's disease exhibited a set of prototypical symptoms including the cardinal signs of anterograde and retrograde amnesia. Initially, the patients would show mild memory lapses. As the disease progressed, the patients would become profoundly forgetful, remembering things said for only a few minutes and then completely losing them. Consistent with the law of regression Ribot had described for retrograde amnesia following head injury, the impairment in Alzheimer's disease was more severe for memories recently acquired than for those acquired earlier in life.

Another disease with prominent loss of memory was first described by Sergei Korsakoff in 1887. His initial report involved a group of patients with an odd combination of peripheral neuromuscular symptoms (polyneuritis) and memory disorder. Many of these patients were chronic alcoholics, who came to the clinic in a global confusional state that gradually resolved, leaving an outstanding selective impairment in memory as the outstanding prominent symptom. The characterization of the memory loss in Korsakoff syndrome was similar to that for the early stage of Alzheimer's disease. These patients could follow a train of conversation, but, when distracted even for a brief period, they lost both the contents of the conversation and the memory that it had taken place. The patients also showed the signs of retrograde amnesia, including the temporal gradient in which remote memories were more preserved than recent ones.

Consolidation and normal human memory

In a monograph published in 1900 Georg Muller and Alfons Pilzecker reported a large number of experiments performed on normal human subjects. They had adapted Ebbinghaus's method for learning "nonsense syllables," short and pronounceable but meaningless character strings, presenting a list of them in pairs and then asking subjects to recall the second item in each pair upon subsequent probing with the first item. A major finding involved the observations of a strong tendency for subjects to spontaneously become aware of the training pairs during the retention phase, even when they tried to suppress rehearsal. They called this phenomenon "perseveration" and linked it to the additional observation that errors made during recall involved items in the same list much more often than those from separate lists. Also, both phenomena of perseveration followed a regular time gradient—they were much more prominent for a few minutes after original learning than later. Muller and Pilzecker speculated that the perseveration reflected a transient brain activity that might play an important role in establishing and strengthening the word associations. They postulated that if this were the case, then the disruption of perseveration should have a deleterious effect on recall.

To test their hypothesis Muller and Pilzecker evaluated the effects on recall performance of interpolated material given in between the initial presentations and the recall test. They tested the effects of presenting an additional list in between training and recall on an initial list, finding that indeed recall was poorer if an additional list was presented, as compared to the results with no intervening material. They called this phenomenon "retroactive interference." They varied the nature of the interpolated material by assessing the effects of presenting pictures instead of another verbal list, and found that this distraction was also effective in producing retroactive interference. Furthermore, they varied the timing of presentation of the interpolated material, and found that delaying the distraction by more than a few minutes diminished its interfering effects considerably. These studies led them to the conclusion that there is a brain activity that normally perseverates following new learning and that this activity serves to consolidate the memory.

These findings were shortly after linked to the reports of retrograde amnesia in patients with brain insult or damage. Thus, temporally graded amnesia was explained as a disruption of the perseveration process caused by a direct functional interruption of the underlying brain activity. In 1903 William Burham described the effect of brain trauma as disrupting a natural physical process of organization associated with a psychological process of repetition and association, processes that required time to mature.

Succeeding decades of progress

In the following chapters we explore in greater detail all of the issues raised in this chapter. The plan for the remainder of the book is to follow up on each of the four central themes, one at a time. This might seem to suggest that these issues are entirely independent, but this is very much *not* the case. The discovered characteristics of conditioned reflexes guided much of the succeeding work that unsuccessfully addressed the issue of compartmentalization of memory in the cortex. Conversely, the results of succeeding studies on the nature of cognition in memory also strongly influenced the ultimately successful advances in the compartmentalization of memory functions. And succeeding studies on both the basis of cellular connections and cognitive mechanisms have led to a more sophisticated understanding of processes underlying memory consolidation. So, while I will proceed to separate these themes as a heuristic, the research that guides them, the issues themselves, and the findings on each of them are strongly interrelated.

Part I of the book updates you on our understanding of the cellular and molecular bases of memory. Chapter 2 reviews the basic anatomy of physiology of neurons, and shows how these basic principles can be put to use in explaining how memory works in relatively simple nervous systems. Chapter 3 describes parallel successes in understanding the cellular bases of a form of plasticity characteristic of mammalian brain areas, and summarizes research indicating that this form of neural plasticity may be the fundamental mechanism of learning in many more complex brain systems.

The Part II of the book builds on the discussion of the nature of cognition in memory. I will update you on how the controversy between behaviorists and cognitivists played out in the middle of the twentieth century, and then how it was resolved by discoveries in neuroscience. In particular I consider a major discovery in the neurology of memory, a case study of amnesia that ultimately showed that memory could be isolated as a cognitive function and that laid the groundwork for resolving the controversy between cognitivist and behaviorist views of memory. Then I elaborate on our understanding of a memory system that mediates "cognitive" or, as it is called today, "declarative" memory. Chapter 4 reviews the evidence from studies of amnesia in humans, and chapter 5 covers the additional evidence from animal models of amnesia. Chapter 6 summarizes complementary evidence from observations on brain activity during declarative memory in humans and animals.

In Part III, I summarize progress on the issue of compartmentalization. In Chapter 7, I begin by describing how the controversy over cortical localization became a central issue in research on memory *per se*, and I show how this controversy was resolved by our modern understanding of cortical modules in information processing and memory. Then I summarize the current psychological, anatomical, and physiological evidence about multiple memory systems in the brain. Chapter 8 introduces substantial direct evidence for the existence and initial localization of multiple memory systems in the brain. Chapter 9 elaborates the anatomy and workings of the full system that mediates declarative memory. Chapters 10 and 11 elaborate on two major systems, one for procedural (habit and skill) learning and the other for emotional memory.

In Part IV, I consider progress on the issue of memory consolidation. In Chapter 12, I describe how modern research has distinguished between two different kinds of consolidation, a short-term cellular fixation process and a long-lasting reorganization process. This chapter reviews the evidence for modulation of memory fixation and considers brain mechanisms that mediate memory reorganization.

Finally, Chapter 13 returns to an emphasis on a particular part of the cerebral cortex, the prefrontal area, and how this area along with other cortical areas works to orchestrate memory. Throughout the text you will see that the issues laid out a century ago are as relevant today as when they were introduced. But now we are truly beginning to resolve the anatomy and mechanisms of memory at a level of sophistication that could not have been envisioned so long ago.

Summing up

There are four main themes in studies on the neurobiology of memory: *connection, cognition, compartmentalization,* and *consolidation.*

Connection concerns the most basic level of analysis of memory function, the fundamental nature of the circuitry of the brain including the elements of information processing and how they communicate with one another in the service of memory. Neurons are independent elements of information processing that are connected via synapses. In the simplest circuits, neurons connect sensory inputs to motor outputs to mediate reflex arcs. However, most reflex circuitries involve more complex arrangements that offer considerable coordination and control over behavior. There are also conditioned reflexes that involve the association of an arbitrary stimulus and an unconditioned stimulus, such that the conditioned stimulus comes to produce a conditioned response that is similar in form to the unconditioned or reflexive response. Conditioning is thought to be mediated by an enhancement or elaboration of the connections between neurons involved in reflex arcs.

Cognition refers to the nature of memories at the highest level of analysis, the psychological level. The central issue in the understanding of the psychological nature of memory involves the debate between behaviorism, which espouses that all learning can be reduced to conditioned responses, and cognitivism, which argues that more complex phenomena such as insight and inference are required to explain complex learned behavior. Over most of the twentieth century evidence for both views has been accumulated.

Compartmentalization refers to the notion that memory as a whole is distributed widely in the brain, and at the same time, there are different kinds of memory that are accomplished by specific brain modules, circuits, pathways, or systems. Gall first proposed the first detailed function mapping of the cerebral cortex, which he called "organology." However, his flawed methods led to incorrect assignments of function–structure relations. Later neurologists discovered case studies of humans with specific cortical damage and consequent specific deficits in language. Also, physiologists demonstrated that specific cortical areas in monkeys had identifiable delimited functional roles in sensory or motor processing.

Consolidation is a hypothetical phenomenon derived from the observation that memories are initially labile and later become resistant to loss, suggesting an extended process during which memories take on a permanent form. The existence of consolidation has been shown in studies on patients with damage to the brain showing a temporally graded retrograde loss of memories, that is, intact memories for material acquired remotely prior to the damage and lost memories for materials learned recently prior to the damage. The existence of consolidation can also be observed in normal humans by interposing interfering materials briefly, but not delayed, following initial learning.

READINGS

Eichenbaum, H., and Cohen, N.J. 2000. *From Conditioning to Conscious Recollection: Multiple Memory Systems in the Brain.* New York: Oxford University Press.

Finger, S. 1994. *Origins of Neuroscience: A History of Explorations into Brain Function.* New York: Oxford University Press.

Finger, S. 2000. *Minds Behind the Brain.* New York: Oxford University Press.

Lechner, H.A., Squire, L.R., and Byrne, J.H. 1999. 100 years of consolidation—Remembering Muller & Pilzecker. *Learn. Mem.* 6:77–87.

McGaugh, J.L. 2000. Memory—a century of consolidation. *Science* 287: 248–251.

Milner, B., Squire, L.R., and Kandel, E.R. 1998. Cognitive neuroscience and the study of memory. *Neuron* 20:445–468.

Polster, M.R., Nadel, L., and Schacter, D.L. 1991. Cognitive neuroscience analyses of memory. A historical perspective. *J. Cog. Neurosci.* 3:95–116.

Tolman, E.C. 1948. Cognitive maps in rats and men. *Psychol. Rev.* 55:189–208.

Zola-Morgan, S. 1995. Localization of brain function: The legacy of Franz Joseph Gall (1758–1828). *Annu. Rev. Neurosci.* 18:359–383.

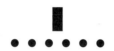

CONNECTION:
THE CELLULAR AND MOLECULAR
BASES OF MEMORY

The parallel anatomical, physiological, and behavioral studies of Cajal, Sherrington, and Pavlov provided an immensely strong foundation for the conditioned reflex as a central model of the basic memory circuit. And this model became the centerpiece of the biological instantiation of the learning mechanism for behaviorists. In succeeding decades further major advances in our understanding of the basic elements of neural connections would be made. In particular, one major discovery was that the nature of transmission of information between neurons is chemical.

The key experiment was performed by Otto Loewi in 1921. He was familiar with current work that had shown that chemical agents could stimulate and modulate the actions of the autonomic nervous system. The general view was that communication across neurons was by an electrical impulse, but the notion that there might be chemical transmission was being considered seriously. Loewi devised an experiment that would provide proof of a chemical mechanism. He removed the heart of a frog and bathed it in a neutral solution, where he stimulated the still attached vagus nerve, producing a well-known inhibition of contractions in the heart. Loewi then removed some of the bathing solution and placed it into a chamber holding another frog heart for which the vagus nerve had been removed. The second heart also slowed, demonstrating that a chemical agent that had been produced in the stimulated heart caused the inhibition. Loewi also performed the complementary experiment, showing that other stimulation that produced an acceleration of the first heart resulted in the release of a chemical agent that also accelerated the second (nonstimulated) heart.

It turns out that the inhibitory agent is the neurotransmitter acetylcholine, the major neurotransmitter of the parasympathetic system, and the accelerating agent is noradrenaline, the major neurotransmitter of the sympathetic system. Since the discovery of neurotransmitters, two major lines of research have refined our understanding of the mechanisms of chemical communication between neurons. First, the pioneering work of Bernard Katz in the 1950s showed that neurotransmitters are released at the synaptic ending of the axon in small packets of molecules called synaptic vesicles. Second, a long list of other neurotransmitters and neuromodulators has now been described, allowing for a range of effects that can be accomplished via neurotransmission.

In addition, interest in the molecular and cellular basis of synaptic modification has intersected with the issue of memory consolidation. In the 1960s and 1970s considerable effort was placed on showing that protein synthesis was required for permanent modifications of cells for lasting memory. Many studies showed that interfering with the synthesis of proteins, using drugs that prevent specific stages of gene expression, blocked the establishment of long-term memory without affecting short-term memory. Moreover, these drugs were effective in blocking later expression of memory even if they were given a few minutes after training, but not if treatment was delayed by an hour or more. The results of these experiments paralleled the time course of effects of other types of interference or brain insult that characterized the earlier studies demonstrating memory consolidation. In addition, the studies on protein synthesis inhibition provided a much more specific mechanism, suggesting that gene expression leading to proteins is a critical part of the consolidation process. As you will see in Chapters 2 and 3, this search has now narrowed substantially toward investigations on particular types of neurotransmitters that are activated during learning and on the identification of specific molecular pathways of subsequent gene expression.

The following two chapters review the state of our understanding about the cellular mechanisms of memory. In Chapter 2, I summarize our knowledge about the basic anatomy and physiology of neurons. Then I show how these basic anatomical and physiological elements are modified to mediate memory within model systems in invertebrate species. Chapter 3 builds on these observations, introducing a mammalian model system for cellular plasticity that shares many of the features of the invertebrate models and expands on them and other mechanisms within more complex circuitries. Then I consider how well this model works in accounting for cellular mechanisms of real memory in mammals.

2

• • • • • •

Neurons and
Simple Memory Circuits

STUDY QUESTIONS

What are the elements of neuronal structure?

How do the electrical properties of neurons arise?

What distinguishes different forms of neural conduction and transmission?

Why are simple invertebrate systems useful for understanding the cellular mechanisms of memory?

What are the molecular and cellular bases of simple forms of learning, including habituation, sensitization, and classical conditioning?

Neurons encode memories by modifications in the strength of the functional connections. In this chapter I summarize some of the key fundamental concepts about the anatomy and physiology of neurons, including the molecular basis of the unusual electrical properties of neurons, different forms of electrical conduction, and transmission of information between neurons. Then I show how these concepts can be put to work toward understanding the cellular bases of basic forms of learning. Three elemental forms of learning that are accomplished within the circuitry of relatively simple animals have served as model systems for the study of memory. These studies have provided a clear understanding of the mechanisms of neuronal plasticity that mediate habituation, sensitization, and classical conditioning mediated within well-identified circuits of a marine invertebrate.

Neuron structure

As recognized at the time of Cajal, neurons are composed of four main elements, the dendrites, the soma or cell body, the axon, and the synapse (Fig. 2–1). There are typically many dendrites and they are often highly branched, such that most neurons receive inputs at the synaptic connections with axons of many other neurons. Each neuron has only one cell body, although the axons of many other cells can contact the cell body directly and these contacts are particularly effective. Each neuron also has only one axon, although in many situations the axon can branch extensively to make a large number of contacts onto one or more other neurons. These basic anatomical facts dictate that neurons receive and integrate information from a substantial number and variety of inputs, and then sum them up to a single main output that can affect one or many cells that are next in the circuit.

The synapse is a complicated structure, composed of two main parts, the presynaptic and the postsynaptic elements. The presynaptic element is an enlargement of axonal ending that contains specialized machinery for the process of neuronal transmission. This machinery includes cellular organelles that produce energy and elements that are involved in the recycling and packaging of neurotransmitters into synaptic vesicles. In addition, there are specialized docking stations for the vesicles from which the neurotransmitter is released. There is a narrow separation between the presynaptic element and postsynaptic cell membrane of the neuron to which it is connected; this separation is known as the synaptic cleft. When released from the presynaptic element, neurotransmitters must diffuse

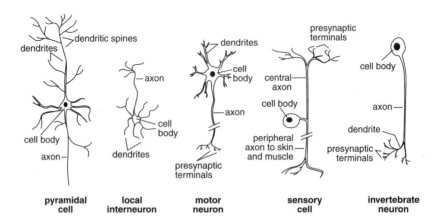

Figure 2–1. Examples of different types of neurons and their major components.

across the synaptic cleft to reach specialized receptors in the postsynaptic element. There are many different kinds of receptors, including distinct types of receptors for the same neurotransmitter, providing for a variety of effects of transmission on the target cell's activity. The structure of these receptor molecules and mechanisms of their activation are only now becoming known.

Within the overall design described above, the elements of neurons can take many configurations suited to specific applications in different parts of the nervous system (Fig. 2–1). A prototypical *principal neuron* is the pyramidal cell of the cortex and hippocampus. These neurons have a long branching dendrite that extends upward from the cell body and receives inputs from other regions, as well as multiple dendrites that branch laterally from the cell to receive inputs from local neurons. The axon extends downward and branches. It may connect with other local cells or extend many millimeters to another brain region. *Interneurons* are neurons that receive inputs and send their outputs within a local brain region. *Motor neurons* of the spinal cord have many branching dendrites that extend in all directions, and a single long axon that extends very long distances to innervate skeletal muscles. Its axon branches extensively and has specialized presynaptic terminals to make contact with muscle cells. *Sensory cells*, conversely, have specialized endings of their dendrites to receive information from specific sensory organs. Some of them may have the cell body displaced such that it is connected to a single main dendritic and axonal element. There are many other variations on these patterns.

The physiology of neurons

As I describe the physiology of neurons, it should be kept foremost in mind that communication in the nervous system involves three main stages that are mediated by different physiological mechanisms (Fig. 2–2). Two of these stages involve electrical mechanisms for *conduction* of neuronal signal over substantial distances through the dendrites and axon, and the third involves chemical mediation of *transmission* of the signal between neurons. The initial phase of conduction, known as *electrotonic conduction*, typically begins at the postsynaptic site, and proceeds to the cell body. This type of electrical conduction is remarkably fast, but dissipates over relatively short distances. The second type of electrical conduction, called the *action potential*, is initiated by a special mechanism at the cell body and conducted down the axon to the presynaptic elements. This type of electrical conduction is relatively slow compared to passive conduction, but involves a mechanism that maintains the signal over very long distances. When the action potential

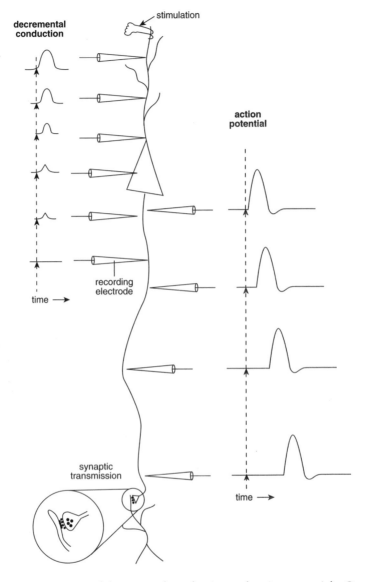

Figure 2–2. Comparison of decremental conduction and action potentials. On the left are idealized waveforms of synaptic potentials recorded at successive loci indicated by the site of the recording electrode. Note that the latency after stimulation until onset of the potential is very short for all recordings. On the right are idealized waveforms of action potentials recorded at successive loci indicated by the sites of recording electrodes. Note that the latency increases substantially between recordings, showing the slow conduction of action potentials as compared with electrotonic conduction.

reaches the presynaptic element, the molecular processes of synaptic transmission are initiated and carry a chemical signal across the synaptic cleft to the presynaptic elements of the next cell. In the following sections, I summarize and compare the different forms of electrical conduction and then describe the mechanisms of synaptic transmission.

The resting potential

To understand the mechanisms of electrical conduction it is important to appreciate that nerve cells, as well as other types of cells throughout the body, have a natural electrical potential known as the *resting potential*. This potential arises from two features common to most living cells (Fig. 2–3). First, there is a natural concentration of molecules inside the cell

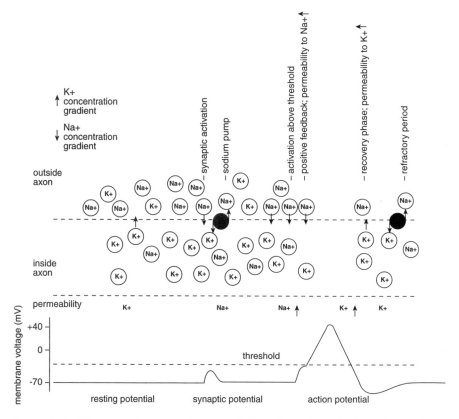

Figure 2–3. Schematic diagram of ions and their flow through the cell membrane (dashed lines) associated with the resting potential, synaptic potential, and action potential.

membrane relative to the fluid outside the cell (called the extracellular fluid), and many of these molecules are polarized in that they have a positive or negative charge. Major contributors to the high intracellular (i.e., inside) concentration are large protein molecules that have a negative charge that is balanced out by small positively charged molecules such as sodium (Na^+) and potassium (K^+) in the intracellular fluid. Second, the membrane that surrounds the cell and contains its contents is typically somewhat permeable in that it contains pores or channels that allow the diffusion of molecules between the inside and outside of the membrane. These two situations conspire to create a situation in which a potential difference between the inside and outside of the cell membrane is established.

The potential difference across the membrane arises because of two natural and competing forces that are consequences of these properties of neurons. One of these forces comes about because of the difference in concentration of molecules inside and outside the membrane. The accumulation of large molecules inside the cell creates a substantial *concentration gradient,* such that the interior fluid of the cell is much more concentrated than the fluid of the exterior of the cell. If the membrane pores or channels were indifferently permeable to all molecules, the difference in concentration would disappear as molecules from the inside diffused out until the concentration on both sides of the membrane was equal. However, the membrane channels are actually quite selective, typically allowing small molecules such as Na^+ and K^+ to flow, and even the passage of those molecules is tightly regulated. Indeed, in the natural resting state, the cell membrane is mostly permeable only to K^+. Because of this selective permeability and because there is typically much more K^+ inside the cell than out, some K^+ flows from inside to outside following the concentration gradient, and this creates a situation where the inside of the cell has a net negative charge due to the loss of some positively charged potassium molecules. If the concentration gradient was the only force involved, K^+ would continue to flow outside the cell until its concentration was equal on both sides.

This overall potential difference, with the inside negatively charged and the outside positively charged, invokes the second force that affects the resting potential. The interior-to-exterior charge difference constitutes an overall *electrostatic gradient* across the cell membrane that tends to repel positively charged molecules from the positively charged exterior. At the same time, because the interior of the cell has become negatively charged, there is an overall attraction of positive charges to the inside of the cell. Because the cell membrane is selectively permeable to K^+, and so it is the only molecule that can pass, the combination of repellant force from the outside and attractive force from the inside draws some K^+ molecules back into the cell. If the electrostatic gradient was the only force involved, K^+ would flow back into the cell until there was no charge difference.

Thus, there are two competing forces on the K^+ molecules. The concentration gradient pushes K^+ outside, whereas the electrostatic gradient pulls K^+ inside. These two forces eventually reach an equilibrium in which K^+ molecules leave the cell to decrease the concentration gradient only somewhat, resulting in an overall net electrostatic gradient in one direction and a concentration gradient of equal force in the opposite direction. This final electrostatic gradient is called the resting potential, and its magnitude is typically about -70 millivolts (inside relative to outside the membrane). The exact magnitude of this potential depends on many factors, including the concentrations of K^+ and other molecules for which the cell membrane is typically less permeable.

Electrotonic conduction

In the natural situation the resting potential is disturbed when chemical processes at the synapse result in a change in the permeability to a molecule, typically Na^+ (Fig. 2–3). Unlike K^+, Na^+ is more concentrated outside the cell membrane. This is because there is an active mechanism, embedded in the cell membrane, that pumps Na^+ molecules from the inside to the outside of the cell. This pump is metabolically expensive, consuming as much as 40% of the energy needs of a neuron. But it is a very valuable mechanism for the conduction of signals.

When synaptic transmission results in a transient increase in permeability to Na^+ at the receptor site, Na^+ follows its concentration gradient and flows into the cell. Because Na^+ is positively charged, this results in movement of the membrane potential in the positive direction, from -70 millivolts to something closer to zero, with the magnitude depending on the strength of the synaptic transmission. This relative positive charge gradient spreads passively and almost instantaneously, like electricity, decreasing the polarization of the membrane for some distance along the dendrite toward the cell body. However, as this *depolarization* spreads, it also diffuses across the membrane surface and so diminishes in size. Thus, electrotonic conduction is fast but it is also *decremental*, in that it decreases in magnitude so that a smaller depolarization reaches the cell body (see Fig. 2–2). The size of the potential depends critically on the distance it must travel, such that synapses on very distant dendrite branches are usually much less effective than those near the cell body.

The action potential

Something truly magical happens at one end of the cell body, and it involves a mechanism that defines the special physiology of the neuron. This special property, which involves a dramatic alteration in the membrane permeabilities, typically occurs only in axons. At the postsynaptic site in dendrites and in most of the cell body, the membrane does not generally change its permeabilities substantially. So, potentials created at the synapse are propagated only by electrotonic conduction of the transient perturbation of the resting potential at the synapse when transmission occurs. As described previously, this perturbation is conducted rapidly, at the speed of electricity, but it also decrements rapidly along the length of the dendrite. So electrotonic conduction is not a mechanism that would support long-range communication of signals down the axon for distances of up to a meter or more, as required in some pathways of the brain.

At the end of the cell body where the axon originates, the membrane takes on a profound new quality, one that allows it to change its permeabilities in a large and very useful way. At this locus, called the initiation zone, the channels in the membrane change their permeability when they are depolarized to a specific threshold, and hence they are called *voltage-gated channels*. The mechanisms of these channels in mediating the action potential were first discovered by Alan Hodgkin and Andrew Huxley in the 1940s. They showed that depolarization of the axon membrane above the threshold, typically about a 15–20 millivolt depolarization, results initially in an increase in permeability selectively to Na^+ molecules. As was the case at the synapse, Na^+ is in greater concentration outside the axon, and therefore an increase in Na^+ permeability results in an influx of positively charged sodium molecules, and consequently a further depolarization of the cell membrane. This sets up an unusual "regenerative" situation, a positive feedback mechanism by which the initial depolarization above threshold causes an influx of Na^+, which further depolarizes the cell, which causes more Na^+ channels to open, which allows more Na^+ in, which additionally depolarizes the cell, and so on. When does this regenerative loop end? Sooner or later, the membrane becomes fully permeable to Na^+ and it will reach its equilibrium potential, that is, its balance between concentration and electrostatic gradients. Thus, the maximum potential is a fixed number for a given cell (whose value depends on factors such as the initial inside and outside Na^+ concentrations, and the temperature). Because the pump makes the Na^+ concentration greater outside the cell, its equilibrium is reached when the inside of the membrane reaches an overall positive value, typically about 40 millivolts.

Importantly, once the threshold of depolarization is achieved, this regenerative process runs itself inevitably and precisely to the equilibrium potential for Na^+. The magnitude of the action potential is much larger than the potentials associated with decremental conduction, and its appearance is "all-or-none." Either the threshold for activation of the voltage-gated channels is not reached, and very little potential is obtained and dissipates rapidly, or threshold is reached, and the mechanism regenerates itself up to the full value of the equilibrium potential for Na^+. Furthermore, when an action potential is generated in the initiation zone, the potential spreads electrotonically. This spread would decrement, but over a short distance would be more than sufficient to take the adjacent voltage-gated channels of axon membrane to threshold. This would regenerate the full magnitude of the action potential at that neighboring locus, and that potential would itself spread, reinitiating a full-blown action potential at its neighboring loci, and so on, continuing to reduplicate the action potential through the length of the axon. This simple regenerative mechanism, therefore, not only insures that the action potential achieves its full size at each locus but also insures its propagation for the full length of the axon regardless of the distance involved.

The action potential also includes a mechanism for recovery. Shortly after the Na^+ channels are activated, voltage-gated channels for K^+ also open. During the resting phase, K^+ channels were open to some extent, allowing the establishment of the resting potential. In addition, just after the initiation of the Na^+ current, other K^+ channels are activated, allowing even greater permeability to this molecule. Because K^+ is more concentrated on the inside of the cell, it flows out, and does so especially strongly because the Na^+ onrush has made the inside of the cell move to a positive potential. The result of this series of events is that the rise in the membrane potential to a positive state is short-lived. The membrane potential rapidly returns to its initial level (indeed to even below that level—an overshoot—because of the especially high K^+ permeability). At that point the membrane has more or less reachieved its normal potential but the molecular balance is not the same as its initial status. There is a lingering high concentration of Na^+ inside the cell, and extra K^+ has left the cell. The pumping mechanism sets this imbalance right, but during this recovery period a new action potential cannot be initiated, and so the cell is said to be in a *refractory period*.

Synaptic transmission

When the action potential reaches the end of the axon, at the presynaptic site, another mechanism takes over to mediate synaptic transmission (Fig. 2–4). The spreading of the action potential to the membrane of the presynaptic element activates voltage-gated channels in that area for a different molecule, calcium (Ca^{2+}). Calcium is more highly concentrated on the outside of the cell, in the synaptic cleft, and so the depolarization of the presynaptic element results in a substantial influx of Ca^{2+} into the presynaptic element. It takes time for these channels to open, in part accounting for the delay in synaptic transmission of signals, but Ca^{2+} is the critical catalyst to initiate synaptic transmission. It appears that Ca^{2+} plays a central role in facilitating the docking of synaptic vesicles at specific sites in the end of the presynaptic membrane. When this docking has been accomplished, the vesicle fuses with the end of the cell membrane and re-

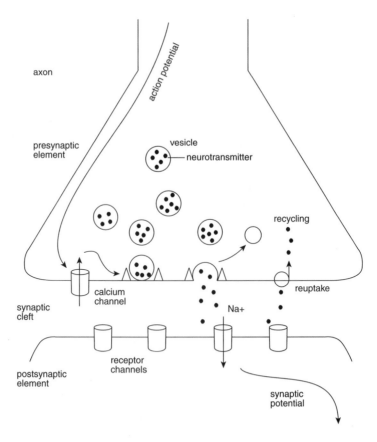

Figure 2–4. Schematic diagram of events in synaptic transmission.

leases its contents, the neurotransmitter, into the synaptic cleft. Quickly the vesicular material is recaptured and recycled, to be filled again with neurotransmitter.

Meanwhile, the neurotransmitter diffuses across the synaptic cleft and finds its way onto and binds with specific receptors. The receptors briefly bind the neurotransmitter, and in doing so, activate channels that control the permeability of the postsynaptic membrane to local molecules. The binding is typically transient, interrupted by an unbinding and diffusion of the neurotransmitter, or by other molecules that destroy the neuro-transmitter. The neurotransmitter or its breakdown products are not allowed to remain in the synaptic cleft for long, however. They are reabsorbed by the presynaptic membrane and recycled.

One main action of these receptors is to initiate changes in the post-synaptic membrane already described, the opening of Na^+ channels to initiate an *excitatory* postsynaptic potential that can be propagated electronically along the dendrite. However, there are many types of neurotransmitters and many types of receptors, even for the same neuro-transmitter molecule. This provides considerable capacity for regulation of the duration and type of potential produced at the postsynaptic element. One major variant is the capacity to generate *hyperpolarization*, rather than depolarization, of the postsynaptic element. This is accomplished, at least in some of these *inhibitory* synapses, by transmitter-gated chloride channels in the postsynaptic element. Chloride is a negatively charged molecule that is more concentrated outside the cell membrane. When its channels are activated, the negatively charged chloride molecules flow inside, making the postsynaptic element become even more polarized than normal. This hyperpolarization also flows via electrotonic conduction across the dendrite and can serve to inhibit the generation of an action potential in the activation zone.

Integration of synaptic potentials

In most cases the synaptic potentials that are initiated by synaptic transmission are relatively small, about 5–20 millivolts. As described earlier, these subthreshold potentials decrement in magnitude as they travel to the initiation zone in the axon. Therefore, in most cases, an action potential does not occur as a result from a single activation of one synapse. Instead, the initiation of an action potential typically requires summation of many synaptic potentials. This summation can occur across time if the same synapse is activated repeatedly quickly enough so that the synaptic potentials can build up. Also, summation can occur by the concurrent activation of many spatial distant synapses on the same dendrite or different dendrites. The combination of excitatory (depolarizing) and inhibitory (hyperpolarizing) synaptic potentials offers considerable fine tuning of the likelihood of an action potential. In addition to these forms of temporal and spatial summation, the degree to which individual synapses control the action potential depends to a great extent where on the dendrite it is initiated—synapses close to or on the cell body are most effective, because they will suffer less from the effects of decremental conduction, as described earlier.

These aspects of integration are complemented by a variety of mechanisms that regulate the efficacy of synapses and their consequent contribution to initiation of action potentials. The efficacy of a synapse is determined by the supply of neurotransmitter, and by the amount and duration of Ca^{2+} influx that determines how much neurotransmitter is released. The sensitivity and duration of receptor activation can be regulated by substances in the synaptic cleft, and, indeed, many drugs operate by interfering with or enhancing the operation of receptors. The number and sensitivity of receptors also determine the efficacy of the synapse. As you will see, alterations in each of these parameters provides a mechanism for changes in synaptic efficacy that underlie memory storage.

Cellular biology of simple memory circuits

To provide examples of how the cellular and molecular mechanisms of neural conduction and transmission become important in memory, the remainder of this chapter summarizes a program of study on the behavior and physiology of a relatively simple invertebrate species. Invertebrates are superb animals in which to study the cell biology of nervous function because their nervous systems involve many fewer neurons than those of most vertebrates, and many of their neurons are quite large and unique. These qualities allow researchers to individually identify exactly the same set of cells in each animal, and to study virtually all of the major cells involved in a functional circuit.

In pioneering studies, Eric Kandel and his colleagues have examined the behavioral, anatomical, and physiological properties of simple forms of memory in *Aplysia*, a large sea snail. Most of their studies have focused on one particular reflex circuit, called the gill withdrawal reflex. When the snail is quiescent, it extends its gills from the abdominal region, as well as a fleshy continuation of the gill called the siphon. Ordinarily the siphon serves to assist the flow of aerated water over the gills as they function in respiration. However, the gills are a delicate organ, one that is easily damaged. Therefore, when there are signs of danger, the snail can withdraw the gill and siphon. In the laboratory, a mantle shelf that ordinarily completely covers the gill and siphon can be retracted, and then when the animal is relaxed, the gill and siphon are extended. The defensive reflex is initiated by a gentle stroke of the siphon with a paint brush. This results in the rapid withdrawal of the gill under the mantle shelf.

This reflex has been studied extensively, using behavioral paradigms that examine three simple forms of learning, *habituation, sensitization*, and *classical conditioning*. For each form of learning the anatomical circuit of the relevant neurons has been characterized, and the cellular and molecular mechanisms that underlie learning have been explored. A review of the findings of these studies provides a solid introduction to central principles of the cellular mechanisms that mediate learning.

Habituation

Perhaps the simplest form of learning is habituation. All of us use habituation every day to help us learn *not* to attend or respond to irrelevant stimuli. For example, if you ever moved from a small to a big city, your attention to the noise of traffic may have initially made it difficult for you to sleep through the night. Each time a car blew its horn or a siren went off, you woke up. However, after several days, you probably came to ignore the noises, that is you habituated to them, and your sleep was undisturbed by them.

Rapid and lasting habituation can also be observed in the gill withdrawal reflex of *Aplysia*. Following elicitation of the reflex and subsequent relaxation, if the siphon is stimulated again the reflex is smaller, and following several repetitions it becomes quite reduced in magnitude. Furthermore, following only 10 stimulations, the reflex may remain habituated for only 15 minutes. But, after 4 days of such training, the habituation can last weeks. The longer-lasting habituation is a very simple form of learning, to be sure, but it has the lasting property that indicates it is indeed a form of long-term memory.

Now the researchers sought to characterize the circuit of nerve cells involved in the reflex and to determine the mechanism of lasting habituation. A highly schematic sketch of this circuit that shows just one of each type of cell is provided in Fig. 2–5. It turns out that all the relevant cells of the circuit are in a single ganglion, or cluster of cells in the abdomen. There are about 40 sensory cells that innervate the siphon skin, and these connect with six motor neurons that innervate the gill musculature. The neurotransmitter for this synapse is glutamate, and this will become important later. There are also clusters of both excitatory and inhibitory in-

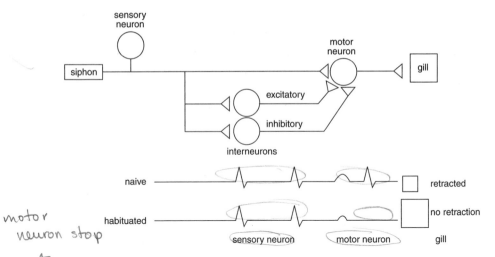

Figure 2–5. Schematic diagram of an idealized circuit for habituation in *Aplysia*, and recordings of action potentials at successive stages in the circuit.

terneurons, cells that receive input from the sensory cells and innervate the motor neurons. When the stimulus is initially applied to the siphon, the sensory neurons are excited, and these excite the interneurons and gill motor neurons. These inputs converge and cause the motor neuron to discharge action potentials repeatedly, producing a vigorous withdrawal response.

Following repetitions of the siphon stimulation, the sensory neurons still produce action potentials, indicating that the habituation is not mediated by a sensory adaptation or any other change in the responsiveness of the sensory elements (Fig. 2–5). However, the magnitude of the synaptic potential in the interneurons and motor neurons is reduced, such that the likelihood of generating an action potential in the motor neuron, and the number of them generated, is smaller. Eventually, even though the sensory neuron is still responding vigorously, no action potentials are produced in the motor neurons. This means that the locus of the memory is to be found in the physiology of the connections between the sensory neurons (as well as the excitatory interneurons) onto motor neurons. This was confirmed by closely examining the synaptic potentials in the motor neurons and confirming that the magnitude and longevity of their depression closely mirror that of the behavioral response.

Now, Kandel and colleagues asked what stage in the process of conduction or transmission was affected by habituation. They found that the receptors in the postsynaptic site were equally sensitive, so the locus of the depression had to be presynaptic. Indeed, they found that the depression was due to a decrease in the number of synaptic vesicles released for each action potential. They then used an electron microscope to examine the number and locations of synaptic vesicles in the presynaptic element before and after habituation, and found that the number of available vesicles did not decrease but fewer of them became docked onto release sites in habituated animals. Furthermore, following extended training, physiological assessments indicated that many fewer sensory neurons had effective connections with motor neurons, and anatomical examination showed that the number of synaptic contacts between sensory neurons and interneurons and motor neurons was substantially reduced. These findings showed that memory can be mediated by changes in synaptic efficacy, both through intracellular mechanisms that control transmitter release and through changes in anatomical connectivity.

Sensitization

A second simple form of nonassociative learning observed in *Aplysia* is sensitization. This kind of learning is, in a way, the opposite of habituation in that it involves an *increase* in reflex magnitude as a result of stimulation. In this case though, the circuit involves a combination of two inputs such that strong stimulation of one input sensitizes, or makes more vigorous, responses to the other input. An everyday example is when we encounter a fearful stimulus, such as a loud noise, we become for some time more likely to startle, or startle more vigorously, to many other sounds as well.

In *Aplysia*, sensitization has been studied using a protocol in which initially the tail of the animal is stimulated with an electric shock, which results in an increase in the robustness of the gill withdrawal to siphon stimulation. A single tail shock produces sensitization that lasts for minutes, whereas a series of 4–5 tail shocks produces sensitization that lasts for a few days. The circuit that mediates this form of learning involves the same set of cells involved in habituation, plus sensory neurons that innervate the tail and additional interneurons (Fig. 2–6). Thus, one way or another, the same set of cells can mediate both habituation and sensitization, two different forms of learning. In the case of habituation, the synaptic depression that occurs is said to be *homosynaptic*, because the mediating events occur within the same pathway that constitutes the reflex itself. However, in the case of sensitization, there must be a facilitation that is mediated by a *heterosynaptic* mechanism because it involves modulation of the reflex pathway by another set of cells, in this situation in the tail sensory pathway.

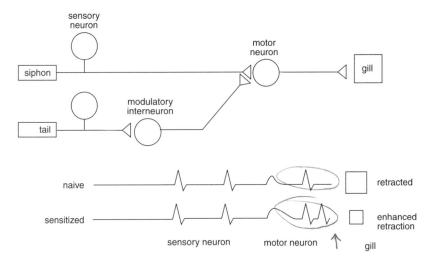

Figure 2–6. Schematic diagram of an idealized circuit for sensitization in *Aplysia*, and recordings of action potentials at successive stages in the circuit.

The central events that underlie sensitization do not involve direct modifications of the siphon sensory neuron, as was the case in habituation. Rather, the tail shocks activate sensory neurons for the tail, which in turn activate modulatory interneurons that synapse onto the cells bodies and presynaptic elements of the siphon sensory neurons. These modulatory neurons affect the strength of synaptic signal produced by the siphon sensory neurons, and so use an indirect mechanism to support the facilitation of reflexes. Specificially, the facilitation is due to forms of modulation that act to increase the number of synaptic vesicles released by the siphon sensory neuron onto its targets, resulting in a substantial increase in the response of the gill motor neurons.

The key to the modulation of sensory neuron synaptic potentials lies in a distinction between two types of receptors (Fig. 2–7). As described before, the conventional receptors, called ionotropic receptors, are found in postsynaptic elements, are transmitter-gated, and allow charged molecules to flow briefly inducing the postsynaptic excitatory and inhibitory potentials. There is also a second class of receptors, called metabotropic receptors. These are activated by transmitters or other molecules, but do not open channels and directly cause changes in the membrane potential. Rather, they produce other changes in the cell that can have lasting effects on its responsiveness.

The changes resulting from metabotropic receptor activation typically involve a cascade of molecular events. Thus, when a neurotransmitter binds

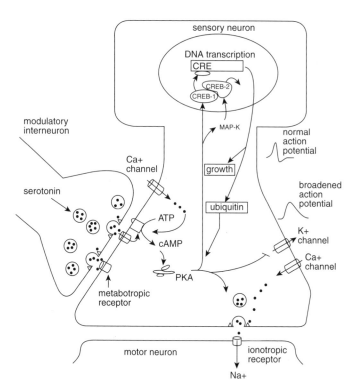

Figure 2–7. Schematic diagram of cellular events that mediate long-term changes in synaptic efficacy of the presynaptic site in *Aplysia*.

onto a metabotropic receptor, an enzyme is activated which in turn alters the concentration of an intracellular signaling molecule called a *second messenger* (distinguishing it from the neurotransmitter as the "first" messenger). In this and many other situations the second messenger is cyclic adenosine monophosphate (cAMP), which is synthesized by the enzyme from the common metabolic molecule adenosine triphosphate (ATP). The action of cAMP is to turn on a number of cellular processes through activation of a special protein called cAMP protein kinase, also known as PKA. In turn, PKA mediates its effects by adding a phosphate group to a variety of proteins, activating them to play any of a variety of roles in cell regulation. Thus, the second messenger signaling system is different from the primary synaptic mechanism in having a variety of long-lasting effects.

In the case of sensitization in *Aplysia*, the specific neurotransmitter of the modulatory interneurons is serotonin, which acts on the metabotropic receptors of the sensory neurons to increase their intracellular cAMP,

seritonin ⇒ cAMP → PKA phosphorylate proteins
Ca²⁺ enter → K⁺ out Na⁺ out ⇒ ↑ neurotransmitters

which in turn activates PKA. This was found by showing that direct application of serotonin is sufficient to activate cAMP, and direct intracellular injection of cAMP is sufficient to enhance transmitter release by the sensory neuron, and to induce the facilitation of the reflex. Furthermore, intracellular infusion of the main subunit of PKA also produces the facilitation, and inhibiting the action of PKA blocks the facilitation. Thus, the full cascade of events associated with the second messenger is both sufficient and necessary for mediation of sensitization. Furthermore, a key specific effect on the physiology of the synapse has been identified. Both cAMP and PKA (or some of its subunits) act to close one of the K^+ channels in the presynaptic membrane of the sensory neuron, reducing the action of this channel in terminating the action potential. This results in a broadening of the action potential, opening the Ca^{2+} channels of the presynaptic element for a longer period, and allowing a greater amount of Ca^{2+} to enter the presynaptic element. The increased Ca^{2+} concentration in the presynaptic element increases the number of vesicles docked per action potential, increasing the release of neurotransmitter, which, of course, leads to a greater response of the motor neurons.

Classical conditioning

Habituation and sensitization are considered very elementary forms of learning, because they do not involve the acquisition of an association between stimuli, but rather a change in responsiveness to repeated stimulation of one kind. The simplest form of associative learning is classical conditioning, the kind of learning that was the focus of the pioneering studies of Pavlov described in Chapter 1. In this form of learning two different stimuli are presented in close temporal proximity, such that typically a form of stimulation that does not ordinarily produce a response is presented before another stimulus that does produce the response. After multiple pairings the first stimulus acquires the ability to produce the response. In that sense, classical conditioning involves the acquisition of an association between the first, or conditioned stimulus, and the second, unconditioned stimulus. In Pavlov's dogs the conditioned stimulus was a tone, that did not initially elicit salivation. It was presented repeatedly prior to injection of food into the mouth (the unconditioned stimulus), which did directly elicit salivation. After several pairings, the tone came to elicit the conditioned response of salivation.

In the *Aplysia* model, a protocol for classical conditioning was established using an elaboration of the habituation and sensitization paradigms and their neural circuits (Fig. 2–8). Added to the already described ele-

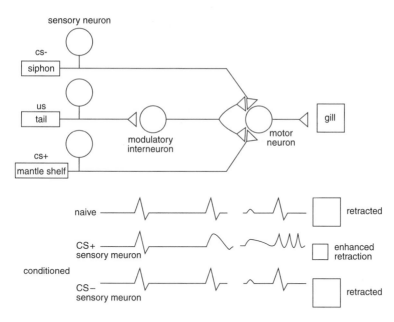

Figure 2–8. Schematic diagram of an idealized circuit for classical conditioning in *Aplysia*, and recordings of action potentials at successive stages in the circuit.

ments is an additional reflex pathway from the sensory neurons of the skin on the mantle shelf that connect to the same set of motor neurons that withdraw the gill. This pathway is essentially the same as the pathway from the siphon to the gill, and offers the ability to differentially condition one of those paths, and not the other, consistent with the selectivity of associations in classical conditioning in mammals. In this differential classical conditioning protocol, then, on some trials the mantle shelf is lightly stimulated and then the tail is shocked. The mantle shelf stimulation is referred to as the positive conditioning stimulus (CS+) and the tail stimulation is the unconditioned stimulus (US). On other trials, the siphon is stimulated and no tail shock is given, and this stimulation is referred to as the CS−. The animals come to have vigorously enhanced withdrawal responses to the mantle stimulation, the conditioned response (CR), but not to the siphon stimulation, that is, they become differentially conditioned to the mantle conditioned stimulus.

As is the case in mammalian examples of classical conditioning, timing is everything. In this case strong tail stimulation simply produces a generalized sensitization. But in the case of classical conditioning, the protocol produces differential conditioning for the paired stimulus. How is this accomplished within the cells of this circuit? The critical steps occur both in the presynaptic and postsynaptic elements of the reflex circuit. At the presynaptic element, it turns out that when an action potential reaches the site, the influx of Ca^{2+} not only induces transmitter docking and release, but Ca^{2+} also binds to the protein calmodulin. The calcium–calmodulin complex binds to the enzyme (adenyl cyclase) that generates cAMP. Additionally, bound to calmodulin, the adenyl cyclase becomes more sensitive to activation by serotonin, consequently releasing a greater amount of cAMP and subsequently enhancing the influx of Ca^{2+}. Thus, the critical timing involves first a priming step in which the CS+ (mantle shelf stimulation) generates calcium–calmodulin bound to adenyl cylase, and then the closely following US (tail stimulation) acts via the modulatory interneurons to induce cAMP and PKA responses—the closely timed combination produces especially large cAMP responses only in the conditioned stimulus sensory neurons.

In addition, there is a change in the postsynaptic element that also mediates the conditioned response. As you should recall, the neurotransmitter for the reflex pathway is glutamate. This neurotransmitter activates two types of ionotropic receptors on the postsynaptic elements. One is a conventional receptor that regulates Na^+ influx. The other is a special receptor, called the N-methyl-D-aspartate (NMDA) receptor, that regulates Ca^{2+} flow. Under normal operation of the reflex, and under habituation and sensitization, the NMDA receptor is blocked by another charged molecule, magnesium (Mg^{2+}). However, NMDA receptors have the unusual property of being modulated by the voltage of the cell membrane such that when the membrane is depolarized the magnesium block is eliminated and Ca^{2+} can flow into the cell. During the protocol for classical conditioning this is accomplished when the CS+ activates the conventional ionotropic receptors, allowing Na^+ influx and producing the typical synaptic depolarization. This transiently unblocks the NMDA channels, so that if a US occurs briefly afterward, facilitating the synapse so that the motor neuron generates a long train of action potentials, the NMDA receptor opens allowing in Ca^{2+}. This results in a cascade of molecular events that results in lasting modifications of the postsynaptic element. The NMDA receptor and its role in memory in mammalian systems is considered again in greater detail in the next chapter.

Substrates of permanent memory traces in cellular mechanisms

The sensitization and classical conditioning studies so far described have focused on the local mechanisms within synaptic elements that mediate short-term memory. To create long-lasting memories, it has long been recognized that additional mechanisms are likely required—mechanisms that rely on structural changes involving the growth of existing synapses or the addition of new synapses. These changes surely involve protein synthesis. Early experiments showed repeatedly that inhibition of protein synthesis, at any stage in the activation of the genes to the production of protein molecules, blocks the formation of memories. Furthermore, the role of protein synthesis in memory formation is a somewhat prolonged one, as demonstrated in studies showing that inhibition of protein synthesis for several minutes after learning also blocks later expression of memory. Following that period, however, inhibition of protein synthesis does not block memory, showing that the process is completed in due course.

What are the mechanisms that connect the activation of intracellular mechanisms at the synapse to the production of proteins and the fixation of memory? There is evidence that the first steps begin with the molecular cascade already described (see Fig. 2–7). For example, in the sensitization protocol described earlier, single stimulations with serotonin result in the release of a small amount of cAMP, sufficient to generate small amounts of PKA that have local effects. But the amount of PKA is not sufficient to diffuse in quantity to the nucleus of the cell where the genetic machinery lies. However, repeated stimulations raise the concentration of cAMP to a level where it interacts with the PKA to break up its form into separate functional units. One type of unit, called the catalytic subunit, then diffuses in sufficient quantity to the nucleus to activate the genetic decoding machinery.

When the active unit of PKA translocates to the nucleus it phosphorylates (adds a phosphorous-containing molecule) to several factors that activate the transcription of RNA from the DNA code (see Fig. 2–7). The most relevant of these for our purposes is a protein called cAMP-response element binding protein (CREB). One form of CREB, called CREB-1, binds to a special element on DNA called CRE and switches on the genes that code for molecules critical to the fixation of memory. This was confirmed in experiments showing that inhibiting the binding of CREB-1 prevents sensitization whereas infusing phosphorylated CREB-1 into the sensory neuron produces lasting facilitation. This combination of findings indicates that CREB-1 is both necessary and sufficient for the fixation of this simple form of memory.

In addition, there are mechanisms for fine tuning the process of fixation. In particular, within the same sensitization paradigm, another form of CREB, called CREB-2, has been identified. CREB-2 appears to suppress CREB-1 and therefore acts as an inhibitory transcription regulator, that is, a repressor. Evidence indicates that CREB-2 is regulated by a different protein kinase called mitogen-activated protein kinase, or MAP kinase. MAP kinase acts by preventing CREB-2's blockade of CREB-1, and thus activation of MAP kinase facilitates CREB-1 and memory. This was shown in an impressive demonstration of enhanced learning in *Aplysia*. Whereas a single stimulation of the sensory neuron ordinarily produces only a short-lasting sensitization, following a treatment that blocked CREB-2, the facilitation was lasting.

The precise set of genes activated by the CREB mechanism, and their specific actions in mediating memory fixation, are not well understood. Because of the rapidity of the gene expression following stimulation, it has been suggested that the critical steps may involve a special class of genes called immediate-early genes that are activated quickly and transiently. Within the *Aplysia* sensitization model, there is evidence that one of these genes may control the production of an enzyme called ubiquitin hydrolase, which appears to diffuse back toward the synapse where it helps release the active subunits of PKA and consequently produce a lasting alteration in synaptic physiology.

In addition, there must be a production of as yet unknown molecules that regulate growth of synapses. It has been shown, for example, that long-term sensitization results in a major increase in the number of synaptic terminals of the sensory neurons. Dendritic processes also grow to accommodate the increase in synaptic contacts. Thus, there has to be a coordination of presynaptic and postsynaptic growth that would mediate long-lasting changes in efficacy of the reflex.

Other "simple" systems

Parallel observations on other model systems indicate that the cellular events and molecular cascade described for *Aplysia* are conserved in evolution. In particular, one prominent model based on another invertebrate often used in genetic studies provides substantial converging evidence of the scheme outlined above. These studies involve a kind of olfactory learning in fruit flies. In this behavioral paradigm, groups of animals are placed in chambers that contain a particular odor and then shocked briefly. On other trials, the same animals are placed in a different chamber that contains another odor and no shock is given. Finally, the animals are placed in an apparatus that allows the animal to migrate between the two familiar chambers and they typically express memory as a preference for the safe chamber. Several different mutant flies have been tested in this protocol, and a number of them turn out to have specific amnesic deficits.

One of these flies, called *dunce*, had a defect in the gene that regulates cAMP and had a severe learning deficit. Another with a defect in adenyl cyclase, the enzyme that synthesizes cAMP from ATP, is called *rutabaga* (one of several named after vegetables, as a reflection on their intelligence), and other flies with defects in genetic regulation of PKA also show deficient memory capacity.

Recently, in this model, the role of CREB has also been examined. These studies found that a genetic manipulation that led to overexpression of a CREB repressor blocked the fixation of memory. More strikingly, and similar to the studies on *Aplysia*, overexpression of a CREB activator reduced the training required to have lasting memory. Usually a single training trial with each odor is sufficient to produce only a short-lived memory. However, when the CREB activator was overexpressed, a single training trial was sufficient to fixate the memory.

Summing up

Neurons are composed of three main elements: dendrites that are specialized for receiving signals from other cells, the cell body, and the axon that is specialized for conduction of the neural impulse. In addition, there are specialized areas of these cellular components that mediate communication between cells, called synapses, each composed of a presynaptic element where neurotransmitters are stored and released and a postsynaptic element where there are receptors that recognize the neurotransmitter and generate signals in the postsynaptic cell.

There are two electrical mechanisms for conduction of the neuronal signal over substantial distances through the dendrites and axon. The initial phase, called *electrotonic conduction*, typically begins at the postsynaptic site and proceeds to the cell body, and involves passive and fast, but decremental conduction of an electrical signal. The later phase is called the *action potential*, which typically begins at the origin of the axon, and involves active and relatively slow, but faithful conduction of a signal over long distances. Neural transmission occurs at the synapse and involves the action potential causing the fusion of synaptic vesicles and release of neurotransmitter from the presynaptic element. The neurotransmitter activates voltage-gated channels in the postsynaptic receptor site, which depolarizes the postsynaptic cell in excitatory synapses and hyperpolarizes the postsynaptic cell at inhibitory synapses.

These basic mechanisms of neuronal physiology are important to understanding the nature of neural plasticity that underlies memory. These and other aspects of the molecular physiology of neurons have been put to use in simple invertebrate systems to understand three fundamental types of learning: habituation, the decrementing of responsiveness to repeated sensory stimulation without reinforcement, sensitization, the incrementing of responsiveness to sensory stimulation following strong stimulation, and classical conditioning, the association of an arbitrary external stimulus with a stimulus that produces a reflexive response.

The findings from the studies of relatively simple invertebrate learning models have provided fundamental insights about the representation of memories in the brain of all animals. These basic insights can be summed up as follows: First, Cajal was right in his conjecture that alterations in synaptic efficacy provide the basic cellular mechanism for memory. Second, the nature of the chemical mechanisms involved in memory are not unique "memory molecules," but rather involve a set of adaptations of natural molecular mechanisms by which synaptic activity is regulated. Indeed, the most common mechanisms involve clever uses of ubiquitous molecules, such as cAMP and the genetic code regulators. Third, the changes that mediate memory do not involve special "memory cells," but rather the same cells that perform sensory, modulatory, and motor functions in the reflex pathway. Fourth, and closely related to the last point, the cells of the nervous system seem to be highly adaptable. It takes very few activations of the right type to induce an adaptation of the cellular mechanisms to support memory, and not many more to incite the permanent fixation process. Fifth, and finally, several mechanisms are employed in memory formation at the cellular level, allowing for different forms of memory to be encoded within the same cells, and allowing for a variety of ways to fine tune the memory and its time course at the various stages in a cascade of cellular events.

READINGS

Bear, M.F., Connors, B.W., and Paradiso, M.A. 2000. *Neuroscience: Exploring the Brain*. New York: Williams & Wilkins.

Carew, T.J. 1996. Molecular enhancement of memory formation. *Neuron* 16:5–8.

Squire, L.R., and Kandel, E.R. 1999. *Memory: From Mind to Molecules*. New York: Scientific American Library.

Tully, T., Bowling, G., Chistensen, J., Connoly, J., Delvechhio, M., DeZazzo, J., Dubnau, J., Jones, G., Pinto, S., and Regulski, M., et al. 1996. A return to the genetic dissection of memory in Drosophila. *Cold Spring Harbor Symposium in Quantitative Biology* 61:207–218.

3
• • • • • •

Cellular Mechanisms of Memory: Complex Circuits

STUDY QUESTIONS

What is LTP?

Why is LTP a good model for the plasticity that underlies memory?

What are the cellular mechanisms for the induction of LTP?

What are the molecular mechanisms for the preservation and expression of LTP?

What is the evidence that something like LTP occurs during learning?

What is the evidence that the mechanisms of LTP are required for learning?

The previous chapter showed how understanding cellular and molecular mechanisms can provide clear insights into the bases for memory in relatively simple nervous systems. Indeed, to the extent that the most important aspects of the relevant circuitry have been included in those model systems, it might not be too vain to conclude that we truly *understand* how memory works in those circuits.

In the present chapter, we aim higher: Can we also understand the nature of learning and memory in more complex systems, such as those of mammals, through a characterization of cellular and molecular properties in the key brain areas involved in memory functions? There is certainly a long history of the expectation that a simple reflex modification mechanism will be conserved across species and in complex as well as simple systems. Pavlov and Sherrington, from distinct behavioral and physiological perspectives, recognized that modification of synaptic function—synaptic plasticity—is the basic substrate of the conditioned reflex mechanism in mammals. In 1949 Donald Hebb broadened this notion beyond that of stimulus and response associations, outlining a cascade of events that begins with synaptic plasticity as the fundamental associative mechanism and extends to the development of "cell assemblies" that represent specific percepts, thoughts, and actions, in all species including humans.

Modern neuroscience since Hebb's time has made tremendous advances in understanding synaptic plasticity mechanisms and their possible role in memory using mammalian model systems. This chapter reviews some of the recent progress toward a full characterization of one particular form of synaptic plasticity observed in the mammalian brain called long-term potentiation (LTP). LTP is a laboratory phenomenon, but its mechanisms are now quite well understood. It can be induced in many brain structures that are involved in memory, and there is substantial evidence that the same cellular mechanisms that mediate LTP are required for lasting memory. Therefore, this chapter reviews the state of our understanding of this important phenomenon as a likely candidate for memory coding in mammalian systems.

Hippocampal long-term potentiation as a model memory mechanism

Long-term potentiation is most commonly studied in the hippocampus, a brain structure that you will come to know quite well in this book. The hippocampus is a complex structure, but it is easy to find in the brain, and its inputs, outputs, and intermediate pathways are largely segregated, making it an excellent model system for studying its circuitry. We now know a lot about the initial steps in the molecular and synaptic basis of LTP, particularly as seen in the hippocampus. The elucidation of these mechanisms has been facilitated greatly by the development of the *in vitro* hippocampal "slice" preparation in which thick transverse sections of the hippocampus are taken from the brain and kept alive in a Petri dish (Fig. 3–1). This preparation lacks the complex influences of the normal inputs and outputs of the hippocampus, but provides an especially clear access to cells and intrinsic connections of the hippocampal circuit. Most of these studies have focused on area CA1 of the hippocampus, where the in vitro preparation allows multiple input and output pathways to be preserved intact and to be manipulated independently for recording and stimulation (Fig. 3–2A).

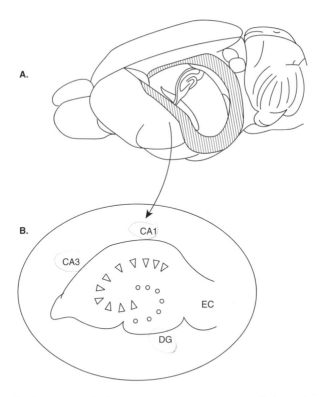

Figure 3-1. The hippocampal slice preparation. *A:* A view of the rodent brain. The hippocampus is a large structure inside the cerebral hemispheres. A slice is taken in a plane transverse to the long axis of the hippocampus. *B:* The hippocampal slice in vitro, with indications of its major subdivisions, CA1, CA3, DG = dentate gyrus, EC = entorhinal cortex.

The phenomenon of LTP was first discovered by Terje Lomo, a PhD student working in Oslo. Lomo was exploring the physiology of the circuitry of the hippocampus, and in particular he was examining the phenomenon of frequency potentiation, an increase in the magnitude of responsiveness of cells following a series of rapidly applied activations. Lomo observed that repetitive high-frequency electrical stimulation (called tetanus) of one pathway resulted in a steeper rise time (slope) of the excitatory synaptic potential to a subsequent single pulse. He also observed that following a tetanus there was recruitment of a greater number of cells reaching the threshold for an action potential, reflected in a greater "population spike," the spike observed when many cells fire together (see examples in Fig. 3–2B). Lomo found that the tetanus-induced changes in the synaptic and cellular responses to single pulses lasted for several hours,

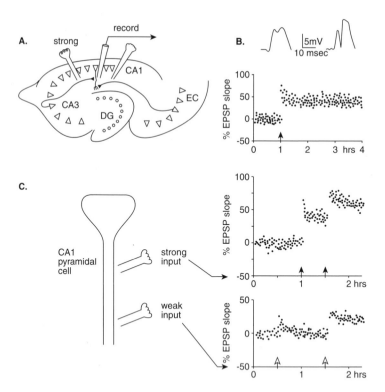

Figure 3–2. Hippocampal long-term potentiation (LTP). *A:* Illustration of a horizontal section through the hippocampus showing the pathways by which pyramidal cells in CA1 are stimulated by either a strong input from CA3 or a weak input from the entorhinal cortex (EC). *B:* Excitatory postsynaptic potentials (EPSPs) recorded after single pulse stimulations of the strong path before (left) and after (right) tetanus. Below is the standard method for tracking the changes in the EPSP slope over a period of hours. *C:* Associative LTP. A schematic diagram of a CA1 pyramidical cell and loci of strong and weak stimulation, and measurements of the EPSP slopes following single pulses of each type of input. The weak input stimulation alone (open arrow at 0.5 hr on lower graph) produces only a transient change, but strong stimulation alone (filled arrow at 1 hr) produces LTP. Combined strong and weak stimulation (both arrows at 1.5 hr) result in LTP at both synaptic sites (data from Bliss and Collingridge, 1993).

leading him to distinguish this phenomenon from short-lasting facilitations. And so, he called it "*long-term potentiation.*" In subsequent years several investigators have characterized the basic properties of the synaptic and cellular components of LTP, creating considerable excitement about this phenomenon as a model for lasting history-dependent synaptic change. The findings have spawned a veritable cottage industry within the field of neuroscience.

What fascinated researchers at the outset were the remarkable parallels between properties of LTP and memory. In 1989 Richard Morris identified five fundamental properties that make LTP such an attractive model of memory. First, LTP is a prominent feature of the physiology of the hippocampus, a brain structure universally identified with memory. Subsequent work has made clear that the hippocampus is not the only site of LTP, but its functional role as a component of one of the brain's major memory systems would seem to demand that it possess a memory mechanism.

The second and third properties have to do with temporal characteristics. LTP develops very rapidly, as one would require of a plausible memory mechanism, typically within 1 minute after a single stimulus train delivered with the proper parameters. Moreover, like a good memory, LTP can be long-lasting. In in vivo preparations it can be observed for hours after a single stimulation train, or for weeks or more after repetitive stimulations that might act as "reminders."

Fourth, LTP has the sort of *specificity* one would require of a memory mechanism: Only those synapses activated during the stimulation train are potentiated. Other neighboring synapses, even on the same neurons, are not altered. This phenomenon parallels the natural specificity of our memories, in which we are able to remember many different specific episodes with the same person (e.g., one particular date you had, out of many, with a given individual) or object (e.g., where you parked your car today rather than last week), and thus would be a key requirement of any useful cellular memory mechanism. In addition, the property of specificity may be key to the magnitude of the storage capacity of brain structures. Each cell can participate in the representation of multiple memories, each composed of distinct subsets of its many synaptic inputs.

Fifth, and perhaps most definitively important for memory, LTP is *associative* in that potentiation occurs best when multiple inputs are stimulated simultaneously during the tetanus (Fig. 3–2C). This phenomenon has been demonstrated most elegantly in studies that employ activation of separate pathways that synapse on the same hippocampal neurons. In these studies the two pathways involve the combination of a "weak" input, designated as one that does not produce potentiation at any stimulation level, plus a "strong" input for which a threshold level of stimulation suffices to produce LTP. Associativity is observed when the weak input is activated at the same time as the strong input, resulting in LTP of the weak as well as the strong pathway. The time window for this sort of association was initially thought to be quite brief, on the order of a few milliseconds, and thus quite limited in the extent to which it could support Pavlovian conditioning, which usually involves hundreds of milliseconds separation between conditioned stimulus (CS) and unconditioned stimulus (US). However, there is new evidence that a form of associativity may be possible within a broader, and more behaviorally meaningful, time window. An intriguing 1997 study by Frey and Morris indicated that activity at hippocampal synapses that produces only a short-lived potentiation can nonetheless create a synaptic "tag" that lasts a few hours. Subsequent strong activation of a neighboring pathway within that period leads to lasting potentiation of both the "strong" pathway and the previously "tagged" synapses. Thus, LTP could serve to associate or integrate patterns of activity over a time window that has obvious behavioral significance.

The property of associativity is especially appealing because it offers a cellular model of the mechanism for structural change in neural connections, a change that would increase synaptic "efficacy," the strength of the postsynaptic response resulting from a presynaptic activation. When Hebb proposed his theory of cell assemblies (see Part III), he recognized the need for alterations in the cells so that a whole assembly could be reactivated to recall a memory. He suggested that the essential trigger for changing synaptic efficacy involved the repeated activation of a presynaptic element AND its participation in the success in firing the postsynaptic cell. The simultaneous activation of many inputs of the hippocampus during a tetanus provides a perfect situation to accomplish the co-occurrence of presynaptic and postsynaptic activity. Furthermore, the property of associativity, by permitting the ability to integrate patterns of activity, simultaneously satisfies the induction requirement of LTP—that there be a combination of presynaptic and postsynaptic activation—and offers a fundamental mechanism for encoding associations between functionally meaningful activation patterns.

Cellular basis for the induction of hippocampal LTP

Many studies have shown that the induction of LTP in area CA1 requires two fundamental synaptic events—activation of presynaptic inputs and depolarization of the postsynaptic cell. Both are ordinarily accomplished within a single high-frequency stimulus train—the initial stimulation depolarizes the cell for a relatively prolonged period during which the following stimulations provide simultaneous postsynaptic activations. However, high-frequency stimulation is not required *per se*. Instead, for example, direct depolarization of the postsynaptic cell by injection of current through an intracellular electrode, combined with low-frequency presynaptic input, will suffice. Conversely LTP induction can be blocked by preventing depolarization, or by hyperpolarization of the postsynaptic cell. These findings show that the conditions of Hebb's postulate about the critical conditions for cellular events are both necessary and sufficient to provide a synaptic mechanism for memory.

Molecular bases for the induction and maintenance of hippocampal LTP

The molecular mechanism that underlies the major type of LTP induction in CA1 involves special properties of a combination of synaptic receptors, some of which should be familiar from your reading of Chapter 2 (see Fig. 3–2). Considerable evidence points to the amino acid glutamate as the primary excitatory transmitter in the hippocampus and elsewhere where LTP is found. There are several types of glutamate receptors, most prominently divided into those that are excited by N-methyl-D-aspartate (NMDA receptors, already introduced in Chapter 2) and those that are activated by a-amino-3-hydroxy-5-methyl-4-isoxazolepropionate (AMPA receptors). These two types of receptors can be dissociated functionally by pharmacological manipulations. In particular, the NMDA receptors are selectively and competitively blocked by the antagonist D-2-amino-5-phosphono-valerate (AP5). A major discovery in revealing the mechanism of LTP was that AP5 has little effect on excitatory postsynaptic potentials (EPSPs) elicited by low-frequency stimulation, indicating that AMPA receptors, and not NMDA receptors, mediate normal synaptic transmission in the hippocampus. In contrast, AP5 completely blocks LTP following high-frequency stimulation trains, indicating that glutamate activation of NMDA receptors is critical to this form of synaptic plasticity.

Discoveries about two major differences between NMDA and AMPA receptors in their regulation of postsynaptic ion permeability in CA1 offer an explanation of the role of these receptors in LTP (Fig. 3–3). First, activation of AMPA receptors increases the permeability of the postsynaptic membrane to both sodium (Na^+) and potassium (K^+) ions, but does not alter cell permeability to calcium (Ca^{2+}). By contrast, activation of NMDA receptors increases permeability to Ca^{2+} as well as to Na^+ and K^+ ions. Second, unlike for AMPA receptors, ion flow through NMDA receptors is highly dependent on the voltage state of the postsynaptic cell at the time of NMDA receptor activation. In the resting state, NMDA receptor channels are blocked by another doubly charged ion, magnesium (Mg^{2+}), which prevents the flow of the other ions even in the presence of glutamate at the receptor. However, when the membrane of the postsynaptic cell is depolarized, Mg^{2+} is expelled from the receptor channel, al-

A. Normal synaptic transmission

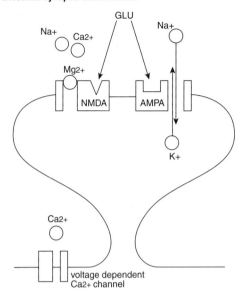

B. During depolarization

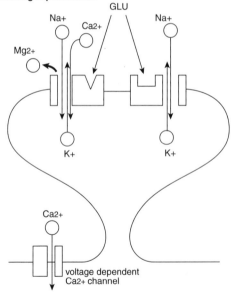

Figure 3–3. Molecular mechanism of the induction of long-term potentiation (LTP). GLU = glutamate; See text for explanation (adapted from Nicoll et al., 1988).

lowing glutamate to bind and the ions including Ca^{2+} to flow. Thus, the effect of the initial activations in the high-frequency stimulus train is to activate the AMPA receptors, depolarizing the postsynaptic cell membrane. This unblocks the NMDA receptor channels so that succeeding stimuli activate the NMDA receptor, allowing Ca^{2+} to enter the postsynaptic cell.

The entry of Ca^{2+} to the intracellular space is a key step in the induction of LTP. This is shown in at least three lines of evidence. First, LTP is prevented when Ca^{2+} is bound by intracellular injection of a calcium chelator (a molecule that binds up calcium). Second, LTP is triggered by intracellular injection of a caged Ca^{2+} compound that releases calcium molecules. Third, the entry of Ca^{2+} into the postsynaptic cell following stimulation trains has been directly imaged using a sophisticated technique called confocal fluorescence microscopy. There is evidence, however, that Ca^{2+} entry does not, by itself, lead to lasting synaptic potentiation; rather, some sort of NMDA receptor activation seems to be required. One possibility under scrutiny is that glutamate also activates metabotropic receptors that mediate release of intracellular stores of Ca^{2+} as an amplification mechanism.

The succeeding steps in the permanent maintenance of LTP are less well understood, and can only be provided in outline form at this time (Fig. 3–4). The leading view is that the role of Ca^{2+} is to activate kinases, enzymes that phosphorylate proteins, transforming them into their active

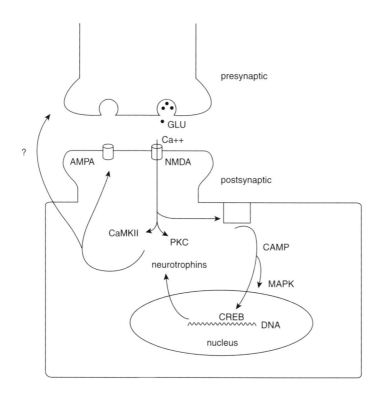

Figure 3–4. Model of the molecular mechanisms of short-term and long-term processes following long-term potentiation induction.

configuration, and some of these will be familiar from your reading about invertebrate systems in Chapter 2. Specific candidates of the critical kinases in the hippocampus include type II Ca^{2+}/calmodulin-dependent kinase (CaMKII), Ca^{2+}/phospholipid-dependent protein kinase C (PKC), and mitogen-activated protein kinase (MAPK).

CaMKII is a very attractive candidate because it is present in large quantities in the postsynaptic area and its initial activation depends on Ca^{2+}. Tetanus stimulates its production, and pharmacological inhibition and genetic elimination of CaMKII block LTP. Furthermore, following activation, CaMKII undergoes an autophosphorylation by which it becomes independent of the transient Ca^{2+} influx to remain phosphorylated. This prolonged activation could mediate long-lasting consequences, one of which might be the conversion of inactive (so-called silent) AMPA receptors into active ones. PKC is also strongly implicated by experiments showing that its activation results in marked potentiation of the EPSP that occludes further potentiation by stimulation trains. Furthermore, intracellular injection of PKC enhances synaptic transmission, and application of PKC antagonists block LTP. MAPK is activated by phosphorylation following LTP or stimulation that results in intracellular Ca^{2+}, and inhibition of MAPK prevents later steps in gene expression.

In addition to modifying existing proteins, there is evidence that the maintenance of LTP also depends on new protein synthesis in the hippocampus. Experiments using protein synthesis inhibitors indicate that proteins synthesized from preexisting mRNA are required for lasting LTP. In addition, there is also evidence that the maintenance of LTP depends upon the cAMP-responsive transcription factor CREB. One possible mechanism for CREB involves the Ca^{2+} influx activating adenylyl cyclase, which in turn activates cAMP. This could in turn activate PKC, leading to the phosphorylation of many proteins, including CREB. The phosphorylated form of CREB is known to modulate the transcription of genes so as to increase the expression of several proteins. There is some evidence indicating that genetically altered mice who lack a form of CREB have deficient LTP maintenance.

One possible target of new protein synthesis in the hippocampus is the production of neurotrophins, molecules long known as regulated by neural activity and having the capacity to promote morphological change and increased connectivity. Stimulation trains capable of inducing LTP increase the gene expression for some neurotrophins in the hippocampus. In turn, some neurotrophins potentiate glutaminergic transmission in CA1, and these effects occur within minutes and last for several hours or longer.

Where is the synaptic alteration?

A major unresolved question is whether the locus of lasting synaptic alteration following LTP is presynaptic or postsynaptic. Of course, changes at both sites are entirely possible. The evidence on both sides of this issue is considerable, and it may not be possible to fully resolve the issue with current methods available to study the hippocampal preparation. Recent attempts to resolve the question have focused on *quantal analysis*, a protocol that involves reducing presynaptic release to a statistical phenomenon. This method allows estimation of the magnitude of the postsynaptic response to a single quantum of transmitter, presumably corresponding to release of a single synaptic vesicle. During LTP there is a decrease in the percentage of failures of postsynaptic response and a decreased variability of responses to presynaptic stimulation, both consistent with an increase in the probability of presynaptic release. However, there is also observed an increase in the amplitude of the response to a single quantum of transmitter, which is consistent with an increase in postsynaptic receptor efficacy. Thus, the current evidence from quantal analyses are consistent with both loci as being involved in plastic change.

Conceptual considerations have also weighed in on this controversy. Possible cellular mechanisms for postsynaptic modification are straightforward to envision, as just discussed. By contrast, because the initial effects of combined pre- and postsynaptic activity evoke cellular mechanisms localized in the postsynaptic cell, an ultimate change in presynaptic physiology would require production and transport of some sort of retrograde messenger, a signal that travels from the activated postsynaptic site to the presynaptic site. Several candidates for the retrograde messenger have been proposed [e.g., arachidonic acid, nitrous oxide (NO), carbon dioxide (CO)], but so far, none has received more than fragmentary support.

Hippocampal long-term depression

If there was only a form of plasticity that *increased* synaptic efficacy, eventually all synapses would become "saturated," that is, raised to a ceiling level of efficacy, and no further learning could occur. So most investigators think that, in addition to the potentiation of synapses, there must be a mechanism of depotentiation or *long-term depression* (LTD) of synaptic efficacy. LTD also can enhance the relative effect of LTP at neighboring synapses, improving the signal-to-noise contrasts, as well as also increasing the range of synaptic coding patterns by a population of synapses providing input to a single postsynaptic cell.

In general, the learning rule for LTD involves activity-dependent plasticity with a direct violation of the Hebb rule for LTP. Thus, LTD has been described under conditions where there is either presynaptic activity or postsynaptic activity, but not both. One can activate presynaptic elements with single pulses at a very low rate that produces no activation, or only weak activation, of the postsynaptic cell. Or one can induce presynaptic activity in the absence of postsynaptic firing, by activating presynaptic elements weakly and out-of-phase with strong stimulation to converging synapses of the same postsynaptic cell. Alternatively, LTD also results from activation of the postsynaptic neuron, without activation of the presynaptic element. This form of LTD can be induced either by stimulation of separate converging synapses on the same postsynaptic cell or by inducing an action potential in the axon that is conducted backward to the cell body (called antidromic activation). All of these forms of LTD have been observed at one pathway or another in the hippocampus, but it remains to be seen if they obey the same induction and maintenance rules and are available at all sites in the hippocampus.

Anatomical modifications consequent to LTP

Most researchers believe that lasting changes in neural connectivity ultimately require altered morphology of synapses. Although this research area has been plagued by technical issues of the proper means of preserving tissue for examination with the electron microscope, there is now substantial evidence that LTP does result in structural alterations in synaptic connections consistent with increases in synaptic efficacy. Most of these data focus on the protruding heads of dendritic spines that are the excitatory synapses of the dentate granule or CA1 pyramidal cells, the same sites that involve NMDA receptor dependent LTP. In the dentate gyrus, the reported structural changes suggest an increase in spine surface area and in the area of the opposing pre- and postsynaptic membranes. In some reports the changes in spines occurred without any appreciable increase in the number of synapses, suggesting an interconversion of spine shapes in which LTP results in increases in synaptic contact area by expansions of the pre- and postsynaptic cell membranes surrounding one another. Studies on CA1 have provided strikingly parallel results, changes in spine dimensions consistent with the overall rounding of spines, although these changes may be transient. Recent studies using newly available high resolution optical methods have detected growth of new spines on postsynaptic dendrites in CA1 shortly after induction of LTP. In addition, lasting changes in spine number have been reported in CA1, and these changes have been characterized as reflecting the transformation of synapses into types with protracted necks as well as sessile types. The coordination of increased presynaptic and postsynaptic active contact, as observed in studies on both the dentate granule and CA1 pyramidal cells, seems to obviate the question of whether the fundamental basis of LTP is pre- or postsynaptic in origin.

LTP beyond the hippocampus

LTP was first discovered in the hippocampus, and it is easily studied there because of the laminar separation of synaptic inputs and outputs. However, there are now reports of potentiation of synaptic efficacy in widespread areas of the brain and LTP is rapidly becoming viewed as a universal plasticity mechanism. Among the areas where LTP, and/or LTD, have been demonstrated are several areas of the neocortex, piriform cortex, amygdala, striatum, cerebellum, and even the spinal cord.

Perhaps best characterized of the nonhippocampal areas is the visual cortex, which has been studied extensively by Mark Bear and his colleagues. In the rat visual cortex, Bear's research group developed an in vitro visual cortex slice preparation in which they would stimulate layer IV input cells and record from layer III principal cells that receive inputs from the layer IV cells (Fig. 3–5). They recorded EPSPs before and after

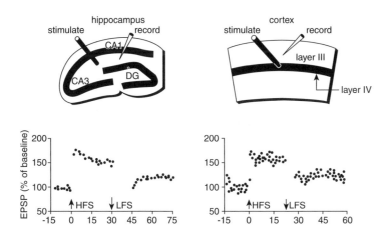

Figure 3–5. Induction of long-term potentiation (LTP) and long-term depression (LTD) in hippocampal and cortical slices. The plots show that in both preparations an increase in the excitatory postsynaptic potentials (EPSP) (LTP) is produced by short bursts of high-frequency stimulation (HFS), and in both preparations a decrease in the field EPSP (LTD) is produced by low-frequency stimulation (LFS) (data from Bear, 1996).

tetanization of the input cells, and found that stimulation of the input layer results in LTP and LTD in principal cells with the same protocols effective for producing these phenomena in the hippocampus. Thus, they demonstrated bidirectional activity-dependent modification of visual cortex synapses such that low-frequency stimulation results in synaptic depression, whereas high-frequency stimulation produces potentiation, just as in the hippocampus. Both forms of synaptic modification are synapse specific and depend on NMDA receptors. Intracellular injections of current that produce postsynaptic depolarization or hyperpolarization paired with low-frequency synaptic activation produce synaptic enhancements or decrements, respectively.

LTP and memory

LTP captures an exciting physiological phenomenon, one that is seen, deservedly, as the most prominent model of synaptic plasticity that might underlie memory. As Charles Stevens once put it, this mechanism is so attractive that it would be a shame if the mechanism underlying LTP turned out not to be a memory mechanism. But there should be no doubt about the fact that LTP is not memory—it is a laboratory phenomenon that involves massive coactivations never observed in nature. The best we can hope is that LTP and memory share a common mechanism. In recent years disappointing evidence has emerged, amidst the more positive findings, regarding all main lines of evidence that have been offered to connect LTP and memory.

Here I attempt just to summarize the history of the research on the possible linkage between LTP and memory. Several relatively direct approaches have been pursued in attempting to demonstrate that LTP and memory share common physiological and molecular bases. Most prominent are demonstrations of changes in synaptic efficacy consequent to a learning experience ("behavioral LTP"), and, conversely, attempts to prevent learning by pharmacological or genetic manipulation of the molecular mechanisms of LTP induction. Examples of each approach are presented here, and discussed in light of the inherent limitations they have in convincingly connecting LTP and memory.

"Behavioral LTP"

Do conventional learning experiences produce changes in synaptic physiology similar to the increases in EPSP and cellular responses that occur after LTP? Seeking changes in synaptic physiology consequent to learning is an ambitious and optimistic approach because one might well expect the magnitude of synaptic change observed in gross field potentials to be van-ishingly small following any normal learning experience—a virtual "nee-dle in a haystack." In addition, it is most likely that learning involves changes in synaptic efficacy in both the positive and negative directions, that is, both LTP and LTD. Thus, learning would likely result in changes in the distribution of potentiated and depressed synapses with little or no overall shift, and consequently no change, or even an overall negative change, in the averaged evoked potentials commonly used to measure LTP.

Addressing the first of these concerns by using powerful and extended experience as the learning event, the initial reports showed enhancement of excitatory synaptic potentials and population spikes after different types of learning experience. The early studies include ones in which several as-pects of synaptic physiology were observed to change in the perforant path-way response in rats who had been exposed for prolonged periods to an "enriched" as compared to "impoverished" environment. The "enriched" rats lived in a large housing area with littermates, with continuous social stimulation and various forms of environmental stimulation through their opportunity to investigate and interact with many objects placed in their shared cages, whereas the "impoverished" rats had solitary housing, the absence of stimulating objects, and a small living space. In one particu-larly illustrative study of this type, hippocampal slices were taken from these rats and were tested for various aspects of synaptic and cellular re-sponsiveness. It was found that rats who had lived in the enriched envi-ronment, compared to those restricted to the impoverished environment, had an increased slope of the synaptic potential and larger population ac-tion potentials, implying more cells recruited, but no change in other phys-iological parameters. These changes are entirely consistent with the pat-tern of increased synaptic efficacy observed following LTP. These changes were not permanent, however. They disappeared if the enriched-condition animals were subsequently isolated for 3–4 weeks prior to the analyses.

Recent observations by Joseph LeDoux and his colleagues offer con-firming evidence for a connection between the phenomena of LTP and en-hanced transmission of relevant sensory inputs in a different neural circuit that supports a specific kind of learning. In this case the learning involved a form of classical (Pavlovian) conditioning in which rats become fearful of tones that have been paired with foot shocks (see Chapter 11). The rel-evant anatomical pathway involves auditory inputs to a subcortical struc-ture in the thalamus called the medial geniculate nucleus, projections from there to another subcortical area called the lateral amygdala nucleus, and then projections from there to other parts of the amygdala which control the expression of fear responses (Fig. 3–6A; this pathway is described in

A.

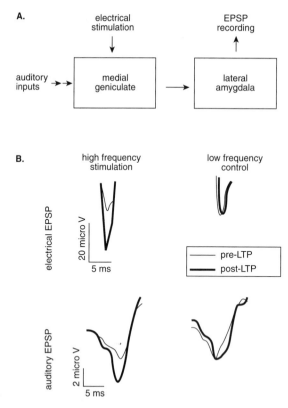

Figure 3–6. Common mechanisms for long-term potentiation (LTP) and sensory processing. *A:* Anatomical pathway for natural auditory stimulation or electrical stimulation of the medial geniculate nucleus and recording in the lateral amygdala. *B:* Examples of excitatory postsynaptic potentials (EPSPs) evoked by auditory stimulation or electrical stimulation of the medial geniculate before and following high- or low-frequency medial geniculate electrical stimulation that produces LTP in the lateral amygdala recording; note that the same stimulation at low frequency does not produce any potentiation of the EPSP. The induction of LTP in that pathway also results in a large increase in the EPSP response to auditory stimulation in the same pathway (data from Rogan and LeDoux, 1995).

more detail in Chapter 11). In one study they used high-frequency electrical stimulation of the medial geniculate nucleus to induce LTP within the lateral nucleus of the amygdala. Consequently they found an enhancement of synaptic responses within the same area of the amygdala to natural auditory stimulation (Fig. 3–6B). In a complementary study they found the converse evidence that fear conditioning enhances early sensory-evoked responses of neurons in the lateral amygdala.

These findings are illuminating in two ways. First, they support the view that there is nothing special about the hippocampus when it comes to LTP. Second, the approach taken by LeDoux and colleagues points toward a potentially more decisive and therefore possibly more fruitful way to link LTP and memory. The pattern of changes in auditory-evoked synaptic potentials, including the magnitude, direction, and longevity of increased responses, paralleled those parameters for electrically induced synaptic potential, showing us that natural information processing can make use of the very cellular and molecular mechanisms set in place by conventional, artificially induced LTP. Conversely, the observation of increased neuronal sensory responses following conditioning shows us that, like LTP, real learning can enhance information processing relevant to the task.

In subsequent studies the same group has also now shown that repeated pairings of auditory stimuli and foot shocks that train rats to fear the tones also alter evoked sensory responses to the tones in the same way as LTP in that pathway (Fig. 3–7). Thus, in rats with properly timed pairings, tones produce evoked potentials of greater slope and amplitude, just as electrical stimulus trains do when applied to this pathway. No enhancement of field potentials is observed with unpaired tone and foot shock presentations, even though this conditioning control leads to as much of a behavioral response (freezing) as paired presentations (even the unpaired control rats learn to freeze to the environmental context where shocks are received—see Chapter 11). Furthermore, this behavioral LTP is enduring, lasting at least a few days, as long as the behavioral response during extinction trials. Thus, LeDoux and colleagues' approach takes us beyond mere similarities between LTP and memory, bringing into contiguity the identical neural pathways and experimental procedures that define LTP and sensory processing in memory.

A different set of studies on the rat motor cortex by John Donoghue and his colleagues demonstrates the generality of this approach to other brain areas and other forms of learning. In these experiments, rats were trained to reach with one particular paw through a small hole in a food

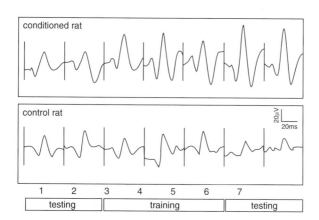

Figure 3–7. Changes in auditory field potentials in the amygdala following fear conditioning. Note the sustained increase in the size of the auditory-stimulation-induced excitatory postsynaptic potentials (EPSP) following paired tone–shock combinations versus no change in the EPSP size under control conditions where tones and shocks were not consistently paired (data from Rogan et al., 1997).

box in order to retrieve food pellets. Initially, the rat's reaching movements are labored and often the food pellets are dropped. However, over the course of one or two hour-long practice sessions, the rats refine their motor coordination and ultimately obtain pellets at a rapid asymptotic rate. Following this kind of motor coordination training, Donoghue and colleagues removed the brain and measured the strength of connections among cells within the area of the motor cortex that controls hand movements. They accomplished this using an *in vitro* preparation of the appropriate brain section and evoking EPSPs in a principal cell layer of the motor cortex by stimulating horizontal fibers that connect neighboring cells to one another (Fig. 3–8). They found that for the same or lower input stimulation intensity, the magnitude of the EPSPs on the side of the brain that controlled the trained paw (i.e., in the contralateral or opposite hemisphere) were consistently larger than those on the side of the brain that controlled the untrained paw. Furthermore, they also found it difficult to induce LTP by electrical stimulation in the trained hemisphere, but not in the untrained hemisphere. Thus, training produced an anatomically localized increase in synaptic efficacy that occluded the capacity for LTP. These observations show in a compelling way that synaptic potentiation results from motor learning, and the real plasticity phenomenon shares common resources with the artificial one, providing strong evidence for common cellular mechanisms of LTP and learning.

Blocking LTP and memory

The major limitation of the preceding approach is that the experiments only provide correlations between aspects of LTP and memory. The con-

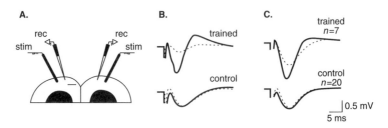

Figure 3–8. Effects of motor skill learning on evoked excitatory postsynaptic potentials (EPSPs) in the motor cortex. *A:* Placement of stimulating and recording electrodes in the two sides of the motor cortex slices. *B:* (example) and *C:* (group average) EPSPs recorded from trained animals and untrained controls. The dark lines represent recordings from the trained hemisphere and dotted lines recordings from the untrained hemisphere (from Rioult-Pedotti et al., 1998).

verse approach is to draw cause-and-effect links between the phenomenology of LTP and of memory by blocking LTP and determining if memory is prevented. Perhaps the most compelling and straightforward data
on a potential connection between the molecular basis of LTP and memory have come from experiments where a drug or genetic manipulation is
used to block LTP and, correspondingly, prevent learning. Here again there
was the need for optimistic assumptions. It had to be assumed that the
drugs were selective to plasticity and not normal information processing
in the brain, and that they would knock out a critical kind of plasticity.
These assumptions were accepted based on the observation that drugs such
as AP5, which selectively blocks the NMDA receptor, prevent hippocampal LTP while sparing normal synaptic transmission. Thus, to the extent
that the role of the NMDA receptor is fully selective to plasticity, one
might predict these drugs would indeed block new learning without affecting nonlearning performance or retention of learning normally accomplished prior to drug treatment.

Consistent with these predictions some of the earliest and strongest evidence supporting a connection between LTP and memory came from studies on spatial learning by Richard Morris and his colleagues. Morris developed a maze learning task in which hippocampal function is required.
In this task, the maze involves a swimming pool in which the water is
made opaque by the addition of a milky powder, and an escape platform
is submerged just under the water at a predetermined location. Rats are
good swimmers, but prefer to find and climb onto the platform. Typically,
they are trained to find the platform from any of four starting positions
around the periphery of the maze, and they show learning by shortening
the time required to escape from all starting points. At the end of training, their memory is assessed using a probe test where the platform is removed, and rats exhibit good memory by swimming in the vicinity of the
former escape locus.

Initially Morris and his colleagues showed that AP5-induced blockade
of NMDA receptors prevents new spatial learning in the water maze. Drug-
treated rats swim normally, but do not reach the same level of rapid escape as normal rats. Indeed, the drug-treated rats often adopt a strategy
of swimming at a particular distance from the walls of the maze, which
reduces their escape latency to some extent without knowing the exact location of the platform. In the probe tests, normal rats show a distinct preference for swimming in the vicinity of the former escape locus, but drug-
treated rats show little or no such bias, indicating the absence of memory
for the escape location (see Chapter 5 for further discussion of this task).
Additional experiments showed no effect of AP5 on retention when train-

ing was accomplished prior to drug treatment. This could be fully predicted because NMDA receptors are viewed as required only for the induction of LTP and not for its maintenance (see Molecular bases for induction and maintenance of hippocampal LTP). Furthermore, the deficit was limited to spatial learning, known from other work to be dependent on the hippocampus, and not to a simple visual discrimination, known to be NOT dependent on hippocampal function.

Additional research by Morris and his colleagues has also shown how NMDA receptor dependent LTP might play a continuing role in updating one's memories. To accomplish this they developed a new version of the water maze task in which the location of the escape platform is moved every day, and animals are given four trials to learn the new location. Across a series of training days the rats became skilled at the task such that they consistently found the platform very rapidly on the second trial it was presented. Subsequent to initial drug-free training, animals were tested with different memory delays inserted between the first and second trial on each day (Fig. 3–9A). On some days, AP5 was infused into the hippocampus, and on other days a placebo was given. AP5 treatment resulted in a deficit on trial 2 performance (Fig. 3–9B). Moreover, this deficit was dependent on the time interval between trial 1 and trial 2, such that no impairment was observed with a 15 second intertrial interval, but significant deficits ensued if the intertrial interval was extended to 20 minutes or longer. These data suggest that memory for specific episodes of spatial learning remains dependent on NMDA receptors and LTP, even after the animals have learned the environment and the general rules of the spatial task.

Genetic manipulations of LTP and memory

Other research has used targeted genetic manipulations to show that blocking the cascade of molecular triggers for LTP also results in severe memory impairments. In one of the early studies of this type, mice with a mutation of one form of CaMKII had deficient LTP and were selectively impaired in learning the Morris water maze. Despite the fact that the genetic manipulation was effective throughout development, the hippocampus appeared normal in architecture and was normal in its basic physiological responsiveness. Since that time, selective memory impairments have been reported in several different types of knockout mice with deficiencies in LTP, with a special emphasis on knockouts of CREB.

The manipulation of biochemical mechanisms by interference with specific genes allows investigators to identify critical molecular events at a very high level of specificity. For example, one study by Alcino Silva and

A.

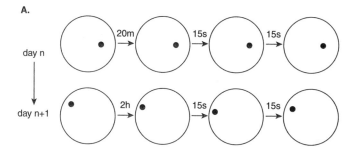

B.

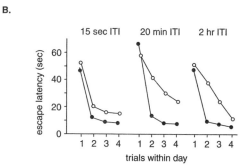

Figure 3–9. Matching-to-place version of the Morris water maze task *A:* Example test sessions. On each session the animal is given four trials with the escape platform in a novel location. Note that the first intertrial interval is variable, and the others are constant at 15 sec. *B:* Effects of infusion of AP5. After initial training on the task, rats treated with AP5 or placebo were tested on a series of four-trial sessions with the escape platform in a novel location each day. On some test sessions the interval between trials 1 and 2 was 15 sec. On these sessions rats given AP5 performed as well as normal subjects in showing a substantial reduction in the latency that indicated intact memory On other sessions the interval between trials 1 and 2 was 20 min or 2 hr. On these sessions normal animals also showed good retention, but AP5 rats showed substantially less reduction in their escape latencies, indicating memory impairment. The later intertrial intervals were all 15 sec, and all animals show substantial latency decreases over these brief intervals. Filled circles = controls; open circles = AP5 (data from Morris and Frey, 1997).

his colleagues showed that substitution of a single amino acid in CaMKII that prevents its autophosphorylation results in severe learning and memory deficits. In addition, other new genetic approaches are providing greater temporal- as well as region-specific blockade of gene activation. In another recent study by Susumu Tonegawa and his colleagues, the genetic block was limited to postdevelopment activation of the genes for the NMDA receptor specifically in the CA1 subfield of the hippocampus, which selectively blocked LTP in that region. Despite these highly selective temporal and anatomical restrictions, the mice with this mutation were severely deficient in spatial learning as well as in other types of memory dependent on hippocampal function. A complementary recent study showed that a mutation that results in overexpression of NMDA receptors can enhance several kinds of memory dependent on the hippocampus. There is also growing evidence that interference with other events involved in the LTP molecular cascade, specifically PKC and MAPK, also have deleterious effects on memory. Thus, it is likely that the full set of cellular events that mediate LTP will also be shown to play critical roles in memory.

Blocking LTP and plasticity of hippocampal firing patterns

The studies described previously provide strong evidence in favor of the view that pharmacological and genetic manipulations that prevent hippocampal plasticity selectively block a critical stage in memory formation. However, skeptical neuroscientists are always concerned that a particular drug or genetic manipulation could have its deleterious effects not on memory directly, but rather on the normal information processing in brain structures that play a role in task performance. In general the best evidence offered in pharmacological and genetic studies involves the observation that the drugs or genetic manipulations do not affect synaptic transmission as revealed in evoked potential protocols. However, it is important to realize that large-scale evoked EPSPs never actually occur during normal information processing. So the data available from these studies do not allow us to conclude that other more complex, and more relevant, patterns of hippocampal information processing are fully normal under the influence of drugs such as AP5.

A newer generation of combined electrophysiological and pharmacological-genetic studies is providing evidence critical to this question. Several studies have how examined the nature and persistence of spatial representations of single hippocampal neurons and neuronal populations in animals with compromised capacity for LTP. These studies involve genetically altered mice or rats with pharmacologically blocked LTP and recordings of so-called place cells, hippocampal neurons that fire when the animal is in a particular location in its environment (see Chapter 6 for a detailed explanation of place cells). One of these studies found that mutant mice expressing an active form of CaMKII that impairs one form of LTP and spatial learning have impoverished and unstable hippocampal spatial representations. Hippocampal cells of these mice initially develop spatially specific firing patterns, albeit in fewer cells, and the spatial specificity of these patterns is reduced. Perhaps most important, unlike normal mice who have very stable hippocampal spatial representations, the spatial firing patterns in mutant mice are lost or changed if the animal is removed from the environment and later replaced even within a few minutes. Acute pharmacological blockade of NMDA receptors in rats also resulted in instability of the spatial firing patterns of hippocampal neurons, without affecting the incidence or spatial specificity of previously acquired spatial firing patterns. The drug did not prevent the initial establishment of hippocampal spatial firing patterns or their short-term retention between repeated recording sessions separated by brief intervals. By contrast the maintenance of a newly developed spatial representation across days was severely compromised.

The consequence of LTP blockade for the network processing of hippocampal spatial representations has also been examined. One study examined the spatial firing patterns of groups of neighboring hippocampal neurons in mice with the CA1-specific knockout of NMDA receptors. They also reported that these cells had diminished spatial specificity, and characterized a reduction in the coordinated activity of neurons tuned to overlapping spatial locations. Furthermore, they tied these findings to the spatial memory impairment by showing how the loss of coordinated activity in mutant hippocampal place cells leads to a poorer prediction of sequential locations during navigation behavior. Another study characterized hippocampal spatial representations in mice with knockouts of CaMKII or CREB. Similar to the other studies, they observed diminished spatial selectivity in both mutants, as well as diminished stability of the spatial representations when some of the environmental cues were altered. CaMKII mutant mice could not recover their spatial representations when the environmental cues were returned to their original configuration. However, the CREB-knockout mice, in whom spatial learning and LTP are partially preserved, showed they could recover their spatial representations in the original environment. These results suggest that the network processes that bind together single neuron representations of spatial cues are particularly dependent on LTP. Further investigations on the coding of space by hippocampal networks offer a particularly promising direction for relating synaptic plasticity processes to memory functions.

Blocking LTP and memory outside the hippocampus

Other studies suggest that the cascade of molecular events that is invoked by LTP may also mediate cortical plasticity that underlies memory. A particularly good example of this work involves a set of studies by Yadin Dudai and his colleagues focused on taste learning mediated by the gustatory cortex of rats. When rats are exposed to a novel taste and subsequently become ill, they develop a conditioned aversion specifically to that taste, and this learning is known to depend on the gustatory cortex. Blockade of NMDA receptors by infusion of the antagonist AP5 produces an impairment in taste aversion learning, whereas the same injections given prior to retention testing, or into an adjacent cortical area, had no effect. Thus, it is likely that modifications in cortical taste representations depend on LTP. Furthermore, blockade of protein synthesis in the gustatory cortex by infusion of an inhibitor prior to learning also prevents development of the conditioned taste aversion. By contrast, the same injection given into a neighboring cortical area or given to the gustatory cortex hours after learning has no effect. Consistent with this finding, MAP kinase as well as a downstream protein kinase were activated selectively in gustatory cortex within 10 minutes of exposure to a novel taste and activation peaked at 30 minutes, whereas exposure to a familiar taste had no effect. Conversely, a MAP kinase inhibitor retarded conditioned taste aversion. This combination of findings provides complementary lines of evidence that strongly implicate the NMDA mediated plasticity and subsequent specific protein synthesis as playing a critical role in cortical modifications that mediate this type of learning.

Summing up

In mammalian systems, the most popular model for the cellular and molecular mechanisms that underlie memory is long-term potentiation (LTP) and its sister phenomenon long-term depression (LTD). Both phenomena follow Hebb's rule in that increases in synaptic efficacy (facilitation of synaptic transmission) marking LTP occur as a consequence of repeated activation of a presynaptic element and its participation in the success in firing the postsynaptic cell, whereas decreases in synaptic efficacy (decrements in synaptic transmission) marking LTD occur as a consequence of the absence of correspondence between activation of a presynaptic element and postsynaptic cell activation.

An understanding of the molecular and cellular mechanisms of some forms of LTP is emerging. The induction of one prominent form of LTP involves the activation of NMDA receptors, which occurs when a non-NMDA receptor is initially activated to depolarize the postsynaptic cell, causing the release of a magnesium block of the NMDA receptor allowing the transmitter glutamate to activate that receptor. This results in an influx of calcium which begins a molecular cascade of events that both stabilizes the changes in the postsynaptic cell and induces gene expression and permanent cellular modifications.

Does LTP equal memory, and do we now understand memory in mammalian systems? There is certainly no consensus among researchers that LTP and memory are the same thing, or even that the case for common mechanisms is strong and closed. As described here, there are compelling lines of evidence favoring this view. There is evidence that LTP enhances learning-related information processing, and conversely that learning results in enhancement of synaptic potentials in circuits relevant to particular forms of memory. Correspondingly, there is evidence that blocking LTP with drugs or genetic manipulations can result in a pattern of amnesia reflected both in memory impairments and instability of relevant neural representations. So, while there is also some contradictory evidence, not outlined here, at least a provisional case for shared mechanisms has emerged.

In the simpler invertebrate systems discussed in Chapter 2, the circuits that mediated forms of habituation, sensitization, and classical conditioning were mostly identified. So, the additional evidence about cellular changes and their molecular mechanisms seems to offer fairly comprehensive framework for an understanding of memory in those systems. In reading this chapter, though, you were introduced to fragments of a few of the brain circuits involved in learning in mammalian systems, and to a few of the different kinds of learning in which they participate. You have not yet seen the full circuitry involved in any of these systems. Nor have you yet heard about why they mediate different forms of learning, or about how many systems and forms of learning exist. Even for the hippocampus itself, you have only been provided with a glimpse of its role in memory and the nature of the information represented within its circuitry. Completing these stories is a major aim of the remainder of this book.

At this point, you should be impressed with the conservation of fundamental cellular and molecular mechanisms of memory across species and brain systems. In all the examples discussed, changes in synaptic efficacy are central. And these changes seem to be subserved by a relatively small set of pervasive molecular mechanisms that reveal a cascade of events that leads from short-term modulation to permanent structural alteration of synapses. Within simpler, well-understood circuitries, this cascade provides a more or less comprehensive picture of memory accomplished. Within more complex circuitries, a higher level of analysis will be required to reach a full understanding of the systems, circuits, and codes for memory.

READINGS

Bear, M.F. 1996. A synaptic basis for memory storage in the cerebral cortex. *Proc. Nat. Acad. Sci. U.S.A.* 93:13453–13459.

Bliss, T.V.P., and Collinridge, G.L. 1993. A synaptic model of memory: Long-term potentiation in the hippocampus. *Nature* 361: 31–39.

Malenka, R.C. 1994. Synaptic plasticity in the hippocampus: LTP and LTD. *Cell* 78: 535–538.

Morris, R.G.M. 1989. Does synaptic plasticity play a role in information storage in the vertebrate brain. In *Parallel Distributed Processing: Implications for Psychology and Neurobiology,* Morris, R.G.M. (Ed.). Oxford: Clarendon Press, pp. 248–285.

Morris, R.G.M., and Frey, U. 1997. Hippocampal synaptic plasticity: Role in spatial learning or the automatic recording of attended experience? *Phil. Trans. R. Soc. Lond.* 352: 1489–1503.

Rioult-Pedotti, M.-S., Friedman, D., Hess, G., and Donoghue, J.P. 1998. Strengthening of horizontal cortical connections following skill learning. Nat. Neurosci. 1:230–234.

Rogan, M.T., Staubli, U.V., and LeDoux, J.E.. 1997. Fear conditioning induces associative long-term potentiation in the amygdala. *Nature* 390:604-607.

Silva, A.J., Smith, A.M., and Giese, K.P. 1997. Gene targeting and the biology of learning and memory. *Annu. Rev. Gene.* 31:527–547.

Steele, R.J. and Morris, R.G.M. (1999) Delay dependent impairment in matching-to-place task with chronic and intrahippocampal infusion of the NMDA-antagonist D-AP5. *Hippocampus* 9:118–136.

Stevens, C.F. 1998. A million dollar question: Does LTP = memory. *Neuron* 20: 1–2.

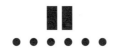

COGNITION:
IS THERE A "COGNITIVE" BASIS
FOR MEMORY?

William James may have best captured the essence of the distinction between the behaviorist and cognitivist views of memory in his turn of the twentieth century text, *The Principles of Psychology*. While acknowledging that habits (learned reflexes) could be chained to mediate even rather complicated and coordinated, sequences, such a form of representation lacked the flexibility and consciousness that characterized real memory. He qualified true memory as "the knowledge of an event, or fact, of which in the meantime we have not been thinking, with the additional consciousness that we have thought or experienced it before" (p. 648). Even in acknowledging that conditioning could revive an image or copy of a prior event, such a revival would not really be a true memory—to be a true memory, the image must not only be conceived of as in the past, but as in one's own past, and the memory must contain one's own experience with the item. This, James argued, would come about only by retrieving memories within a network of associated information, and bringing this network-memory up to the realm of consciousness. But, other than suggesting this would require a vastly complicated brain process, James was at a loss to offer details on the mechanisms of conscious recollection.

By contrast, the behaviorist school that emerged in the Golden Era promised tight experimental control and a detailed understanding of the elements of learning within the context of findings emerging from Pavlov's physiological studies. So ignoring James's admonitions, the behaviorists held sway in the thinking of most learning theorists for several decades. Nevertheless, battles between the "behaviorists" and "cognitivists" would continue for that entire period. A major early challenge came from Yerkes, who, based on his extensive observations of problem solving in great apes, concluded that higher animals did not learn by random trial and error with reinforcement guiding behavior, but rather exhibited ideation and insight. A greater degree of success in challenging the reductionist approach was achieved by two later experimentalists, Edward Tolman and Fredric Bartlett, working with rats and humans, respectively.

Tolman and the "cognitive map"

In the 1930s and 1940s Edward Tolman was more successful in challenging behaviorism precisely because he developed operational definitions for mentalistic processes including "purposive behavior" and "expectancy." Moreover, he rigorously tested these ideas using the same species (rats) and maze learning paradigms that were a major focus of prominent behaviorists. Tolman and his students performed several experiments pitting these views against one another in analyses of maze learning by rats. Their studies focused on whether rats could demonstrate "insight" by taking a roundabout route or shortcut in a maze when such strategies were warranted, and were inconsistent with a previous reward history that favored a different route. For example, in an experiment that demonstrated detour taking in rats, Tolman used an elevated maze that involved three diverging and then converging routes from a starting place to a goal box (Fig. II-1). During preliminary training the rat could take any route, and came to prefer the shortest. When this route was blocked (at block A) most rats would prefer to switch to the next shortest route. Only when this route was also blocked would they take the longest path. In the critical test phase, a new block was introduced at the point where the two shorter paths converged (block B). Rats began by running down the shortest path (path 1) as usual. But instead of immediately selecting the next shortest path (path 2), as they had done during the preliminary phase when the shortest route (path 1) was blocked, most rats immediately selected path 3.

In addition to this "detour" ability, Tolman also provided evidence that rats could take shortcuts. In this experiment rats were trained to approach a goal via a single circuitous route, then the maze was substituted with many direct paths, some leading toward and others away from the goal locus. Most rats ran to the path that took them directly to where the entrance of the food box had originally been located. These studies provided compelling operational evidence of Tolman's assertions that rats had inferential capacities revealed in the flexibility of the behavioral repertoire that could be brought to bear in solving problems for which behavioral theory had no explanation.

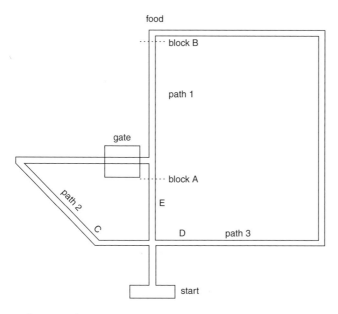

Figure. II-1. Schematic diagram of the maze Tolman used to test the ability of rats to infer a detour.

Thus, Tolman's basic premise was that learning generally involved the acquisition of *knowledge* about the world, and in particular about relationships among stimuli and between stimuli and their consequences, and that this knowledge led to expectancies when the animal was put in testing situations. His views contrasted sharply with those of the behaviorists on three key features of learning. First, the behaviorists argued that the contents of memory involve habits that can be characterized as acquired stimulus–response reflex sequences. But for Tolman learning involved the creation of a "cognitive map" that organized the relations among stimuli and consequences that would guide behavioral solutions to obtain desired consequences.

Second, for the behaviorists reinforcement was the central driving force of learning. Thorndike's "law of effect" attributes all learning to the principle that behaviors that lead to a positive reinforcement strengthen stimulus–response connections and are thus more likely to be repeated. Alternatively, Pavlov had proposed that learning involved the association of conditioned and unconditioned stimulus through temporal contiguity. In Pavlov's paradigm, that key association was between the bell, as conditioned stimulus, and the taste of food as unconditioned stimulus; through the learned association the bell comes to substitute for the food taste in evoking salivation. For Tolman, however, reinforcers served simply as more information on which to confirm one's expectancies about when, where, and how rewards were to be obtained—learning itself was driven not by reinforcement but by curiosity about the environment and seeking of knowledge for expectancies about its predictive structure. Reinforcers would certainly determine what behavior might eventually be emitted, but were not necessary for establishment of the representation.

Third, for the behaviorists the responses emitted are precisely the motor commands that are the end point of stimulus–response reflexes. The range of behavioral responses then is fully determined as the motor patterns that were elicited and reinforced during learning itself. But to Tolman, learning and performance were fundamentally independent events. That is, what an animal knew about the world and what it was going to do about it were surely related (through its expectancies), but were not the same thing, as the behaviorists held. Thus, Tolman argued, animals could use their cognitive maps and expectancies to guide the expression of learned behavior in a variety of ways not limited to repetition of the behavioral patterns exhibited and reinforced during learning. These aspects of expectancy, insight, and flexibility will prove to be important aspects of modern views of memory.

It would be too strong to say that Tolman's arguments were sufficiently compelling to cause learning theorists to abandon the reductionist views. Indeed, as shown by the success of B.F. Skinner's successes in the 1950s and 1960s, the behaviorist school still played out a long run in research laboratories, in the development of some clinical approaches to abnormal behavioral patterns in people, and in the popular press.

Frederic Barlett and the "schema"

Around the same time as Tolman was carrying out his classic studies on maze learning in rats, the British psychologist Frederic Bartlett published a treatise on human memory. And just as Tolman's theory challenged stimulus–response behaviorism, Barlett's work stood in stark contrast to the then established and better known rigorous methods introduced by Ebbinghaus, which guided the pursuits of most of his contemporary psychologists. However, Bartlett's insights about the structure and richness of memory have proven to be critical for modern views of memory. His work was central in bringing the field of memory research back to issues about the nature of the more complex forms of memory that support conscious recollection. Bartlett differed diametrically from Ebbinghaus in two major ways. First, his interest was in the mental processes used to remember. He was not so interested in the probability of recall, as dominated Ebbing-haus's approach, but in what he called "effort after meaning," the mental processing taken to search out and ultimately reconstruct memories. Second, Bartlett shuddered at the notion of using nonsense syllables as learning materials. By avoiding meaningful items, he argued, the resulting memories would necessarily lack the rich background of knowledge into which new information is stored. Barlett's main strategy to study recollection was called the method of repeated reproduction. His best known work examined recollections of a South American Indian folk tale written in a syntax and prose style that were quite different from the culture of his British experimental subjects. In particular the story contents lacked explicit connections between some of the events described, and the tale contained dramatic and supernatural events that would evoke vivid visual imagery on the part of his subjects. These qualities were, of course, exactly the sort of thing Ebbinghaus worked so hard to avoid with his nonsense syllables. But Bartlett focused on these features because he was primarily interested in the content and structure of the memory obtained.

Bartlett did not use rigorous operational definitions or statistical measures, but his analyses were compelling nonetheless. Bartlett concluded that remembering was not simply a process of recovering or forgetting items, but rather that memory seemed to evolve over time. Items were not lost or recovered at random, as Ebbinghaus might predict. Rather, material that was more foreign to the subject, or lacked sequence, or was stated in unfamiliar terms, was more likely to be lost or changed substantially in both syntax and meaning, becoming more consistent with the subject's common experiences. These and many other examples led Bartlett to develop an account of remembering known as "schema" theory, in which a schema is an active organization of past experiences in which, during remembering, one constructs or infers the probable constituents of a memory and the order in which they occurred. He proposed that remembering is therefore a *reconstructive* process and not one of mere *reproduction*, as Ebbinghaus preferred. In Bartlett's terms, remembering required the ability to "turn round" on one's own schemata, using consciousness to search within the simpler learned sequences for rational and consistent order and to reconstruct them anew consistent with one's whole life of experience. In this way Bartlett gave consciousness a function beyond merely being aware. It played a central role in the reconstructive act of remembering, making it consciously mediated, running contrary to current psychological views that would banish references to consciousness.

Ultimately, behaviorist-versus-cognitivist controversy on the nature of memory would be resolved by observations from neuroscience. This work involved examinations of amnesic patients, people who were suffering severe memory loss as a result of specific brain damage. While debilitating, it turns out that the memory capacity lost was selective to aspects of conscious recollection described by James and Bartlett, and had properties shared with Tolman's characterizations of the cognitive map. Other capacities that the behaviorists might recognize as intact stimulus–response learning were spared, even in severe cases of amnesia in humans. Parallel studies on animals with experimental brain damage in the same brain areas implicated in human amnesia provided additional insights into the anatomical psychological bases and fundamental psychological mechanisms of cognitive memory. In addition, related physiological observations provide an understanding of the coding elements that underlie the cognitive mechanisms in conscious memory. These findings are the focus of this section.

READINGS

Bartlett, F.C. 1932. *Remembering*. London: Cambridge University Press.

James, W. 1890. *The Principles of Psychology*. New York: Dover Publications (1950 edition).

Tolman, E.C. 1932. *Purposive Behavior in Animals and Men*. Berkeley: University of California Press (1951 edition).

4

• • • • • •

Amnesia—
Learning about
Memory from Memory Loss

STUDY QUESTIONS

Who is H.M. and why is he so valuable to memory research?

What nonmemory abilities are spared in amnesia?

What memory capacities are spared in amnesia?

How is the kind of memory lost in amnesia best characterized?

Over 50 years of experimentation on the course of normal learning did not resolve the debate between behaviorists and cognitivists. But studies on the loss of memory in humans, the phenomenon of amnesia, provided a pair of breakthroughs that has led to an understanding and validation of both the behaviorist and the cognitivist views.

The first major breakthrough came with the 1957 report by Scoville and Milner on the most famous neurological patient ever, a man known by his initials H.M. This patient had been severely epileptic for several years. In an effort to alleviate his disorder, the medial temporal lobe area was removed, and indeed the surgery did reduce the frequency of his seizures considerably. However, following the surgery this patient became severely amnesic, and yet showed hardly any other neurological deficits. Because of both the severity and the selectivity of his memory deficit, the findings on H.M. changed everything about how we think about the brain and memory. Before H.M. the search for memories was focused on the cerebral cortex—in H.M. the critical damage was in areas underneath the cortex. Before H.M. the generally held view was that memory and other perceptual and cognitive functions were not anatomically separable—H.M. showed a clear dissociation between fully intact perception and cognition versus severely impaired memory. The observations on the pattern of his impairment directly addressed the nature of cognitive processes in memory; these findings are discussed in this chapter in detail. The discovery of a "pure" memory deficit following selective brain damage also addressed how memory is compartmentalized in the brain, and that topic is discussed in the next section of this book. In addition, a prominent component of H.M.'s amnesia is a temporally graded retrograde memory impairment, like that of Ribot's patients introduced in Chapter 1, and the implications of these findings for the phenomenon of consolidation are discussed in greater detail in Chapter 12.

The initial observations did not at first provide clarification about the nature of cognitive processes in memory. H.M.'s loss of everyday memory was "global," that is, it appeared to encompass all kinds of memories, and in this broad scope did not directly reveal anything about the memory processes that underlie the deficit. Yet, even from the outset, exceptions to H.M.'s global amnesia were noted—he was able to learn new motor skills. In addition, another hint of an exception to the otherwise pervasive scope of amnesia came from the observation that prior exposure to picture or words could facilitate later identification of those items from fragmentary information. But these spared capacities at first seemed meager compared to the devastation of his overall memory capacity.

A deeper understanding about the exceptions came in 1980 when Neal Cohen and Larry Squire made a second major breakthrough in understanding the nature of the memory processing deficit behind amnesia. They described a complete preservation of the acquisition, retention over several months, and expression of a perceptual skill in amnesic patients. The behavioral paradigm they explored involved an improvement in fluency during reading of mirror-reversed words. Ordinarily one is slow in deciphering a word that is presented "backward," that is, with each of the letters reversed as if seen in a mirror. However, with practice one improves considerably at this general skill, even when none of the particular words are repeated. Cohen and Squire found that this kind of learning was fully normal in a set of amnesic patients.

In addition, when normal subjects were presented the same mirror-reversed words a second time, they showed an extra level of facilitation in reading them beyond that explained by the general skill acquisition—that is, they showed memory for the particular mirror-reversed words they had seen before. However, the amnesic patients were markedly impaired both in recognizing the familiar words and in recollecting their training experiences. Cohen and Squire were struck by the dissociation between the ability to acquire the general mental procedure of reading reversed text, an ability that appeared fully normal in the amnesic patients, and the capacity to explicitly remember or consciously recollect those training experiences or their contents, which was markedly impaired in the amnesics. They attributed the observed dissociation of these two kinds of memory performance, together with the earlier reported exceptions to amnesia, to the operation of distinct forms of memory. Cohen and Squire suggested that the medial temporal region was specialized for *declarative memory,* the capacity to consciously recollect everyday facts and events, and that other brain regions were sufficient to mediate a collection of learning capacities that they called *procedural memory,* the ability to tune and modify the brain's networks that support skilled performance. Two decades of research have supported this dissociation, and further characterized and distinguished the properties of declarative and procedural memory.

The following sections provide a more detailed overview of the patient H.M., in order to provide a closer perspective on the nature of his amnesia. Then the distinction between declarative and procedural memory is explored further, using several examples from the experimental literature on amnesia.

The amnesic patient H.M.

In 1933, when H.M. was 7 years old, he was knocked down by a bicycle, hit his head, and was unconscious for 5 minutes. Three years after that accident he began to have minor epileptic seizures, followed by his first major seizure while riding in his parents car on his 16th birthday. Because of the epileptic attacks his high school education was erratic, but eventually he graduated in 1947 at age 21 with a "practical" course focus. Subsequently, he worked on an assembly line as a motor winder. However, the seizures became more frequent, on average 10 minor attacks each day and a major one each week, and he eventually could not perform his job. Attempts to control the seizures with large doses of anticonvulsant drugs were unsuccessful, leading to consideration of a brain operation. There was no evidence of localization from electroencephalographic (EEG) studies. Nevertheless, because of the known epileptogenic qualities of the medial temporal lobe areas, an experimental operation was considered justified as an effort to ameliorate his devastating seizure disorder. In 1953, when H.M. was 27, Dr. William Scoville performed the bilateral medial temporal lobe resection.

The surgical approach to this area is difficult, because the relevant tissue lies inside the part of the temporal lobe near the midline, almost in the center of the brain. The surgical procedure involved making a hole above the orbits of the eyes and lifting the frontal lobes. From this approach the anterior tip of the temporal lobe could be visualized, and the medial part resected. Suction was used to remove all of the tissue bordering the lateral ventricle, including the anterior two-thirds of the hippocampus, as well as the amygdala and surrounding cortex very selectively (Fig. 4–1).

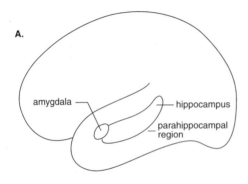

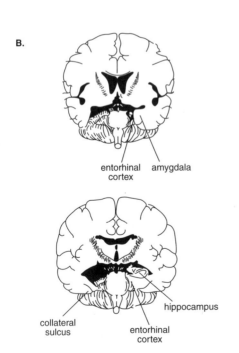

Figure 4–1. A: Position of the hippocampus, amygdala, and surrounding cortex in the human brain. *B:* Sections through the human brain showing reconstructions of the area of medial temporal lobe removal in the patient H.M., based on MRI scans. Top: A more anterior section showing the area of removal that involved the amygdala (left side) compared to the intact area (right side). Bottom: A more posterior section showing the area of removal that involved the hippocampus (left side) as compared to the intact area on the right. In H.M. the lesions were bilateral (from Corkin et al., 1997).

The operation reduced the frequency of seizures to a point that they are now largely prevented by medication, although minor attacks persist. However, one striking and totally unexpected consequence of the surgery was a major loss of memory capacity. Because of the combination of the unusual purity of the ensuing memory disorder, the static nature of his condition, his cooperative nature, and the skill of the researchers who have protected and worked with him, H.M., is probably the most examined and best known neurological patient ever studied.

After recovery from his operation, H.M. returned home and lived with his parents. There he did household chores, watched TV, and solved cross-word puzzles. Following his father's death he attended a rehabilitation workshop and became somewhat of a handyman, doing simple and repetitive jobs. Eventually his mother and then another relative could no longer care for him, so he was moved to a nursing home where he still resides, participating in daily social activities of the home, as well as watching TV and solving difficult crossword puzzles. He is characterized as a highly amiable and cooperative individual. He rarely complains about anything, and has to be quizzed to identify minor problems such as headaches. He never spontaneously asks for food or beverage, or to go to bed, but he readily follows directions for all of his daily activities. His temper is generally very placid, although this author recalls one day when H.M. was depressed about "having not done anything with his life." However, when assured that he was indeed a very important person, his mood returned to its normal rather upbeat state, and he told one of his famous stories about once considering a career in neurosurgery. He is aware of his memory disorder, but is not consistently concerned about it. Sometimes when given a rather difficult memory question he reminds the tester, "You know I have a memory problem." The severe magnitude of his memory disorder has continued unabated since the time of the surgery.

Some of the most compelling examples of the severity of H.M.'s amnesia come from anecdotes of those who have worked with him. I recall my first encounter with H.M., while transporting him from the nursing home to M.I.T. for a testing period in 1980. On the way to the nursing home, I had stopped at a nearby McDonald's for lunch, and had left a coffee cup on the dashboard of the car. When I retrieved H.M., I sat him comfortably in the back seat and we began the trip to Boston. After just a few minutes H.M. noticed the cup and said, "Hey, I knew a fellow named John McDonald when I was a boy!" He proceeded to tell some of his adventures with the friend, and so I asked a few questions and was impressed with the elaborate memories he had of that childhood period. Eventually the story ended and H.M. turned to watch the scenery passing by. After just a few more minutes, he looked up at the dashboard and remarked,

"Hey, I knew a fellow named John McDonald when I was a boy!" and proceeded to relate virtually the identical story. I asked probing questions in an effort to continue the interaction and to determine if the facts of the story would be the same. H.M. never noticed he had just told this elaborate tale, and repeated the story more or less exactly as before. A few minutes later the conversation ended, and he turned to view the scenery again. However, just minutes later, once more H.M. looked up to the dashboard and exclaimed, "Hey, I knew a fellow named John McDonald when I was a boy!" I helped him reproduce, as well as he could, the same conversation yet again, then quickly disposed of the cup under the seat. . . .

The selective nature of H.M.'s memory disorder

H.M.'s disorder is highly selective in two important ways. First, his impairment is almost entirely selective to memory, as distinguished from other higher-order perceptual, motor, and cognitive functions. Second, even within his memory functions, the disorder is selective to particular domains of learning and memory capacity. Some of the details concerning these two aspects of his preserved and impaired capacities are discussed next.

H.M.'s perceptual, motor, and cognitive functions are intact

The results of extensive testing of sensory functions showed that H.M.'s perceptual capacities are entirely normal. He performs well within the normal range on tests of visual acuity, adaptation, and other commonly tested visual-perceptual functions. He can recognize and name common objects. He has some loss of touch and fine motor coordination revealed in sophisticated tests, but these are not noticed in his generally good performance on tasks that require coordination in his daily environment. H.M.'s intelligence was above average in standard IQ tests just before the operation. After the surgery his IQ actually rose somewhat, perhaps because of the alleviation of his seizures. H.M.'s language capacities are largely intact, although he exhibits slight deficits in the fluency of his speech, and his spelling is poor. He appreciates puns and linguistic ambiguities, and communicates well and freely. His spatial perceptual capacities that do not depend on memory are mixed. For example, he has some difficulty copying a complex line drawing, and cannot use a floor plan to walk a route from one room to another in the M.I.T. testing facility. On the other hand, he does well on other complex spatial perceptual tasks, and can draw and recognize an accurate floor plan of his former house.

By contrast, H.M. has almost no capacity for new learning, as measured by a large variety of conventional tests. He was not given standard memory tests prior to the operation. After the surgery his scores on standardized scales indicated a severe memory disorder. In particular, he scores zero on components of the test that assess the persistence of his memory for short stories, lists of words or numbers, pictures, or any of a large range of other materials.

H.M.'s memories acquired in childhood are intact, and his immediate memory capacity is normal

H.M. can remember material learned remotely prior to his operation. His memory for the English language seems fully intact. He also retains many childhood memories. By contrast, all memory for events for some period preceding the operation was lost. In addition, H.M.'s immediate or short-term memory is intact. He can immediately reproduce a list of numbers as long as that of control subjects—thus the "span" of his short-term memory is normal. However, the memory deficit becomes evident as soon as his immediate memory span is exceeded or after a delay with some distraction. These aspects of H.M.'s spared memory abilities are discussed further in later chapters.

"Exceptions" to H.M.'s impairment in new learning

The early studies on H.M. also revealed a few "exceptions" to his otherwise profound defect in lasting memory. One of these, called mirror drawing, involved the acquisition of sensorimotor skill. In this task the subject sits at a table viewing a line drawing and one's hand only through a mirror (Fig. 4–2). The line drawing contains two concentric outlines of a star, and the task is to draw a pencil line within the outlines. Errors are scored each time an outline border is contacted. This test may seem simple, but in fact normal subjects require several trials before they can successfully draw the line without committing crossover errors. H.M. showed strikingly good improvement over several attempts within the initial session, and considerable retention of this skill across sessions, to the extent that he consistently made very few errors on the third test day. This success in learning this sensorimotor skill contrasted with his inability to recall ever having taken the test.

In addition, H.M. also showed strikingly good performance in perceptual learning in a task called the Gollins partial pictures task, which involves the recognition of fragmented line drawings of common objects. For each of 20 items, subjects are presented with a series of five cards containing fragments of a realistic line drawing of the same object. The first card of each series contains the fewest fragments of the drawing and the last card contains the complete drawing (Fig. 4–3). Subjects are initially

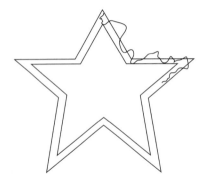

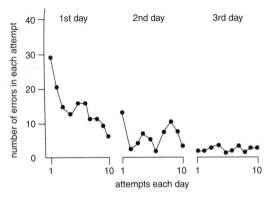

Figure 4–2. The mirror drawing test. *Top:* Sketch of the double-star pattern and the beginning of a typical early attempt at drawing a line between the boundaries. *Bottom:* H.M.'s performance across 10 attempts on 3 successive days (data from Milner et al., 1968).

shown all 20 of the most difficult items and asked to identify the object drawn on each one. Then the second, slightly more complete version of each item is presented with the ordering of the 20 cards randomized, so it is impossible to anticipate an item based on its predecessor. The procedure is continued using successively more complete versions of each item until all are identified. Then, after an hour of intervening activity, the entire test is repeated, and the number of errors (unidentified drawings) is scored. Normal subjects show retention of this perceptual memory reflected in the ability to identify less complete versions of the drawings. H.M.'s scores on the retest were not as good as age-matched controls, but he showed a surprising degree of retention, especially considering he did not remember having taken the initial test.

A broad range of spared learning abilities in amnesia

The observations of Cohen and Squire showing fully intact perceptual skill learning were properly heralded as a revelation about memory processing

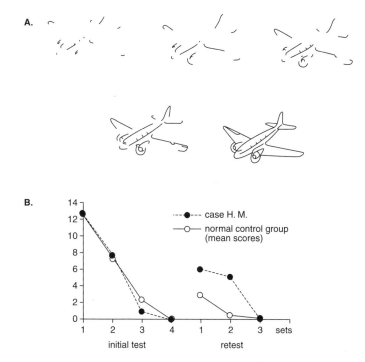

Figure 4–3. The Gollins partial pictures test. *A:* An example of the series of partial figures that compose one item on the test. *B:* Performance of H.M. and normal control subjects measured by the number of errors on the entire series on the initial test and on a delayed retest with the same items (data from Warrington and Weiskrantz, 1968).

functions accomplished by the medial temporal lobe. Subsequently, several laboratories uncovered a variety of examples of spared learning ability in amnesia. Examples from a broad range of those findings are presented next, to provide a view of the scope of preserved learning and memory capacities observed in amnesia. These include a form of perceptual learning called "priming," skill learning, Pavlovian conditioning, and sequence learning.

Priming

Perhaps the most intensively studied form of memory that can be accomplished fully normally in amnesic patients is the phenomenon known as repetition priming, or just "priming." Priming involves initial presentation of a list of words, pictures of objects, or nonverbal materials, and then subsequent reexposure to fragments or very brief presentation of the whole item. In the reexposure phase, learning is measured by increased ability to reproduce the whole item from a fragment (as in the Gollins partial pictures task described earlier) or by increased speed in making a decision about the item.

One example study particularly nicely illustrates a striking dissociation between intact priming and impaired declarative memory performance by amnesic subjects. This experiment used the word stem completion task, a test of verbal repetition priming in which subjects initially study a list of words, then are presented with the first three letters of each word (the word "stem") and asked to complete it. The stimulus words are selected as ones for which the stem can be completed more than one way to compose a high frequency word. For example, the word "MOTEL" is used because its stem "MOT———" can be completed to form either the stimulus word or "MOTHER" (see other examples in Fig. 4–4 top). Priming is measured by the increased likelihood that the subject will complete the stimulus word presented during the study phase. In this experiment, subjects initially studied a list of such words and, to make sure they attended to them, had to identify shared vowels among sets of words or rate the words according to how much they liked them. Then, in the test phase, they were presented with the three-letter word stems and tested for their memory in one of three ways. In the *free recall* condition, subjects were not presented with stems but just asked to recall the studied words. In the *cued recall* condition, subjects were presented with the word stems and told to use them as cues to remember words that were on the list. In the *completion* condition, they were presented with word stems and asked sim-

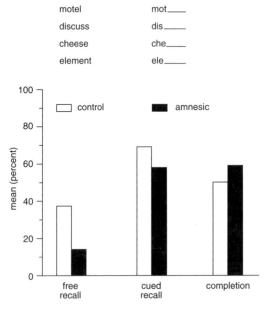

Figure 4–4. Word stem completion test of verbal priming. *Top:* On the left are examples of study words, and on the right, examples of the word stems used for cueing. *Bottom:* Performance of normal control subjects and amnesics on three versions of the test (data from Squire, 1987).

ply to "write the first word that comes to mind." The amnesics were impaired in recall as tested either with cueing or without (Fig. 4–4 bottom). By contrast, they were not impaired on the completion test. A particularly revealing comparison can be made between the performance of amnesics across the different test conditions. They did much better on the cued recall than the free recall condition, but no better on cued recall than on completion. One interpretation of these findings is that performance in cued recall might be entirely supported by priming. By contrast, the normal subjects did much better on cued recall than on priming, suggesting they used the stems to aid an active search in recalling the words.

Intact priming in amnesia is not restricted to nameable objects and verbal material. For example, H.M. also shows normal priming in a task explicitly designed to be refractory to verbalization. In this test H.M. and normal subjects were presented with a set of stimuli each of which consisted of five dots arranged in a unique pattern (Fig. 4–5 top). To establish baseline performance, subjects were asked to draw on the dots any line pattern they wished. Substantially later they were presented with a set of predetermined target patterns and asked to replicate them onto a corresponding dot pattern. After exposure to the entire list plus a distracter task, they were provided with the dot pattern again and asked to complete it any way they wished. Priming scores were calculated based on the incidence of baseline patterns. As shown in Fig. 4–5 (bottom), H.M. showed significant above chance priming for dot patterns, indicating as much memory as the normal subjects. This intact performance stood in contrast to his inability to recognize the same dot patterns when explicitly asked if he had seen them before.

Skill learning

Mirror drawing, described before, is an example of spared capacity for the acquisition of sensorimotor skills. In addition, the intact capacity to learn skills extends to the acquisition of cognitive rules. For example, in one study subjects were presented with strings of letters that were generated by an artificial "grammar" that determined general rules for sequencing and length of the letter strings (Fig. 4–6). They studied these strings by reproducing each item immediately after its presentation. Then subjects were informed that the letter strings were formed by complex rules. Subsequently they were shown novel letter strings one at a time and asked to classify them as "grammatical" or "nongrammatical" according to whether they conformed with the rules. Finally, subjects were tested to determine if they could recognize grammatic letter strings after a brief study phase. Both amnesic and normal subjects were able to correctly classify the letter strings

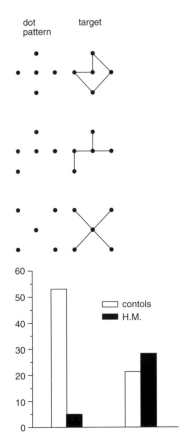

Figure 4–5. Priming for dot patterns test. *Top:* Examples of dot patterns and target completion pattern. *Bottom:* Performance (percentage correct) as measured by recognition of the target and by correct completion in normal control subjects and case H.M. (data from Gabrieli et al., 1990).

on about two-thirds of the trials. By contrast, the amnesic patients were impaired on recognition of studied grammatical items.

Classical (Pavlovian) conditioning

Modern formal studies of classical conditioning in both humans and animals have focused on conditioning of eyeblink reflexes, because these are easy paradigms to control and allow straightforward measures of learning. These studies typically involve repeated pairings of a tone or light as the conditioning stimulus (CS) and an airpuff to the eye as the unconditioned stimulus (US) that produces a reflexive blink. The measure of classical conditioning is the occurrence of eyeblinks during the CS period prior to presentation of the US, that is, conditioned eyeblink responses. Systematic studies comparing amnesic and normal subjects have demonstrated intact classical eyelid conditioning in amnesics, as well as normal extinction of conditioned responses when the CS was presented repeatedly with-

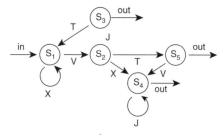

Figure 4–6. Artificial grammar test. A rule system used to string letters into "grammatical" and "nongrammatical" series, and several example items (data from Knowlton et al., 1992).

grammatical	nongrammatical
XXVT	TVT
XXVXJJ	TXXXVT
VXJJ	VXXXVJ
VTV	VJVTX

out the US. The examples of intact eyelid conditioning all involve a procedure known as "delay-conditioning," in which the presentation of the CS is prolonged and overlaps the US. Another procedure, known as "trace-conditioning," involves a brief CS followed by a trace interval during which no stimulus is presented, followed by the US alone. The distinction between these two types of classical conditioning is important because it has been shown that rabbits with hippocampal damage normally acquire the eyelid response with the delay-conditioning procedure but cannot learn under the trace-conditioning procedure. Just like rabbits with hippocampal damage, human amnesics are impaired in trace eyelid conditioning. Moreover, this deficit has been related to the conscious awareness of the stimulus contingencies.

Sequence learning

Another domain of intact learning in amnesia involves the gradual improvement in speed of performance following specific regularities in stimulus–response sequences. A compelling example of intact learning of a specific perceptual–motor habit involves manual sequence learning in a task called the serial reaction time test. On each trial subjects were shown a light at one of four locations on a computer monitor, and had to press one of four keys that corresponded to that light location. On each trial the lights were presented in a consistent pattern, and the entire pattern was presented repetitively in each training session such that subjects could anticipate the position of the next light. As a control, in separate testing blocks the sequence of light positions was randomized. Normal subjects and amnesics decreased their reaction times to press the keys, and did so at an equal rate. Both groups showed minimal improvement when the light position sequence was random, indicating that the improvement on regular sequences involved acquisition of a specific habit and not a general ability to coordinate the pressing of keys for appropriate lights.

Another example of spared learning of a specific habit in human amnesic patients comes from studies of speed reading. Several experiments have shown that amnesics improved their reading times over the course of repeating a story aloud. In these studies there was no general facilitation between stories, indicating that the habit was text-specific. Moreover, this intact capacity does not seem to rely on memory for the content of the story, as demonstrated in an experiment showing that the phenomenon extends to nonwords (pronounceable but meaningless letter strings) as well as text. However, even with nonwords, the facilitation is specific to the sequence of repeated nonwords and is not a reflection of a general learning to read new nonwords.

Characterizing the properties of declarative and procedural memory

There have been numerous attempts to identify the common properties among the types of learning and memory spared in amnesia, and to distinguish them from the common aspects of learning and memory on which amnesics fail. These comparisons have provided insights into the nature and cognitive mechanisms that underlie declarative memory, as well as properties of the domains of procedural memory.

One way to characterize declarative memory is to consider whether there is a set of common or fundamental properties of memory that is spared in amnesia. Some of the earliest findings on H.M. indicated that intact learning in amnesia is limited to motor skills or simple perceptual learning. Other studies have suggested that spared learning always involves the slow incremental acquisition of habitual routines or to specific categories of information.

However, intact learning in amnesia is not limited to general motor skills. Rather, the scope of spared memory in amnesia includes a variety of forms of highly specific new learning. Also, intact learning in amnesia is not limited to simple forms of perceptual learning or other easy tasks, as clearly shown by the improvements in very difficult tasks such as grammar learning and sequence production. In addition, spared learning in amnesia is not limited to types of learning that involve slow incremental improvement, but includes a variety of forms of one-trial learning, such as observed in numerous repetition priming tests. Indeed, priming for single exposures to pictures can be both robust and last at least a week in amnesic subjects. Finally, preserved learning in amnesia is not limited to any particular category of learning materials, as one can see in our broad range of examples, including intact learning for words, nonwords, common objects, tones, nonverbalizable pictures, motor patterns, and spatial patterns. In sum, the domain of intact learning ability is global, and it can be either fast or slow, and include both general skills and highly specific information content. Thus, the common properties among examples of intact memory in amnesia are not to be found in relatively objective parameters such as the modality of information, or the speed or specificity of memory.

Formal characterizations of nondeclarative memory

Several hypotheses have emerged from efforts to characterize the critical features that are common to intact learning in amnesia. Instead of simpler objective parameters such as those listed just previously, these proposals focus on more complex and higher-order properties, and in particular, the form of memory expression, the extent of conscious access to memories, and the structure of the memory representation.

One of the most objective attempts to formalize the general learning abilities of amnesics was provided by Morris Moscovitch in his 1984 list of sufficient conditions for demonstrating preserved memory. He focused on task demands, and argued that amnesics show savings on tests that satisfy three conditions: *(1)* the task has to be so highly structured that the goal of the task and the means to achieve it are apparent, *(2)* the means to achieve the goal are available to the subject (i.e., the response strategies are already in the subject's repertoire), and *(3)* success can be achieved without reference to any particular event or episode. Combining these, he suggested that amnesics will succeed whenever they simply have to perform a task guided by the conditions and strategies at hand. The new memory is revealed in changes of task performance itself, typically either a change in the speed of responding or in a bias of choices that are readily available.

Daniel Schacter made a similar distinction between "explicit" and "implicit" memory. Explicit memory involves conscious recollection generated by direct efforts to access memories. Explicit tests of memory involve direct inquiries that ask the subjects to refer to a specific event of learning or a specific fact in their knowledge. Examples of explicit tests of memory include, "What were the words on the list you studied?" and "Which of these two items did you see before?" The full range of explicit memory tests includes a large variety of direct measures of recall or recognition of word or picture lists, paired associates, story recall, and most of the common tests of memory that are performed so poorly by amnesic patients. Explicit memory expression also includes most everyday instances of memory, such as recalling what one had for breakfast this morning or what the capital of France is. Both examples involve conscious efforts to search for a specific event or fact.

By contrast, implicit memory involves unconscious changes in performance of a task as influenced by some previous experience. Implicit tests of memory involve indirect measures such as changes in the speed of performance or in biases in choices made during performance of a task that can be solved with the information at hand. Examples of implicit memory tests include the full variety of assessments of motor, perceptual, and cognitive skills, habits, conditioning, and repetition priming described earlier at which amnesic patients usually succeed. Notably none of these tests requires the subjects to be aware of their memory, or to "remember," a specific event or fact.

A related proposal is Endel Tulving's distinction between "episodic memory" and "semantic memory." Episodic memory contains representations of specific personal experiences that occur in a unique spatial and temporal context. Episodic memory involves the capacity to reexperience particular events in one's life, what Tulving calls "time traveling." By contrast, according to Tulving, semantic memory is the body of one's world knowledge, a vast organization of memories not bound to any specific experience in which they were acquired. Some investigators have suggested that the pattern of impaired and spared memory capacities in amnesia can be explained as an impaired episodic memory capacity and intact semantic memory. This view readily accounts for the impairment in day-to-day episodic memory ("What did you have for breakfast?"). In addition, episodic memory can strongly facilitate one's performance on many standard tests, such as one's ability to recall or recognize a recently studied list of words. Memory in these situations is stronger in normal subjects because they can refer to their episodic memory for the specific learning experience, in addition to any memory for the materials independent of that specific experience. But, according to this view, amnesics have only the episode-free record and so usually perform less well.

Furthermore, according to this view, amnesic subjects perform well on implicit memory tasks, because the memory demands avoid reference to the temporal or spatial context in which the information was acquired, and do not require the subject to refer to the learning experience directly. In these tests there is typically no advantage conferred on normal subjects in remembering the items. The episodic–semantic distinction shares much with Moscovitch's characterization of successful memory performance whenever amnesics do not have to "conjure up, that is, 'remember,' any previous experience or a newly learned fact." Indeed, the episodic–semantic and implicit–explicit views are fully compatible, to the extent that implicit memory tests always and only require semantic memory.

In support of this view, Tulving et al. described a patient, K.C., with normal intelligence, preserved general knowledge, and fragmentary general knowledge of his past. He also had expert knowledge from work done 3 years before a closed head injury. By contrast, K.C. did not remember a single personal event from his previous life and did not remember new events. He had some capacity to gradually acquire new knowledge, as demonstrated in studies aimed at very gradual accumulation of semantic knowledge by teaching methods that reduce interference associated with making errors. In addition, there are now several cases of childhood brain injury that result in amnesia for everyday life events, but near normal general world knowledge. Some of the latter cases appear to have relatively circumscribed damage to the hippocampus, suggesting specific involvement of this structure in episodic memory.

Disentangling episodic and semantic memory is a difficult problem. Surely these patients forget "facts," such as a list of words, just as rapidly as they forget daily events, such as what they had for breakfast. One study directly addressed the issue of semantic learning in amnesia by attempting to train H.M. on new vocabulary words. H.M. and normal subjects were given implicit test instructions and were directed away from conscious recollection of the events surrounding the learning experiences. Training proceeded in several phases. They first studied word definitions for eight novel vocabulary words created by the experimenters. The subjects were given a recognition test asking them to choose a definition for each word. Then they studied synonyms for the words, and were tested on a sentence completion task where they had to fill in a blank at the end of a sentence with one of the new words. Normal subjects learned the new words readily, completing each phase within a few trials. Despite an exhaustive regimen of testing, H.M. showed virtually no ability to learn new semantic knowledge.

This is not to say that amnesics cannot acquire any semantic knowledge, and indeed there are many examples of highly specific learning even for complex materials. For example, there have been demonstrations of successful learning where subjects were trained to use computer commands and terminology. The training methods used painstaking and very gradual procedures by which the commands were introduced in situations where responses were "error-free" at each stage. These subjects did subsequently show aptitude for learning new computer terms. But the range with which they could use this new learning was highly limited, such that their learning could be expressed only in replications of the precise training conditions. Schacter referred to this characteristic of their successful learning as a "hyperspecificity" of the preserved memory. Such limited applicability is not characteristic of our common use of semantic memory in solving everyday problems across a broad range of one's daily challenges.

Summing up

H.M. was important as much for the selectivity of his deficit as for its severity. Subsequent to the discovery of H.M.'s amnesia, Scoville publicized the findings, and supported Milner, Corkin, and others in their research on H.M., in great part to insure that the operation would not be performed again. H.M. was among a group of patients who underwent the experimental operation for bilateral medial temporal lobe resection. However, all the other patients were severely psychotic, muddling the interpretation of the memory tests. The resection in some of the patients involved only some of the cortex and the amygdala, and these patients' memory was intact. Also, the severity of the amnesic deficit in other patients was related to the amount of hippocampal damage, so it was concluded that the hippocampus and immediately adjacent cortex were the likely critical area for memory.

Combining the data across an enormous range of memory and non-memory assessments, H.M.'s amnesia is characterized by several cardinal features: *(1)* intact perceptual, motor, and cognitive functions, *(2)* intact immediate memory, *(3)* severe and global anterograde amnesia, *(4)* temporally graded retrograde amnesia, *(5)* spared remote memory. At that time, views about memory were most influenced by the notion that different cortical areas contained specific perceptual and memory functions together, such that perception, cognition, and memory were considered inseparable and, by Lashley's proposal, widely distributed in the brain. The case study of H.M. was a breakthrough because it showed that a general memory function could be dissociated from other functions. In addition, the findings of exceptions to severe global amnesia, in successful sensorimotor and perceptual learning, foreshadowed a second major breakthrough that promises to further clarify the nature of hippocampal processing in memory.

Other studies on many amnesic patients have shown that the domain of spared learning in amnesia includes intact repetition priming, skill learning, Pavlovian conditioning, sequence learning, and more. The common features that distinguish the impaired and preserved memory capacities in amnesia have been characterized in several ways, including the distinctions between explicit and implicit memory expression, and between episodic and semantic memory.

Based on considerations from a wealth of data from studies on amnesic patients, the most consistent characterization of the domain of memory impaired in amnesia is captured by the notion of "declarative memory," the memory for facts and events that can be brought to conscious recollection and can be expressed explicitly. Conversely, the most consistent characterization of learning ability spared in amnesia is the notion of "procedural memory," the acquisition of skills and preferences that can be expressed unconsciously by implicit changes in the speed or biasing of performance during a repetition of processing of the learning materials. These characterizations capture all of the features of the distinctions outlined previously. However, they leave unresolved the nature of memory traces that underlie either category of memory. An understanding memory representation at that more fundamental level requires the establishment and exploitation of animal models of different types of memory, because only in such models can the required biological recordings and manipulations be pursued. A consideration of the challenges and successes of animal models of declarative and procedural memory begins in the next chapter.

READINGS

Cohen, N.J. 1984. Preserved learning capacity in amnesia: Evidence for multiple memory systems. In *The Neuropsychology of Memory*, N. Butters, and L.R. Squire, (Eds.) New York: Guilford Press, pp. 83–103.

Cohen, N.J., and Squire, L.R. 1980. Preserved learning and retention of a pattern- analyzing skill in amnesia: Dissociation of knowing how and knowing that. *Science* 210:207–210.

Corkin, S. 1984. Lasting consequences of bilateral medial temporal lobectomy: Clinical course and experimental findings in H.M. *Semin. Neurol.* 4:249–259.

Moscovitch, M. 1984. The sufficient conditions for demonstrating preserved memory in amnesia: A task analysis. In *The Neuropsychology of Memory*, N. Butters, and L.R. Squire (Eds.). New York: Guilford Press, pp. 104–114.

Ogden, J.A., and Corkin, S. 1991. Memories of H.M. In *Memory Mechanisms: A Tribute to G.V. Goddard*, W.C. Abraham, M. Corballis, and K.G. White (Eds.) pp. 195–215.

Schacter, D.L. 1987. Implicit memory: History and current status. *J. Exp. Psychol. Learn. Mem. Cogn.* 13:501–518.

Scoville, W.B., and Milner, B. 1957. Loss of recent memory after bilateral hippocampal lesions. *J. Neurol. Neurosurg. Psychiatry* 20:11–12.

Squire, L.R., Knowlton, B., and Musen, G. 1993. The structure and organization of memory. *Annu. Rev. Psychol.* 44:453–495.

Tulving, E. Schacter, D.L., McLachlin, D.R., and Moscovitch, M. 1988. Priming of semantic autobiographcal knowledge: A case study of retrograde amnesia. *Brain and Cogn.* 8:3–20.

5
· · · · · ·

Exploring Declarative Memory Using Animal Models

STUDY QUESTIONS

What is an animal model of amnesia? Why are such models valuable?

What characteristics of amnesia are well modeled using nonhuman primates?

What characteristics of amnesia are well modeled using rodents?

How good were the initial attempts at each of these models?

What advances led to breakthroughs in each model?

Almost immediately after the early reports on H.M. and other patients suffering the consequences of medial temporal lobe excision, efforts began to reproduce elements of the amnesic syndrome in monkeys, rats, and other animals. The major aim of these early efforts was twofold. First, specific experimental brain damage offered an increase in anatomical specificity over that which occurs in cases of surgeries, accidents, and disease. Increased anatomical specificity of the damage improved the ability of investigators to designate which structures of the temporal lobe are critical to memory. Second, in animals, to a much greater extent than in humans, investigators can control the nature and extent of experience gained prior to the brain damage. Human patients arrive in the clinic with a unique background of learning that differs along many dimensions and to a very great extent among individuals. In addition, the specifics of the history of individual people can only be known to the extent that there is a record of one's history, which is typically rather vague. By contrast, in animals, investigators can dictate all the details of experience the animal brings to the experimental setting where learning will be studied. From many of our considerations so far, it should be obvious that new learning occurs in the context of previously acquired knowledge (one's schema or prior semantic knowledge), and so it is greatly advantageous to know and control the nature and extent of that knowledge.

As in any other situation where an experimental model is desired, it is important at the outset to classify the precise aspects of the human condition that one wishes to model. Fortunately, the properties of a valid animal model of the human amnesic syndrome were clearly outlined in the clinical studies presented earlier: (1) sensory, motor, motivational, and cognitive processes should be intact; (2) short-term memory should be intact. (3) following preserved short-term performance, memory should decline with abnormal rapidity, that is, exceeding the rate of natural forgetting in intact control subjects. (4) the deficit should be global in scope for the to-be-learned materials, that is, the impairment should span sensory and conceptual modalities of new learning. (5) there should be a graded retrograde impairment, such that learning accomplished recently prior to brain damage would be lost, whereas learning accomplished remotely long before the damage should be spared.

Two lines of research in the development of animal models

The efforts to model amnesia associated with damage to the medial temporal lobe followed two parallel approaches, one using monkeys as the experimental subjects and the other using primarily rats. The studies on monkeys began appropriately by reproducing the same pervasive medial temporal damage that was done to H.M. Therefore, this line of research has been most useful in characterizing the nature of the memory mediated by the entire set of structures in the medial temporal lobe. The early studies on rats focused on the hippocampus, leaving out of the experimental ablation other structures that were damaged in H.M. and in experiments on monkeys. Therefore, this line of research has been most useful in characterizing the role of the hippocampus itself. The conclusions derived from these two lines do not entirely overlap, because of differences both in the size and locus of experimental brain damage and in the behavioral tests typically employed in monkeys and rats. The following sections summarize some of the findings from both lines of research.

The development of a model of amnesia in monkeys

The behavioral assays initially used to study the role of the medial temporal lobe in monkeys focused on two type of tasks that were already being used in comparative studies on the cognitive functions of nonhuman primates: visual discrimination and matching to sample. In visual discrimination training, typically there are two stimuli for each problem, usually flat plaques painted with different colors or patterns, or easily discriminated three-dimensional objects (Fig. 5–1A), each placed to cover food wells on a choice platform. One stimulus is arbitrarily assigned as "positive," and displacing the plaque would reveal a hidden reward on each trial. The other stimulus is assigned a "negative" value and never rewarded. The positions of the stimuli are varied randomly across trials, so their spatial position does not correlate with the reward locus. In delayed matching to sample, each trial is composed of three distinct phases (Fig. 5–1B). In the first phase, called the sample phase, a single stimulus is presented. This is followed by a variable delay phase during which the monkey has to remember the stimulus for different periods of time. In the third phase,

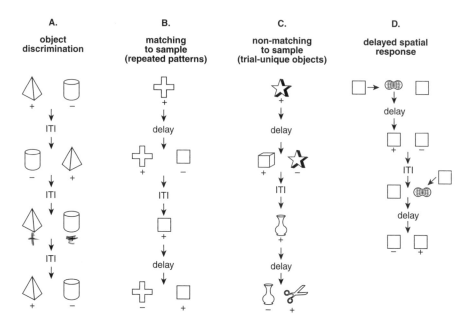

Figure 5–1. Illustration of trials in four memory tests used on monkeys: *A:* Visual discrimination. *B:* Delayed match to sample with trial-repeated stimuli. *C:* Delayed non-match to sample test with trial-unique objects as memory cues. *D:* Delayed spatial response. ITI = intertrial interval.

called the choice phase, two stimuli are presented, one identical to the sample and baited and the other different and not baited. So the requirement of the task is to "match" a choice stimulus to the sample in order to receive the reward. Typically in these early studies, the same two stimuli were two-dimensional patterns reused on every trial, with the sample selected randomly across trials. As described later, there are several important variations on this task, employing different kinds of stimuli, a different "nonmatching" rule by which the subject must select the alternative to the sample item in the choice phase (Fig. 5–1C). Among the variations in stimuli was the use of two identical plain stimuli, and the requirement was for the subject to select the same location it had seen food covered by the plain stimulus on the sample trial. This is called the classic "delayed spatial response" task (Fig. 5–1D).

The early efforts to model amnesia in monkeys using these tests were not impressively successful. The general pattern of results was not inconsistent with the properties of amnesia listed earlier. Also, some of those key properties, including no effect on aspects of the task that did not require memory and normal short-term memory, were very well duplicated in monkeys with medial temporal lobe damage. But the *magnitude* of both the anterograde and retrograde components of the memory deficit were quite modest compared to the apparent almost total loss of memory observed in H.M. Monkeys with substantial removals of all of the medial temporal lobe structures were only mildly impaired on learning new visual pattern, color, object, or auditory discrimination problems. In relearning visual pattern or object discriminations that the monkeys had acquired a few weeks prior to the surgery, deficits were reliably observed. However, the *magnitude* of this retrograde impairment was also disappointing—monkeys with medial temporal lobe damage merely showed less savings from the previous learning and not a complete loss of recently acquired information.

Furthermore, monkeys with medial temporal lobe lesions performed surprisingly well on matching to sample and other delayed response tests. The task was trained preoperatively, and there was a retrograde impairment in reacquisition of the task with short delays. This loss of recent memory was consistent with the characteristics of human amnesia. However, having reacquired the task after the surgery, the monkeys performed well even at memory delay intervals of several seconds. It was a state of affairs that led many to suggest that there might be a true species difference in the role of the medial temporal lobe in memory, such that memory relied much more on hippocampal function in humans than in animals.

Success with a new test of recognition memory

A major breakthrough came with a combination of a novel twist in the procedures used for the delayed matching to sample task combined with a modification in the approach for removing medial temporal lobe structures. The key aspects of the task variant involved the use of new sets of stimulus objects on each trial (the "trial-unique stimulus" procedure) plus a nonmatching reward contingency (Fig. 5–1C). Thus, on each trial, the sample was a novel three-dimensional "junk" object. Then, to obtain a reward during the choice phase, the subject was required to select a different novel junk object over the now-familiar sample object. Because an entirely novel sample is used on each trial, it is appropriate to think of this task as a test of recognition for the newly familiar object. Notably this characterization of the task is quite different from that for the task where the same stimuli are used repeatedly—in such a situation both stimuli are highly familiar, so their potential for recognition would hardly differentiate them.

The distinction between the trial-unique or repetitive stimulus procedures had a profound effect on monkeys' performance in the delayed matching (or nonmatching) task and on the effects of medial temporal lobe damage. Normal monkeys learned the task with the trial-unique procedure exceedingly rapidly. Monkeys with damage to the hippocampal region were impaired in learning the task when the memory delay was short, but they did eventually reach a high performance criterion and continued to perform well when the memory load was low. However, when the delay was extended, a deficit was observed and the severity of the impairment increased as the delay was elongated (Fig. 5–2A). In addition, if a list of items was presented and then memory for each was tested in a sequence of choice trials, a severe deficit was observed.

Monkeys with damage to the medial temporal lobe have a selective memory impairment

The introduction of a new benchmark assessment of amnesia monkeys using the delayed nonmatch to sample (DNMS) task opened up the opportunity to readdress whether this approach would indeed provide a valid model of the fundamental characteristics of human amnesia. Recall that these characteristics include: spared nonmemory functions and short-term memory in the face of rapid forgetting, global scope of amnesia across learning materials, and graded retrograde amnesia.

A central issue is the selectivity of the deficit to memory and the sparing of perceptual, motor, motivational, and attention or other cognitive functions. The DNMS task provides an automatic and ideal control in that

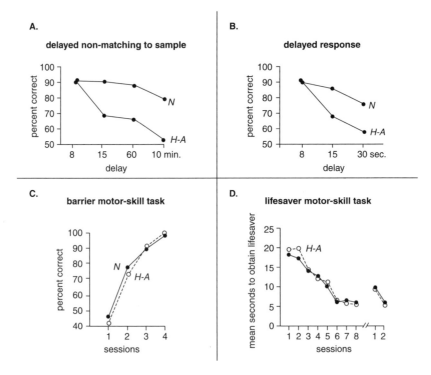

Figure 5–2. Performance of normal monkeys and monkeys with medial temporal damage on different memory tasks. N = normal animals; H-A = animals with hippocampus plus amygdala and cortical damage (data from Squire, 1987).

all of those nonmemory functions are fully required even in the absence of a memory delay. Thus, if monkeys with medial temporal lobe damage perform normally at the shortest delay, it must be that they can attend to, perceive, and encode the object cues, that they can execute the choice responses, that they are motivated to participate in the task, and that they can acquire and retain the nonmatching rule.

Producing a DNMS task with no memory delay at all is problematic because, quite simply, the manually operated apparatus typically used requires 8–10 seconds to exchange sample and choice objects, and deficits in memory can be apparent in human amnesics within 10 seconds. This issue was addressed directly by the development of a computerized version of the DNMS task that employed complex visual patterns presented on a "touch screen" of a video display. Intact subjects required trials to learn the computerized version of the task at the brief delay. Nevertheless, following a medial temporal lobe ablation the rate of learning was fully normal. In subsequent testing with delays up to 10 minutes, normal monkeys showed a gradual forgetting. Monkeys with medial temporal damage performed as well as normal subjects at delays up to 1 second, but at longer delays a deficit became ever more apparent.

Another characteristic of human amnesia is that the deficit can be seen across a variety of learning materials. That is, the impairment is global with regard to the stimulus modality of items to be remembered. Early evidence that addressed this question came from studies of the delayed spatial response task, which is based on memory for a spatial location and not the visual qualities of a particular stimulus. Monkeys with medial temporal damage show the same spared memory at brief delays and increasing impairment at long delays as seen in standard DNMS (Fig. 5–2B).

In addition, this issue was addressed by the development of a tactual variant of the DNMS task. Monkeys were initially trained on the conventional version of the task, and then retrained with the room lights gradually dimmed to complete darkness except for small dim cue-lights signaling the positions of the objects. In this situation the animals had to perceive and encode the objects entirely by tactual cues. Normal monkeys required about twice as many trials to relearn the task in the dark, but performance was excellent in the final preoperative stage of tactual DNMS testing even over long delays. After removal of the medial temporal lobe, relearning at a short delay was substantially impaired, but the animals did eventually succeed and continued to perform well with short delays, as observed with the visual version of the task. More important, the deficit grew as the delay was elongated. Thus, the pattern of sparing of ultimate performance at a short delay and increasing impairment at longer delays was identical to that observed for the visually guided version of the same task, demonstrating that the amnesic deficit extended across specific sensory modalities.

Another central characteristic of the amnesic syndrome is the phenomenon of graded retrograde memory loss. As described in Chapter 4, H.M. and other amnesic patients display a loss of memories backward in time from the moment of brain damage, with the most severe loss in the period just prior to the damage and total sparing of remotely acquired memories, including childhood recollections and general knowledge acquired early in life. However, a major problem in the interpretation of retrograde memory loss in human patients is that the amount and timing of prior learning experiences can only be approximated. Conversely, one of the major advantages of an animal model of amnesia is that one can examine the retrograde loss of memories with a "prospective" design. That is, one can provide measured amounts of learning at specific times prior to brain damage that occurs suddenly. In so doing, one can directly compare the strength of memories acquired at different times in intact animals and one can more accurately measure the period and magnitude of retrograde loss.

Unfortunately, the DNMS task is unsuitable for this kind of study because single exposures to objects do not provide sufficiently strong memories to endure testing weeks or months after learning. To address this issue and develop a task that would be suitable for a study of retrograde memory, experimenters created an object discrimination task where subjects were presented with pairs of novel objects like those used in DNMS testing, and repeatedly reinforced the choice of one object over the other. Normal monkeys learned sets of these pairings rapidly, accumulating 100 successfully acquired problems over 4 months of training. Following completion of the learning series, in half of the animals the hippocampus and nearby cortex were removed and the animals were allowed 2 weeks to recover. Then all the animals were each tested with just one trial on each problem. Normal animals scored well on the most recently acquired problems, and their performance declined a bit, showing some forgetting for problems learned more than 2 months before. By contrast, monkeys with hippocampal damage were substantially impaired, performing at just above that expected by chance, on problems presented within 2 weeks of the surgery. They performed significantly better on remotely learned discriminations, exhibiting normal performance on those acquired 4 months prior to the surgery. This pattern of recent retrograde memory loss and spared remote memory, emphasized most strikingly by worse performance on recent memory than remote memory within the medial temporal group, provides compelling evidence that damage to the medial temporal region results in a graded retrograde amnesia (see Chapter 12 for an extended discussion of this topic).

A domain of spared learning ability in monkeys with medial temporal damage

In addition to the previously described aspects of *impaired* learning and memory following hippocampal damage, there is the critical characterization of a *spared* domain of new learning capacity in H.M. and other amnesic patients. Toward the goal of modeling this phenomenon, there are specific examples that represent a domain of spared learning in monkeys following ablation of the entire medial temporal lobe.

One spared domain that closely parallels intact motor skill learning in human amnesics is the acquisition of manual skills in monkeys. In a study of this kind of learning, experimenters devised two manual skill tests on which monkeys could be trained. One of these involved training the monkeys to reach around a clear barrier to obtain a reward. Another involved challenging the monkeys to obtain a doughnut-shaped candy (a "lifesaver") reward that was presented in the middle of an irregularly bent stiff wire (a coat hanger). To rapidly retrieve the reward the monkey had to improve its manual manipulation of the lifesaver around the turns of the coat hanger. In both tasks monkeys with medial temporal damage improved in performance at the same rate as normal subjects, demonstrating preserved motor skill learning in amnesia (Fig. 5–2C, D).

In addition, monkeys with medial temporal lobe damage perform normally well in the acquisition and retention of single visual discrimination problems that are acquired gradually. This spared learning capacity was described in some of the early studies on medial temporal lobe ablations in monkeys, and was confirmed in studies using the same junk object stimuli employed in DNMS. Notably, the deficit is observed only under conditions where normal learning was slow and gradual (by presenting each pair of object only once per day). In conditions where normal animals learn object discriminations most rapidly (acquisition in a single session with multiple presentations), a deficit is observed. Thus, these findings revealed a common, albeit not universal, aspect of learning by the medial temporal system, that this system acquires information rapidly. Under the conditions where normal acquisition was rapid, animals without that system were disadvantaged. Conversely, under conditions where the rapid learning system conferred no advantage, no learning deficit was observed.

This combination of observations, and several other findings, showed that many of the central features of the phenomenology of human amnesia can be modeled in animals, and specifically in monkeys. This work set the stage for a more detailed examination of which medial temporal lobe structures are critical for memory in monkeys; this work is discussed in Chapter 9. A parallel effort was also ongoing to model amnesia in other animals, particularly rats. The results of this effort are summarized next.

Can declarative memory be modeled using rats?

Scoville and Milner's 1957 report on H.M. had suggested that, among the structures damaged within the temporal lobe, damage to the hippocampus in particular was responsible for the memory deficit. Therefore, following the initial reports on human amnesia, several laboratories developed procedures for ablation of the hippocampus in rats, as well as cats and rabbits. As was the case with monkeys, the first tests to be employed in examining the effects of hippocampal damage were a variety of simple conditioning, discrimination learning, and maze learning tests that were the focus of current research by learning theorists. However, the results using each of these formal tests seemed inconsistent by any simple analysis. The findings were puzzling at best, and certainly did not support a conclusion that hippocampal damage results in severe and global amnesia in rats or other nonprimates. A few of these findings are summarized next to illustrate the confusing state of affairs that ensued from this research.

The earliest assessments of learning and hippocampal function in rodents included two different tests of conditioning animals to avoid noxious stimuli (usually irritating electrical shocks). One of these, called "shuttle-box avoidance," involved training rats to alternate (shuttle) between two adjacent compartments of an alleyway. In one version of this task, each trial began with a buzzer that signaled the rat to shuttle to the alternate chamber before the floor in the currently occupied side was electrified by a mild current. The surprising result was that rats with large ablations of the hippocampus and overlying cortex learned the task in *fewer* trials than normal rats or rats with cortical damage only, and they retained this learning solidly across testing days. Shortly after, and contrasting with the first results, another study reported that rats with hippocampal ablations were *unable* to learn a different sort of avoidance task called "passive avoidance." Initially, hungry rats were trained to approach a chamber that had food. They began each trial in a large compartment, and were then signaled by a door opening to leave that compartment and to approach and enter the small food-containing chamber. After learning to execute the approach behavior immediately upon opening of the door, one day they were shocked while eating and driven out of the reward chamber. Normal rats and rats with hippocampal ablations rapidly learned the initial approach response and, consistent with the earlier experiment, rats with hippocampal ablations had shorter approach latencies and less variability in learning. However, the two groups responded quite differently in the avoidance component of training. After having been shocked just once in the reward chamber, none of the normal rats reentered again. By contrast, each of the rats with hippocampal damage did return to the chamber in which they were shocked. Although there was a learning impairment here following hippocampal damage, the overall pattern of findings did not offer compelling support for a simple amnesic disorder: After outperforming normal rats on the initial learning phase, rats with hippocampal damage showed a deficit in passive avoidance that seemed to reflect an inability to give up the previously acquired response, rather than a failure to learn *per se*. What a confusing state of affairs!

Rats with hippocampal damage also performed perfectly normally, or better than normal rats, in the acquisition of standard Skinnerian conditioning tests in which rats learned to press a bar for food rewards. In addition, the pattern of early findings on the acquisition of simple sensory or spatial discriminations was no easier to reconcile with the deficit in human amnesia than were the findings on approach and avoidance learning. For example, in one of the first of these studies, rats with hippocampal ablations acquired at the same rate as normal animals a visual discrimination in which the stimuli were presented simultaneously. This task employed a Y-shaped maze composed of a start arm and two choice arms: one choice arm was black and the other white, and their left–right positions were randomly changed across trials (Fig. 5–3, left). The rat began each trial at one end of the start arm and then was rewarded for consistently selecting one color choice arm by food placed at the end of that arm.

The opposite result was obtained in another version of the same visual discrimination task where the critical stimuli were presented successively on separate trials (Fig. 5–3, right). On each trial of this test, the rats were

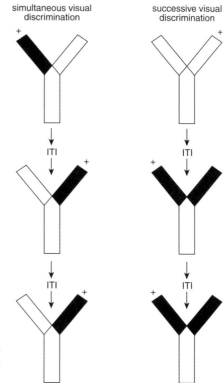

Figure 5–3. A sequence of trials on two different versions of a visual discrimination task using a Y-maze.

presented with one of two mazes, either a maze with two black goal arms or a maze with two white goal arms. The right arm contained food when the goal arms were white, whereas the left arm contained the food when the goal arms were black. In this variant of visual discrimination, rats with hippocampal damage required over twice as many trials as normal rats to reach a learning criterion. However, after a 2-week period, rats with hippocampal ablations showed as good retention as normal rats. As was the case with passive avoidance, although a discrimination learning impairment was observed following hippocampal damage, the overall pattern of results could not be interpreted as supporting a rodent model of global amnesia. Rats with hippocampal damage were not consistently impaired in learning a set of seemingly similar visual discriminations, and there was no impairment in long-term retention in either version of the task.

Many subsequent efforts continued to provide mixed results on the effects of hippocampal damage on simple discrimination learning in rats and other species. There were some kinds of tasks where a disproportionate number of studies showed either impairment or spared learning: Discrimination learning was intact in three times as many experiments as not, although there were also many examples of deficient learning in each situation. This was the case across a broad variety of critical stimuli: nonspatial stimuli including specific visual, auditory, tactile, or olfactory cues, and spatial stimuli including left and right arms of a T- or Y-shaped maze. By contrast, a different result was obtained when animals were required to "reverse" the reward assignments, that is, when they were required to relearn the discrimination for same stimuli but each stimulus had the opposite reward assignment. In these situations animals with hippocampal damage more often showed impairments, although again there were many exceptions. Some researchers suggested that the deficit following hippocampal damage was an impairment in withholding previously learned responses. There was a constituency for this idea, but surely this was not the sort of conclusion that supported a straightforward model of amnesia in animals.

Several new ideas suggested the hippocampus is involved in only one type of memory

In the mid-1970s, several breakthroughs were made in the establishment of a rodent model of amnesia. Parallel to the successful approach in understanding human amnesia, a number of proposals emphasized the critical participation of hippocampus in some aspect of memory and lack of critical involvement in some other aspect of memory processing. Despite major differences in the fundamental processing function assigned to the hippocampus, all the proposals shared two general aspects of their formulations that are very important. First, each proposal espoused the view that the hippocampus plays a selective role in a distinct, higher-order form of memory, whereas hippocampal-independent mechanisms are sufficient to mediate simpler forms of learning and memory. The recognition of multiple forms of memory, only one of which depends on the hippocampus, constituted a major breakthrough of research on rodent memory in that period.

Second, there was substantial agreement on the characteristics of the kind of learning that was successful *in*dependent of hippocampal function. All the proposals that emerged in this period described the capacities of animals with hippocampal damage in a manner consistent with characterizations of "habit" learning. Some characterized learning without the hippocampus as involving dispositions of specific stimuli into approach and avoidance categories, and as involving slow and incremental behavioral adaptation to the stimuli. Others characterized the behavior of animals with hippocampal damage as prone to rigidly adopt permanent assignments of cues and behaviors associated with reinforcement very early. The combination of these qualities remains undisputed in accounting for the success of rats with hippocampal damage in simple approach and avoidance conditioning and in discrimination learning.

Beyond general agreement on what the hippocampus does *not* do, however, the theories differed substantially. In the following section two prominent views are discussed. Both of these proposals received substantial support from a particular key line of experimentation. At the same time each line of experiments challenged the conclusions from the other theory.

A cognitive map in the hippocampus?

In 1978 John O'Keefe and Lynn Nadel proposed that the hippocampus implements the cognitive maps described by Tolman. In a monumental achievement, O'Keefe and Nadel surveyed the extensive research findings on the anatomy and physiology of the hippocampus and on the studies of the effects of hippocampal damage in animals and humans. Each of these areas of knowledge was interpreted as supporting their overall hypothesis that the hippocampus is specifically dedicated to the construction and use of spatial maps of the environment. In their survey of the studies on animals with damage to the hippocampus or its connections, O'Keefe and Nadel emphasized that hippocampal damage typically results in severe impairment in most forms of spatial exploration and learning. Conversely, they noted that impairment of nonspatial learning (such as simple discrimination learning) is less commonly reported. These conclusions were combined with evidence of hippocampal "place cells," hippocampal neurons that signaled the location of the animal in space while it explored its environment (see Chapter 6 for details), leading them to suggest that hippocampal spatial information processing is a critical element of creating maps of space.

It is important to emphasize that O'Keefe and Nadel's analysis went well beyond making a simple distinction between "spatial" and "nonspatial" learning. They proposed that the acquisition of cognitive maps involves a wholly distinct form of cognition from that of habit formation. Cognitive maps involve the representation of places in terms of distances and directions among items in the environment, and are composed as a rough topological map of the physical environment that the animal uses to navigate among salient locations and other important cues. They envisioned cognitive maps as enabling animals to act at a distance, that is, to *navigate* to locations beyond their immediate perception. In addition, cognitive mapping was characterized by a rapid, all-or-none assignment of cues to places within the spatial map. This kind of learning was envisioned as driven by curiosity, rather than reinforcement of specific behavioral responses, and as involving relatively little interference between items because they would be represented separately in a map or in different maps for distinct situations. In short, spatial mapping had most of the qualities of Tolman's cognitive maps, and therefore represented the form of cognitive memory as distinguished from habit learning.

To get a feel for the striking and selective impairment in spatial learning following hippocampal damage in animals, consider the evidence from the water maze test, a spatial memory task that has received widespread use in studies of learning and memory. Originally developed by Richard Morris in 1981, this apparatus involves a large swimming pool filled with tepid water made murky by the addition of milk powder (Fig. 5–4A). An escape platform is hidden just beneath the surface of the water at an arbitrary location. Rats are very good swimmers and rapidly learn to locomote around the pool, but they prefer not to swim and will seek the platform so they can climb onto it. Animals cannot see the platform directly, but instead must use distant spatial cues that are visible above the walls of the pool around the room. On each training trial, the rat begins swimming from one of multiple locations at the periphery of the maze, so that it cannot consistently use a specific swimming course to reach the escape platform. Rats learn to use a spatial navigation strategy to find the platform even after training from a consistent starting

Figure 5–4. The Morris water maze task. *A:* A sketch of the apparatus and two trials of a typical training sequence. In the place navigation version of the task, the rat begins each trial at one of four randomly selected locations and must find a submerged platform (dashed circle) positioned at a constant location. In the cued navigation version, the rat also starts at one of four locations, and the platform is visible (solid circle) and moved randomly across trials. *B:* Performance of rats with hippocampal lesions, cortical lesions, and normal controls in acquiring the water maze task. Place navigation = hidden platform; cue navigation = visible platform. *C:* Performance on the transfer test. Left: Swim path of a control subject; dashed lines indicate quadrant of the maze in which the platform had been located. Right: Swim times of rats in different maze quadrants; black bar corresponds to the training quadrant (data from Morris et al., 1982).

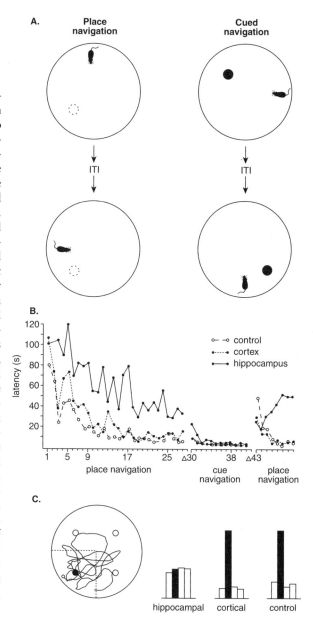

point, as evidenced in their ability after training to locate it efficiently from novel starting points.

Morris and his colleagues showed that hippocampal ablation results in severe impairments in the water maze task (Fig. 5–4B). In the initial trials, all animals typically required 1–2 minutes to find the platform. During the course of repeated trials, normal animals rapidly reduced their escape latency, such that they eventually reached it in less than 10 seconds from every starting point. Rats with hippocampal ablations also reduced their escape latencies, showing some extent of learning. However, they reached asymptotic performance at approximately 35 second latencies, largely due to a reduction of completely ineffective strategies such as trying to climb the walls; however, they never learned to swim directly to the platform location in the manner that normal rats do.

In a subsequent "transfer test" the escape platform was removed and rats were allowed to swim for 1 minute with no opportunity for escape. In this transfer condition, normal rats circled in the close vicinity of the former location of the platform, as measured by a strong tendency to swim within the quadrant of the pool in which it had been located (Fig. 5–4C). Rats with hippocampal ablations showed no preference for the quadrant of the platform, highlighting the severity of their spatial memory deficit. In a different version of the water maze task, when the escape platform could be seen above the surface of the water (cue navigation), both normal rats and rats with hippocampal ablations rapidly learned to swim directly to it. This protocol emphasized the distinction between intact learning to approach the platform guided by a specific local cue, versus no capacity for learning guided by the relation among distant spatial cues. Since Morris and colleagues' original experiment, several studies have confirmed the selective impairment on the spatial version of the Morris water maze task following hippocampal damage, and this task has become a benchmark test of hippocampal function in rodents.

An alternative theory: The hippocampus and remembering recent experiences

In 1979, David Olton and his colleagues proposed an alternative view of the role the hippocampus plays in learning and memory. He argued that the hippocampus is critical when the solution of a problem requires memory for a particular recent experience. He called this "working memory," but note that we will not use this term because it has a different meaning in the current cognitive and neuroscience literatures. In current usage, working memory refers to the ability to temporarily hold information *online* while the subject is working on that information. As described in detail in Chapter 13, this memory capacity has been tied to the function of prefrontal cortex rather than hippocampus. The kind of memory Olton described involved the capacity to remember information that was obtained in a single experience, and to retain and then use it after any delay and over substantial interpolated material, exceeding the properties of working memory. Olton and his colleagues distinguished this kind of memory from "reference memory," which he characterized as memory for information that is constant across trials. Such reference information includes that there is a food reward at the end of each arm, that the rewards are not replaced during a trial but are replaced between trials, etc. On a conceptual level Olton viewed his theory as capturing the distinction raised by Tulving (1972) between "episodic memory" events tied to specific time and place, as contrasted with "semantic memory" for knowledge that is time- and event-independent (see Chapter 4). Accordingly, it is more appropriate to describe Olton's characterization of hippocampal memory as memory for unique episodes.

Olton and colleagues' evidence was generated in great part from experiments using a novel test apparatus called the radial-arm maze. This maze is composed of several (typically eight) runway arms radiating outward like spokes of a wheel from a central platform (Fig. 5–5A), and there are many variants on the number of arms and reward contingencies involved in this task. In the standard version of the task, at the outset of each trial a food reward is placed at the end of each of the arms of the maze. During the course of a trial, the rat is free to enter each arm to retrieve the food rewards. Once retrieved, the food rewards are not replaced during that trial. Rats rapidly learn to approach each arm just once on a given trial. On subsequent trials, all of the arms are baited again just once. The number of arms entered during a trial provides a measure of the ability of the rat to remember which arms it has visited on that particular trial. Notably, this is not a test for memory of spatial locations—typically the spatial cues themselves are never hidden and do not need to be remembered. Instead, the central memory demand is to remember the animal's most recent visits to particular arms of the maze, that is, the recent behavioral episodes as opposed to the many other times each arm has been visited.

In a classic experiment demonstrating the specificity of the impairment following hippocampal damage, Olton and his colleagues compared performance for different maze arms that had distinct reward contingencies (Fig. 5–5B). Some arms of the maze were baited once each trial, following the typical contingency that required memory for specific experiences. In addition, other arms were never baited, and rats were to learn across trials not to enter these arms at all. The latter capacity is another example of "reference memory" emphasizing the fixed nature of the stimulus–response associations for these arms. After initial training of all animals to high levels of performance on both components of the task, half

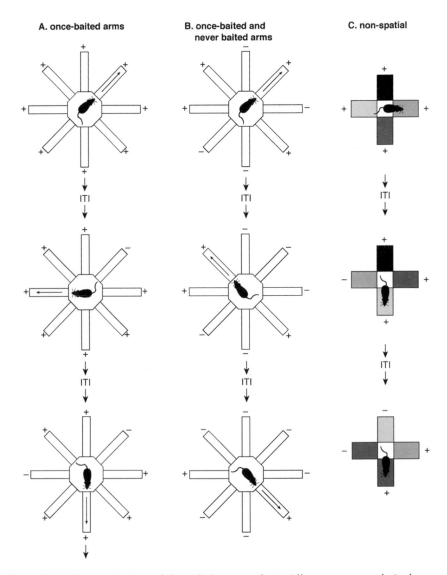

Figure 5–5. Three variations of the radial maze task. *A:* All maze arms are baited once, and the rat must visit each without a repetition. *B:* Only half the arms are baited once and the other half are never baited. Rats learn to visit each baited arm once per trial and never to visit the unbaited arms. *C:* The nonspatial version of the task. Each arm has a different surface on the floor, and the arms are interchanged randomly between trials. Rats learn to visit each cue once per trial.

the animals had the hippocampus disconnected by transection of a major fiber bundle called the fornix. Subsequently in postoperative testing, normal animals continued to perform at very high levels on both the components of the task. By contrast, rats with hippocampal disconnections performed less well than normals from the outset of postoperative testing on both components of the task, but improved rapidly on their reference memory choices. However, they never performed better than chance even with extended training on the arms that required memory for specific experiences.

Olton's proposal was seen as in direct conflict with the cognitive mapping notion, and many succeeding experiments provided support for one or the other proposal. Olton's hypothesis provided the better explanation of one of the early and persistent complexities of data on spatial discrimination, reversal learning, and alternation. Early studies found that hippocampal damage generally does not prevent learning of a simple spatial discrimination on a Y- or T-maze. O'Keefe and Nadel were quick to point out that this maze problem can be solved in two ways, by orienting for a left or right turn or by going to the place of reward. In their view, the hippocampus mediates the place strategy but not the orientation strategy, so that when deprived of hippocampal function the rats have an alternative solution and hence are unimpaired. However, an equally frequent result in the early studies is that rats with hippocampal damage are impaired at spatial reversal learning and are unable to learn to alternate left and right arm selections in Y- or T-mazes, and can show the clear dissociation between intact spatial discrimination and impaired alternation in the same T-maze apparatus outfitted with different types of choice points. It might well be that rats find it easy to adopt an orientation strategy in spatial discrimination, but strongly favor a place strategy in reversal learning and have to use a place strategy in delayed alternation. But it is not the nature of the spatial cues that differentiates these alternatives among these tasks. Rather, it is the demand to use the same cues in different ways for each task that is the critical factor. Olton's memory dichotomy accounts for these results more directly, in that only reference memory is required for the spatial choice never rewarded, but memory for the most recent experience is required for the alternation of choices.

Another line of evidence strongly favoring Olton's theory consisted of experiments extending the role of the hippocampus to memory for specific experiences in the radial maze guided by nonspatial stimuli. The structure of the task was generally the same as in the previous tests of spatial working memory. Each of multiple maze arms was baited just once and perfect performance was measured as the ability of the rat to obtain all the rewards by entering each arm only one time. For the nonspatial version of this task, however, they created a four-arm maze in which the walls and floor of each arm were covered by a distinct set of tactile and visual cues, and distant cues were eliminated by covering the arms with a translucent gauze (Fig. 5–5C). Furthermore, after each arm entry the rat was briefly confined to the central platform while the arms were rearranged to eliminate any consistent arm positions or their configuration. Thus, the rats had to remember entered arms by their distinctive internal (intramaze) cues and ignore any spatial cues about the locations of the arms. After initial preoperative acquisition, normal rats continued to perform the task well but rats with fornix transections failed to reacquire the task even with extended retraining, despite the nonspatial nature of this variant of the task.

The findings on these two theories of hippocampal function leave us in a quandary. O'Keefe and Nadel's theory predicts impairment on any task that requires the use of spatial cues in a cognitive map. It is not entirely clear that performance on the radial maze requires cognitive mapping. But the same spatial stimuli guide performance on both the episodic memory and reference memory versions of the task (Fig. 5–5B). So, the cognitive mapping view would not predict a difference in role of the hippocampus in the two versions of the task. On the other hand, the pattern of deficits on the radial maze tasks indicates that memory for specific prior episodes is critical, and not a demand for the use of spatial cues per se. At the same time, the Morris water maze task is clearly a "reference" memory task. Learning this task requires hippocampal function, a finding that cannot be explained by Olton's hypothesis. Clearly these two theories each capture a critical aspect of hippocampal functioning. However, another fundamental formulation must be pursued to account for both sets of findings. The following section diverges from these maze studies and reconsiders the properties of declarative memory that emerged from studies on human amnesia. Subsequently I return to the findings from the maze studies, as well as other experiments, and offer a reconciliation of the findings within the framework of properties of declarative memory.

Convergence on the relational account of hippocampal function in memory

As discussed in the preceding chapter, characterizations of memory functions of the medial temporal lobe in humans focus on declarative memory, the memory for everyday facts and events that can be brought to conscious recollection and can be expressed in a variety of venues. An approach to investigating this kind of memory can be obtained through a deeper consideration of the fundamental features of declarative memory. First, consider the notion that declarative memory is a combination of "event" or episodic memory and "fact" or semantic memory. How do these two kinds of memory combine to compose declarative memory? We acquire our declarative memories through everyday personal experiences, and in humans the ability to retain and recall these "episodic" memories is highly dependent on the hippocampus. But the full scope of hippocampal involvement also extends to semantic memory, the body of general knowledge about the world that is accrued from linking multiple experiences that share some of the same information. For example, a typical episodic memory might involve recalling the specific events and places surrounding the meeting of a long-lost cousin. Your general knowledge about the relationships of people that compose your family tree and other facts about the history of your family come in great part from a synthesis of the representations of many meetings with relatives and other episodes in which family personalities or events are observed or discussed. Similarly, our episodic memory mediates the capacity to remember a sequence of events, places passed, and turns taken while walking across a city, and a synthesis of many such representations provides general knowledge about the spatial layout of the city.

Second, consider the nature of declarative memory expression. Declarative memory has been characterized as available to conscious recollection and subject to verbal reflection or other explicit means of expression. By contrast, procedural memory has been characterized as the nonconscious acquisition of a bias or adaptation that is typically revealed only by implicit or indirect measures of memory. Thus, declarative memory for both the episodic and semantic information is special in that one can access and express declarative memories via various routes and these memories can be used to solve novel problems by making inferences from memory. For example, even without ever explicitly studying your family tree and its history, one can infer indirect relationships, or the sequence of central events in the family history, from the set of episodic memories about your family. Similarly, without ever studying the map of a city, one can make navigational inferences from the synthesis of many episodic memories of previous routes taken.

These descriptions present a formidable challenge for the study of declarative memory in animals. We do not have the means for identifying episodic memory or monitoring conscious recollection in animals; the very existence of consciousness in animals is a matter of debate. An assessment of verbal reflection is, of course, out of the question, and it is not otherwise obvious how to assess episodic and semantic memory or evaluate "explicit" memory expression in animals. However, these aspects of memory may in fact be accessible if we consider further characterizations that have been offered to distinguish declarative and procedural memory. To the extent that these descriptions do not rely on consciousness or verbal expression, they might be operationalized for experimental analysis in animals.

To this end, in 1984 Cohen offered descriptions that could be helpful toward the goal of operationalizing fundamental properties of declarative memory. He suggested that "a declarative code permits the ability to *compare and contrast* information from different processes or processing systems; and it enables the ability to *make inferences* from and generalizations across facts derived from multiple processing sources. Such a common declarative code thereby provides the basis for access to facts acquired during the course of experiences and for conscious recollection of the learning experiences themselves" (p. 97, italics added). Conversely, procedural learning was characterized as the acquisition of specific skills, adaptations, and biases and that such "procedural knowledge is tied to and expressible only through activation of the particular processing structures or procedures engaged by the learning tasks" (p. 96).

Two distinctions revealed in these characterizations have been employed during development of assessments of declarative and procedural memory that may be applicable to animal studies. First, declarative memory is distinguished by its role in comparing and contrasting distinct memories, whereas procedural memory involves the facilitation of particular routines for which no such comparisons are executed. Second, declarative memory is distinguished by its capacity to support inferential use of memories in novel situations, whereas procedural memory only supports alterations in performance that can be characterized as rerunning more smoothly the neural processes by which they were initially acquired.

These distinctions, plus consideration of the nature of episodic and semantic memory as described in humans, can be extended to make contact with the broad literature on hippocampal function in animals, resulting in a proposal for the representational mechanisms that might underlie declarative memory. Based on a consideration of these characteristics of declarative memory, Eichenbaum and Cohen suggested that the hippocampal system supports a *relational representation* of memories. Furthermore, a critical property of the hippocampal-dependent memory system is its *representational flexibility*, a quality that permits inferential use of memories in novel situations. According to this view, the hippocampal system mediates the organization of memories into what may be thought of as a "memory space."

This theory has been elaborated to make contact with several of the key observations of the theories of memory described earlier.

Within the relational memory theory, the memory space is constructed by an interleaving of episodic memories into a semantic structure in which memories are connected by their common elements. In this scheme the major components of a memory space are the representations of memories as sequences of events that compose specific experiences, that is, distinct episodic memories. Episodic memories, then, are interleaved into the memory space by shared events within related memories. Thus, the construction of family trees and layouts of cities are built up from linking together many episodic memories for specific encounters with family members and for specific trips through a city.

Furthermore, such a memory space supports the kind of comparing and contrasting among memories that allows flexible and inferential use of memories. Within the memory space scheme these capacities are generated by the structure of the relational representation. When one element of the network is activated by a retrieval cue, all memories that contain that item and are sufficiently strongly associated will be activated, including elements of those memories that are elements of yet other related episodic representations. Consequently, memories that are only indirectly associated with the originally activated element would also be activated. Such a process would support the recovery of memories in a variety of contexts outside the learning situation and would permit the expression of memories via various pathways of behavioral output.

Conversely, according to the relational memory account, hippocampal-*in*dependent memories involve *individual representations*; such memories are isolated in that they are encoded only within the brain modules in which perceptual or motor processing is engaged during learning. These individual representations are *inflexible* in that they can be revealed only through reactivation of those modules within the restrictive range of stimuli and situations in which the original learning occurred. One might expect individual representations to support the acquisition of task procedures that are performed habitually across training trials. Individual representations should also support the acquisition of specific information that does not require comparison and consequent relational representation.

The combination of relational representation (a consequence of processing comparisons among memories) and representational flexibility (a quality of relational representation that permits inferential expression of memories) suggests an information processing scheme that might underlie declarative memory in humans and animals as well. Most important, this description of the nature of declarative memory is testable in animals.

Testing the relational memory theory

Large-scale networks for family trees and city layouts are but two examples of the kind of memory space proposed to be mediated by the hippocampus. Within this view, a broad range of such networks can be created, with their central organizing principle the linkage of episodic memories by their common events and places, and a consequent capacity to move among related memories within the network. These properties of declarative memory suggest an approach for the development of animal models. Thus, a way to study the development of a memory space from overlapping experiences, and to make inferences from the network knowledge, is to train subjects on multiple distinct experiences that share common elements and then test whether these experiences have been linked in memory to solve new problems. One can conceive of this approach as applied to various domains relevant to the lives of animals, from knowledge about spatial relations among stimuli in an environment, to categorizations of foods, to learned organizations of odor or visual stimuli or social relationships.

In the remainder of this section some of the evidence supporting the relational account of hippocampal memory function is elaborated. The first set of experiments reexamines discrimination learning, showing once more that learning performance may be severely impaired or completely intact depending on performance demands, showing how a critical demand for relational processing leads to different behavioral outcomes. The second set of experiments examines directly the role of the hippocampus in flexible memory representations and the expression of memory by novel uses of previously acquired knowledge.

The importance of linking multiple distinct experiences

A critical aspect of the relational theory is the interleaving of multiple experiences that share information into a larger network of memories. Therefore, it can be expected that the hippocampus will play a critical role in learning in situations where the task has a strong demand to synthesize multiple overlapping experiences. One such case involves spatial learning, similar to the example of the learning of routes through a city, but involving rats and the Morris water maze task. As described before, in the conventional version of this task, rats learn to escape from submersion in a pool by swimming toward a platform located just underneath the surface. Importantly, training in the conventional version of the task involves an intermixing of four different kinds of trial episodes that differ in the starting point of the swim (see Fig. 5–4A). Focusing on this task demand, the relational memory account offers a straightforward accounting of the pattern of deficits and situations where intact spatial learning is observed. Releasing the rats into the water at different starting points on successive trials strongly encourages the subjects to compare their views along the swim paths as they pass the positions of extramaze stimuli, forcing the animal to consider its relation to the positions of the cues across trials. Indeed, it is difficult to imagine how the task could be solved without synthesizing the information acquired during the different swim episodes into a representation of spatial relations among cues, allowing them to disentangle otherwise conflicting associations of the separate views seen from each starting point. Under these conditions of strong demands to interleave the different types of episodes, animals with hippocampal damage typically fail to acquire the task.

The importance of the demand for interleaving four different types of trial episodes was demonstrated in an experiment that explored acquisition of the water maze when this requirement was eliminated. This experiment used a version of the task where rats were released into the maze from a constant start position on each trial. Initially, animals were trained to approach a visible black-and-white striped platform. Then the visibility of the platform was gradually diminished using a series of training stages that involved a large, visible, white platform, then smaller platforms, and finally sinking the platform below the water surface. With this gradual training procedure, rats with fornix transections learned to approach the platform directly, although they were slower to acquire the response at each phase of training (Fig. 5–6A). In addition, their final escape latencies were slightly higher than those of intact rats, due to an increased tendency for "near misses," trials on which they passed nearby the platform without touching it and forcing them to circle back. But, in contrast to the standard version of this task, animals with hippocampal damage were able to learn the location of the escape platform.

Both sets of rats were using the same extramaze cues to guide performance, as indicated by the results from the standard "transfer" test in which the escape platform is removed and the swimming pattern of the rats is observed for a fixed period. Both normal rats and rats with hippocampal damage swam near the former location of the platform, indicating that they could identify the place of escape by the same set of available extramaze cues rather than solely by the approach trajectory. After several probe tests, these rats were to learn a novel escape location using multiple starting points. Rats with hippocampal damage failed completely. The success of rats with hippocampal damage on the constant start version of the task, contrasted with their failure on the standard, variable

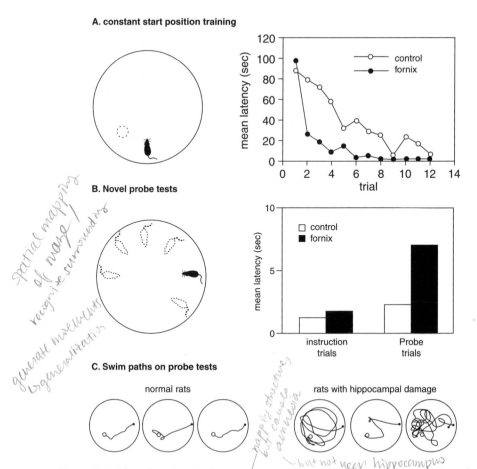

Figure 5–6. Place learning in the water maze. *A:* In the constant start version of this task, the rat always begins from the same location near the escape platform. Note that rats with hippocampal damage (fornix lesions) learn the task more slowly than normal rats, but eventually succeed. *B:* Navigation from novel starting locations. Six novel starting locations were used in the probe testing trials that were intermixed among repetitions of the instruction trial. *C:* Example swim paths for individual normal control rats and rats with hippocampal damage on the probe trial that began from the "east" start location (see black rat in *B*) (data fom Eichenbaum et al., 1990).

start version, indicating that it was not the use of distal spatial cues *per se*, but rather other factors governing how these cues were used that determined the critical involvement of the hippocampus. Rather, the cognitive demand that invoked critical hippocampal function was the requirement to interleave information from multiple experiences on different escape paths taken across trials.

The flexible and inferential expression of spatial memories

Were there differences in the way in which rats with hippocampal damage and normal rats learned and represented the task? This question was addressed by using a series of probe tests, each involving an alteration of the cues or starting points, intermixed within a series of repetitions of the instruction trial. One of the probe tests demonstrated a particularly striking dissociation between the two groups of rats. In this test, the platform was left in its normal place but the start position was moved to various novel locations. When the start position was the same as that used during instruction trials, both normal rats and rats with hippocampal damage had short escape latencies (Fig. 5–6B). On the critical probe trials with novel starting positions, normal rats also swam directly to the platform regardless of the starting position. By contrast, rats with hippocampal damage rarely swam directly to the escape platform and sometimes went far astray, subsequently having abnormally long average escape latencies on these probe trials. This striking deficit in rats with hippocampal damage was demonstrated by a close examination of their individual swim trajectories (Fig. 5–6C). All the normal rats nearly always swam directly to the platform regardless of their starting point. But rats with hippocampal damage swam in various directions, occasionally leading them straight to the platform, but more often in the wrong direction, and they sometimes never found the platform in this highly familiar environment. The observation of a severe deficit in using spatial information acquired successfully to navigate from novel starting points constitutes strong evidence indicating the importance of the hippocampus in the flexible and inferential expression of spatial memories.

Extending the role of the hippocampus in relational representation and representational flexibility to nonspatial learning and memory

The preceding set of experiments provides compelling evidence that the hippocampus plays an important role in spatial learning by supporting the interleaving of multiple overlapping experiences and in using the resulting organized spatial representation to navigate from new locations. Now we consider whether this accounting applies globally to nonspatial as well as spatial memory organizations. One study that examined this issue directly explored the role of the hippocampus in learning an organization of odor stimuli, and in flexible and inferential expression of this organization. This study compared normal rats and rats with selective damage to the hippocampus on their ability to learn a set of odor problems and to interleave their representations of these problems to support novel inferential judgments about them.

To accomplish this an odor-guided version of the so-called paired associate task was developed for rodents, and this task extended the learning requirement to include multiple stimulus–stimulus associations with overlapping stimulus elements (Fig. 5–7). The task was especially designed to take advantage of the superb abilities of rats to learn about odors, and to exploit their natural food foraging behaviors. The stimuli were common household spices, such as oregano, garlic, etc. These stimuli were mixed into ordinary playground sand and presented in small plastic cups. Rewards were a highly preferred sweetened cereal (Froot Loops) buried under the sand. Prior to formal testing the animals were exposed to cups of sand with buried cereal, and rapidly learned to forage through the sand to find the rewards.

Animals were initially trained to associate pairs of odor stimuli with one another. For brevity, the initial pairs will be called A-B and X-Y, where each letter corresponds to a different odor. Each trial was composed of an initial presentation of one of two sample stimuli, A or X. Then that stimulus was removed and the pair of choice odors, B and Y, was presented (Fig. 5–7A). The rule for the choice was as follows: If A was the sample, then B should be selected to obtain a reward; if X was presented, Y contained the reward. Animals were trained on repetitions of these two types of trials (A-B and X-Y) until they achieved a criterion of 80% correct choices. Then they were trained on a second set of paired associates, and this time each association involved an element that overlapped with one of those in the previous pairings, B-C and Y-Z. So now the sample stimuli were B or Y, and the choice stimuli were always C and Z. This problem was also trained to the 80% correct criterion. Then they were trained with all four problems (A-B, X-Y, B-C, and Y-Z) intermixed (Fig. 5–7B). Normal rats learned each set of paired associates rapidly, and hippocampal damage did not affect acquisition rate on either of the two training sets or their combination. It is important to recognize that correct response for each pairing can be learned independently for each problem. That is, unlike the situation with the water maze described before, the solution to each problem does not interfere with solutions to any of the other problems. Therefore, it was not expected that damage to the hippocampus would affect the ability to acquire these problems. However, it was expected that normal rats and rats with hippocampus damage would form qualitative different representations of the problems, and this was examined next.

Following successful acquisition of all the paired associates, subjects were given probe tests to determine whether they organized their repre-

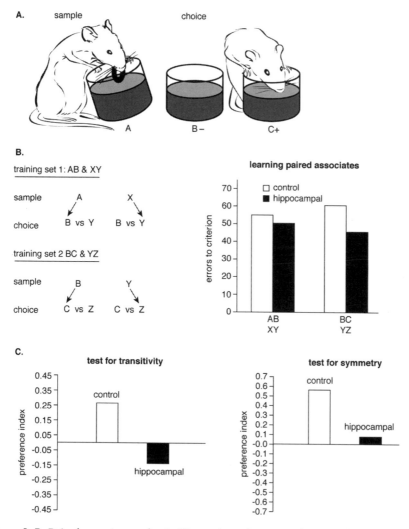

Figure 5–7. Paired associate task. *A:* Illustration of a rat performing the sample and choice trials of the task. *B:* Odors presented in the sample and choice trials in each training set (left) and performance of rats in learning each set. *C:* Performance on the probe tests for transitivity and symmetry. The preference index was calculated as the ratio of the difference in times spent (transitivity) or choice (symmetry) in digging between the two cups and that for the sum on the same measure for the two cups (data from Bunsey and Eichenbaum, 1996).

sentations of the four odor pairs into an efficient scheme that interleaved overlapping odors pairs, or simply learned each problem independently. In the preceding scheme, representations of the pairs A-B and B-C could be organized into a larger network, A-B-C, and similarly X-Y and Y-Z could be organized into X-Y-Z. Two kinds of probe tests were presented to examine whether these larger network representations were formed, and to assess their flexibility.

One test assessed the capacity for "transitive inference," the ability to make a judgment about two odors that are only indirectly related by another, not presented item. In this scheme, note that odor A and odor C were never presented together but can be indirectly related via their shared associate B. Similarly, X and Z are indirectly related via odor Y. In a critical test for transitivity, subjects were presented with trials using the same sample-choice format with trials on A-C and X-Z. However, in these tests no reward was provided, and the time spent foraging in the two choice cups was compared as a measure of their recognition of the appropriate relations between indirectly associated elements. Normal rats also showed strong transitivity, reflected in a preference for odors indirectly associated with the presented sample (Fig. 5–7C). By contrast, rats with selective hippocampal lesions were severely impaired, showing no evidence of transitivity.

The other probe involved a test for "symmetry" of the learned associations, the ability to recognize related pairings regardless of the order in which the items are presented. In this scheme, the subjects were asked to recognize appropriate pairings in the reverse order of that used in training on the second set of problems. Again, the sample-choice format was used, but the pairings were C-B and Z-Y. In the symmetry test, normal rats again showed the appropriate preference in the direction of the symmetrical association. By contrast, rats with hippocampal lesions again were severely impaired, showing no significant capacity for symmetry (Fig. 5–7C). The combined findings show that rats with hippocampal damage can learn even complex associations, such as those in the odor paired associates. But unlike normal animals, they do not interleave the distinct experiences according to their overlapping elements to form a larger network representation that supports inferential and flexible expression of their memories.

A case of naturalistic learning, and natural inferential memory expression

Extending the range of our study of hippocampal involvement in associative learning, the role of the hippocampal region has also been assessed using a type of social olfactory learning and memory, called the social transmission of food preferences. This test is based on observations of rat social behavior in the wild. Rats form large social communities and send out "foragers" to explore for food sources. When forager rats return to the nest, they inform others of new foods by carrying the odor of a new food on their breath. Subsequently, the other rats to whom this information is conveyed seek out that same food. This form of social learning is interpreted within the heuristic that a food recently consumed by the forager is safe, and thus transmitting this information is adaptive in rat social groups.

This behavior can be easily adapted to a formal laboratory test by designating "demonstrator" (forager) and "observer" (subject) rats, and reproducing the elements of the foraging and social communication events (Fig. 5–8). Initially, the demonstrator rat is given rat chow tainted with a food spice, such as cinnamon or chocolate powder. Then the demonstrator is placed in the home cage of the subject for several minutes, during

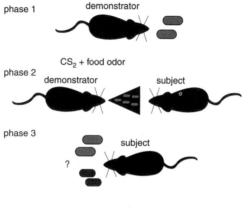

"Natural" odor-guided paired associate learning

phase 1   demonstrator

CS₂ + food odor
phase 2
demonstrator   subject

phase 3
                   subject
        ?

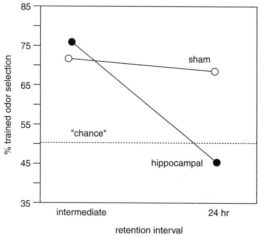

Figure 5–8. The social transmission of food preferences task. *Top:* Protocol for the task. *Bottom:* Performance of intact rats (open circles) and rats with selective hippocampal lesions (filled circles) in immediate and 1-day retention tests (data from Bunsey and Eichenbaum, 1995).

which the two animals socially interact. Then the demonstrator is removed, and the subject must remember the food odor for a variable period. Finally, the subject is presented with two food cups, one with rat chow tainted with the same odor as presented to the demonstrator and the other cup with another food odor that may be equally familiar or novel to the subject. Learning is demonstrated as an increase in the probability that the observer will later select that same food as the demonstrator had eaten over other foods.

Previous investigations of this behavior in normal rats has shown that the mechanism underlying this learning involves an association between two odors present in the demonstrator rat's breath, the odor of the recently eaten food and a natural odorous constituent of rat's breath, carbon disulfide. These studies have shown that exposing the subject to the distinctive food odor alone, or to carbon disulfide alone, have no effect on later food preference. However, exposure to the combination of these two odors using a "surrogate rat," a cotton ball saturated with carbon disulfide, substitutes well for the social interaction in producing the appropriate learned food preference. Thus, the shift in food choice cannot be attributed to mere familiarity with the food odor. Rather, the conclusion from these studies is that the formation of a specific association between the food odor and carbon disulfide, in the absence of any primary reinforcement, is both necessary and sufficient to support the shift in food selection.

Social transmission of food preferences provides a strong example of declarative-like learning in the natural behavior of rats. Learning involves the formation of a specific stimulus–stimulus association in a single training episode. Furthermore, this paradigm provides one of the best examples of a natural form of "inferential" expression of the memory. Thus, note that the training experience involves a social encounter without any feeding, during which the subject is exposed to an arbitrary stimulus and another natural stimulus that acts as a reinforcer. By contrast, the memory testing situation is nonsocial, and involves food selection choices without the presence of the same stimulus that reinforced learning the new food odor. This aspect of the task, expression of memory in a situation very different from the learning event, is strongly consistent with the declarative property of representational flexibility.

The role of the hippocampus has been investigated using this task, assessing both immediate memory and delayed memory for social exposure to the odor of a novel food. The behavior of rats with hippocampal damage during the social encounter is entirely normal. In the memory test, normal rats showed a strong selection preference for the trained food odor, and this memory was robust when tested immediately and after a 1-day retention period (see Fig. 5–8). By contrast, rats with selective damage to the hippocampus showed intact immediate memory, but their performance fell to chance level of food choices within 24 hours. The observation of intact immediate memory, similar to the pattern of spared short-term memory in human amnesics, indicates that the hippocampus is not required for perceptual, motivational, or behavioral components of the social learning or the ability to express the learned food choice preferences. But the hippocampus is required for long-term expression of the memory in a situation that is far outside the learning context.

Summing up

There is a long and mixed history of attempts to model amnesia in animals. Efforts in both monkeys and rats were largely unsuccessful owing to the poor choice of memory tests and the lack of realization that there are different forms of memory, only one of which depends on the medial temporal lobe. However, there have now been many successful demonstrations of the characteristics of human amnesia in both monkeys and rats. In monkeys, major advances were made with the advent of the delayed nonmatch to sample test that provided a novel test of recognition memory. The results using this test plus those of a set of related tests showed that medial temporal lobe damage similar to that in H.M. results in a remarkably similar pattern of impaired and spared memory abilities. In rats, major advances were made following the realization that much of the ambiguity in the pattern of effects of hippocampal damage could be explained by distinctions between impairments in spatial memory versus spared nonspatial memory, and between memory-specific recent experiences versus spared learning guided by habits or dispositions of specific stimuli. However, experiments in support of each of these two accounts are in apparent conflict.

The combined results from both these accounts, and across many other experiments, provide compelling evidence for a comprehensive account of the cognitive mechanisms of declarative memory. Various kinds of learning, spatial and nonspatial, simple and complex, can be accomplished independent of the hippocampus in animals, as indeed is the case in human amnesic patients as well. However, the hippocampus is required to link together the representations of overlapping experiences into a relational representation, and supports the flexible and inferential expression of indirect associations among items within the larger organization of linked memories. This hippocampal function applies across many situations, including navigation within spatial organizations, and nonspatial organizations of specific stimuli (e.g., odors) in logical schemes or in natural social behavior. The next chapter explores the nature of the neural code that accomplishes this networking function of the hippocampus.

READINGS

Cohen, N.J. 1984. Preserved learning capacity in amnesia: Evidence for multiple memory systems. In *The Neuropsychology of Memory*, N. Butters, and L.R. Squire (Eds.). New York: Guilford Press, pp. 83–103.

Cohen, N.J., and Eichenbaum, H. 1993. *Memory, Amnesia, and the Hippocampal System*. Cambridge: MIT Press.

Eichenbaum, H. 1997. Declarative memory: Insights from cognitive neurobiology. *Annu. Rev. Psychol.* 48:547–572.

Mishkin, M,, and Petri, H.L. 1984. Memories and habits: Some implications for the analysis of learning and retention. In *The Neuropsychology of Memory*, N. Butters, and L.R. Squire (Eds.). New York: Guilford Press, pp. 287–296.

Morris, R.G.M., Garrud, P., Rawlins, J.P, and O'Keefe, J. 1982. Place navigation impaired in rats with hippocampal lesions. *Nature* 297:681–683.

O'Keefe, J.A., and Nadel, L. 1978. *The Hippocampus as a Cognitive Map*. New York: Oxford University Press.

Olton, D.S., Becker, J.T., and Handlemann, G.E. 1979. Hippocampus, space, and memory. *Brain Behav. Sci.* 2:313–365.

Squire, L. 1992. Memory and the hippocampus: A synthesis from findings with rats, monkeys, and humans. *Psycho. Rev.* 99(2): 195–231.

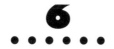

Windows into
the Workings of Memory

STUDY QUESTIONS

What is brain imaging, and how can it be used to study human memory?

What are the characteristics of memory processing that activate the medial temporal lobe in normal human subjects?

What are place cells?

What is the full characterization of events that are encoded by hippocampal neuron firing patterns?

What is a "memory space," and how might it be constructed by the properties of hippocampal neuron firing patterns?

So far this review of our understanding of hippocampal function in memory has focused predominantly on studies of amnesia in humans and on the effects of hippocampal damage in animals. In the present chapter, complementary evidence is presented from other related approaches. These approaches involve monitoring the ongoing operation of the human hippocampus and related brain structures during memory performance, providing a virtual "window" into the inner workings of the normal brain. This is accomplished at two levels of analysis: by using functional neuroimaging methods in normal humans and by recording the activity patterns of single neurons in animals.

With regard to the functional imaging studies, there are now multiple sophisticated methods that are employed, particularly positron emission tomography (PET) and functional magnetic resonance imaging (fMRI). It is beyond the scope of this text to discuss the details of these methodologies, except to say that both involve measurements of blood flow and brain oxygen consumption, which provide good reflections of the level of activation of a brain area encompassing several thousand neurons over a second-to-second time scale. By telling us when, for example, the medial temporal area becomes active, functional neuroimaging studies in humans can inform us about the aspects or kinds of memory in which the hippocampal system is and is not involved, providing a way to assess its functional role.

Single cell recording studies in animals provide an even closer look at the inner workings of the hippocampus. This method involves monitoring the action potentials of individual neurons and so allows a major increase in resolution of cellular activity within different parts of the medial temporal area, and even allows us to distinguish particular types of neurons within a specific brain structure. Also, this method has a greater resolution in time, allowing us to capture millisecond-to-millisecond computations by the fundamental elements of neural processing. Thus, these two approaches have complementary strengths and limitations. The strength of functional imaging is that it allows the simultaneous examination of the entire system, but at only a gross level that tells us which structures are activated to major shifts in task demands. Single cell recording methods allow us to monitor only one part of the system at any time, but offer insights into the fundamental coding properties of the units of neural computation.

Functional neuroimaging studies of the human hippocampal system

Early attempts to observe hippocampal activation in PET or fMRI during one or another memory performance were largely disappointing. Scannning during the study of materials such as word lists, and other tasks for which memory depends on hippocampal function, failed to show increased activation over nonmemory processing of the same materials. However, this turns out to be an artifact of the procedures in analysis of brain images. All imaging techniques involve a *comparison* of activation levels between two conditions, an experimental and a control condition. In memory studies, the experimental condition involves the critical memory demand under study, for example, memorizing word lists. The control condition involves the same perceptual and cognitive demands, except without the critical memory demand. In the word list example, the control might be reading words without having to remember them. The areas associated with memory processing *per se* are defined operationally as those brain regions where the activation level is greater in the experimental condition than in the control condition. However, the evidence described previously, as well as other physiological data that are described later, indicate that the hippocampus is always active in encoding new information for declarative memory. In the example, the control condition where subjects merely read words may invoke quite substantial hippocampal activation associated with remembering the experience of reading the word list. More generally, there is virtually no condition where memory processing is expected to be altogether absent. Thus, the failure to find activation associated with memory in the early studies may be attributed to the lack of a substantial difference in the activations associated during the memory condition (e.g., studying a word list) and apparent nonmemory activities for which memory processing was nevertheless invoked (reading a word list).

Since those early studies, another generation of experiments has taken the issue of control conditions into consideration and in recent years has shown that the human hippocampal system can be seen in action during various memory performances and the results of these studies correspond well to those of the studies of amnesia. Thus, the findings from functional brain imaging generally support the distinction between declarative and procedural memory, and they provide new details on the nature of events that activate the medial temporal area. The following section explores these characteristics of medial temporal activation.

The medial temporal area is involved in "global" information processing

Consider first the range of to-be-remembered materials over which the medial temporal area operates. Studies of patients with bilateral damage to the medial temporal area have shown that amnesia is a *global* memory deficit. As discussed in Chapter 4, amnesic patients have a memory impairment that crosses between different learning materials and sensory modalities, encompassing verbal and nonverbal, spatial and nonspatial materials, regardless of whether they are presented visually, auditorily, etc., indicating that the role of this region in memory is, likewise, *non*specific with regard to material and modality. However, other studies involving patients with *unilateral* damage, that is, involving damage only to the left or right medial temporal lobe region, have shown clear material-specific memory impairments: Verbal memory performance is selectively compromised after *left* medial temporal lobe damage, and nonverbal memory performance is selectively compromised after *right* temporal lobe damage. In other words, there is a *laterality* in the critical medial temporal lobe contribution to memory, corresponding to the different types of learning materials. Furthermore, the nature of processing for which the hemispheres are specialized follows the well-known laterality for nonmemory processing of verbal versus nonverbal materials assigned to the left and right hemispheres, respectively. How well do the findings from functional imaging studies of memory correspond to this picture from studies of amnesia?

Across a variety of functional imaging studies one can see both the globalness of medial temporal processing, considering both hemispheres, and also the material-specificity of left versus right hemisphere processing. Looking across the range of studies that have reported medial temporal activation, one sees that a range of stimulus materials can engage this system. Thus, ignoring the particular hemisphere in which activation occurs, activation in the medial temporal lobe has been reported for words, objects, scenes, faces, and spatial routes, landmarks, or locations. In addition, in studies that compared different classes of materials, clear hemispheric specialization has been seen. The results generally indicate greater left than right activation for words, and greater right than left activation for novel faces or objects. Accordingly, with regard to the scope of the materials processed by the medial temporal lobe, there is good concordance of the functional imaging and the data from studies on amnesia.

Next we consider several general findings on the types of memory processing that have consistently activated the medial temporal area across multiple studies. These include activation by the simple presentation of novel stimulus information, activation by the processing of new stimulus associations, and activation associated with explicit, conscious recollection.

Activation of the medial temporal region by the presentation of novel information

There are now several lines of evidence that have suggested medial temporal lobe involvement in specific aspects of cognitive processing, although some of these are not identical to dimensions that are featured in accounts of amnesia. However, it is important to keep in mind that functional imaging studies are likely to reveal the initial stages of memory processing when the medial temporal area becomes involved, even in situations where its involvement may not be critical to that particular type of processing. A good example involves several reports of engagement of the medial temporal region by the mere presentation of novel information. These studies have found greater activation for the processing of *novel* as compared to *familiar* pictures of complex scenes or objects. In one study, subjects viewed magazine photos of scenes in alternating blocks of trials that included either a series of different scenes, each presented once, or just one scene that was presented repeatedly as a control. Subjects were instructed to study the scenes so they might be able to recognize them later, and they were scanned during this study phase. Greater activation was seen in the medial temporal region for the novel scenes in the experimental condition compared to the single repeated scene in the control condition. In perhaps the most striking example of a novelty detection effect, the right hippocampus was selectively activated by the presentation of novel visual noise patterns, that is, a series of random dot patterns, compared to the presentation of the same patterns a second time (Fig. 6–1A).

These findings have led some investigators to propose that the medial temporal region may be involved in novelty detection per se. However, as you will see later, the medial temporal region is activated also by familiar material under circumstances where the subject is making recognition judgments. So, clearly the detection of novelty *per se* is not the primary function revealed in activation by novel stimuli. Rather, an effect of stimulus novelty on medial temporal activation makes good sense as a reflection of the kind of processing that would underlie declarative memories of the many pictures. The presentation of a brand new scene every few seconds should invoke considerable declarative memory processing as the hippocampus is involved in encoding the information within scenes and the sequence of constantly changing scenes. By contrast, the control condition that involves repeated presentations of a single unchanging scene, minimizes this processing demand. Therefore, the comparison of these two conditions is likely to reveal the differential activation for maximal and minimal processing of new information.

Medial temporal activation associated with processing stimulus associations

The data just described suggest that the hippocampus always becomes engaged when new material is presented, but may become more activated to the extent that processing relations among elements within or across scenes is strongly demanded by the materials or the task. This view could account for why the early studies failed to find medial temporal activation when subjects were presented with highly familiar stimuli such as word lists, as compared to other manipulations of the same materials that also invoke memory processing. The studies that focused on the presentation of several changing scenes as compared to the same unchanging scene may have revealed a difference in the amount of hippocampal activation de-

A. novel visual "noise"

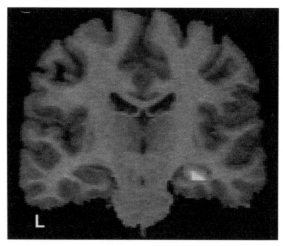

B. the combination of time-specific and personally relevant memory

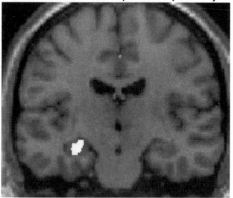

Figure 6–1. Functional imaging of the human hippocampus. *A:* Activation of the right hippocampus during viewing of novel as contrasted with familiar visual noise patterns (from Martin, 1999). *B:* Activation of the left hippocampus during recall of memories that are both temporally specific and personally relevant (from Maguire and Mummery, 1999).

manded by the differential requirement for processing information within and across items that would be encoded in memory.

Consistent with this expectation the strongest support for the medial temporal region activation in processing information across scenes for explicit memory comes from a study by Henke and colleagues in which subjects were shown a series of pictures, each of which showed a person and a house (either the interior or the exterior) simultaneously. Subjects were required to judge if the person was likely to be the inhabitant or a visitor to that house, based on their appearance and that of the house. For example, one pair of pictures showed an elegant lady and an equally elegant sitting room that would constitute an appropriate match. Another example showed a disheveled man and a large mansion, representing an unlikely match. Thus, while the task did not directly demand the subjects to associate the two images, the nature of the judgment encouraged them to make an association between the person and the house. As a control, subjects were shown other pairs of pictures and requested to make separate decisions about the person's gender (male or female?) and view of the house (exterior or interior?). This test requirement encouraged the subjects to encode the house and person separately.

Greater medial temporal activation was observed when the subjects were encouraged to associate the person and the house than when they encoded the same kinds of items separately. These findings suggest that it is not merely the processing of novel pictures that activates the hippocampus. If this were so, one would expect the same level of activation for similarly novel pictures of people and houses. Instead, the findings support the view that the medial temporal region is more activated when there is a greater demand for learning associations or relations between items in single learning episodes, as compared with processing the items separately.

In a related study, Maguire and Mummery examined the activation of medial temporal structures during recollection of different types of materials. They found a large network of brain areas activated during different types of recall associated with different aspects of real-world memory, including whether the memory occurred at a particular time or instead involved time-independent factual information, or was personally relevant or instead involved general knowledge of public events. They found a striking and specific activation of the left hippocampus when what subjects recollected was a combination of personally relevant and specific in time (Fig. 6–1B).

Medial temporal activation associated with conscious recollection

More directly related to declarative memory, other studies have considered whether the medial temporal lobe region is disproportionately engaged in explicit memory, that is, in conscious recollection. In one experiment, subjects first studied word lists and then their memory was later tested in different ways during scanning. At testing, subjects were given word stems and asked to complete the stems either with the first word that came to mind, just as in a typical repetition priming experiment (see Chapter 4), or with a word from the study list, to engage conscious recollection, or with the first word that came to mind that was *not* on the study list, as a baseline condition where the subject stared at a cross-hair on the screen. Medial temporal activation was found for the condition that involved conscious recollection, as compared to either the priming condition, which involved implicit memory instructions, or the baseline condition.

Other studies have related medial temporal activation to successful retrieval of previously stored information, that is, success in the effortful reactivation of stored representations. In one such study, subjects listened to two lists of words prior to being in the scanner. For one list, subjects were to decide whether each word was said by a male or female speaker. This condition was employed to encourage processing at the level of perceptual features of the words and to deemphasize encoding the semantic or conceptual content in the words. For the other list, the subjects had to decide whether each word referred to a living or nonliving thing, in order to encourage conceptual or semantic encoding over perceptual encoding. Subjects were subsequently tested for recognition memory while being scanned, in a series of test blocks that assessed memory separately for perceptually encoded and semantically encoded words.

Greater medial temporal lobe activation was observed for test blocks that involved words from the semantically encoded list compared to the perceptually encoded list. The fact that there was a higher rate of successful recall of semantically encoded words compared to perceptually encoded words suggested that increased medial temporal activation for semantically encoded words was a consequence of the role of this region in successful recall, that is, in successfully gaining access to some memory representation. This connection was seen more formally as a strong positive correlation across subjects and conditions between test performance and medial temporal lobe activation.

Another line of studies has shown that the medial temporal region is activated when subjects are involved in effortful retrieval and manipulation of retrieved geographical information. In these studies experienced London taxi drivers were scanned as they were requested to retrieve information about routes around London. Greater activation of medial temporal structures was seen during recall of route information than during recall of famous landmarks, movie plot lines, or movie scenes. In another study subjects learned to navigate around in a virtual reality environment. Subjects were then scanned while they made judgments about the appearance or relative position of particular places in the environment compared to a control condition involving scrambled versions of the same stimuli. Medial temporal activation was observed bilaterally for both conditions that tested memory of the learned places compared to the control condition.

These functional brain imaging studies indicate that the medial temporal region becomes activated whenever new, complex material is presented. Furthermore, these results indicate that the medial temporal region is maximally activated when processing this material demands encoding new associations or relations among separate items in specific memory episodes. In addition, the medial temporal area is similarly invoked during the act of explicit memory retrieval, that is, during conscious recollection. These findings are entirely consistent with the observations on the pattern of impaired and spared capacities in human amnesia, and thus demonstrate a close correspondence of the data from two different approaches. Furthermore, the combination of activations during both episodic learning and conscious recollection indicates that the medial temporal area is involved similarly in encoding and retrieval phases of declarative memory.

The representation of experience in the activity of networks of hippocampal neurons

The foregoing characterizations of the effects of damage to the hippocampal region (in Chapters 4 and 5), and of activation of the hippocampal region in humans, suggest that its fundamental role is in encoding rich episodic information and conscious and flexible memory expression. What kind of neural representation within the hippocampus would support this functional role? As described in the preceding chapter, on a conceptual level, the form of such a representation might be constituted as a large network that encodes episodic memories and links these memories via their shared features. Can such a scheme be confirmed and elaborated by observations on the elements of the hippocampus, that is, in the firing patterns of single hippocampal neurons?

While any conclusions about the nature of firing patterns in the hippocampus is still quite preliminary, there is an emerging body of data consistent with this scheme. A wealth of evidence indicates that hippocampal neurons encode a broad variety of information, including all modalities of perceptual input as well as behavioral actions, and cognitive operations. In addition, hippocampal neurons seem especially tuned to relevant conjunctions among features that reflect unique episodic information, rather than simple perceptual or motor features. Moreover, hippocampal neural activity is particularly sensitive to modifications with experience such that alterations in the meaning of items or their relationships result in major changes in cellular firing patterns. Combined, these observations provide a bridge to current characterizations of declarative memory being accessible by many routes of expression, including literally one's verbal declarations about the contents of prior experiences. I begin with a conceptual scheme that could accomplish the coding of episodic information and the linking of this information into a larger network or memory space. Then I review the observations from studies on the firing patterns of hippocampal neurons that support this scheme.

A scheme for hippocampal representation in declarative memory

The evidence from both studies on human and animal amnesia and from brain imaging studies on humans points to an important role for the hippocampus in encoding complex information that contributes to our memory for personal experiences, that is, episodic memories, and for our ability to synthesize this episodic information into our body of world knowledge, fact or semantic memory. It is well known that the hippocampus receives information from virtually all sensory domains as well as other information about our internal states and our own behaviors (see Chapter 9). In addition, the hippocampus is remarkable for the extent of interconnectivity among the principal cells in its major processing areas. Also, the studies on hippocampal plasticity outlined in Chapter 3 have indicated that hippocampal neurons are particularly good at encoding conjunctions of diverse inputs. This combination of observations suggests a scheme in which subsets of hippocampal neurons could act as small networks for encoding episodic memories and for linking them together into larger networks that could support the properties of declarative memory.

An outline of such a scheme is presented in Fig. 6–2. The scheme proposes three types or levels of coding by single hippocampal neurons. At the lowest level in this scheme, each hippocampal cell encodes a highly complex set of sensory and other information that composes a single behavioral "event." A single event is brief in its scope, akin to a single photographic snapshot that would include information about any salient stimuli, ongoing behavior, and the location or background in which the event occurred. In this scheme, single hippocampal neurons are viewed as capable of encoding the conjunction of all of this information that composes a single event captured in a brief moment of time.

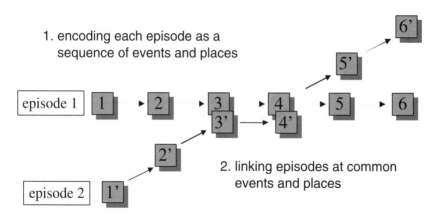

1. encoding each episode as a sequence of events and places

2. linking episodes at common events and places

3. constructing a memory space that supports flexible memory expression

Figure 6–2. Schematic model of a simple "memory space." Events include ongoing behavior and location information, as indicated by individual numbered boxes. Episodes are composed of a sequence of event representations. The memory space is composed of a set of episodes linked by common, nodal events.

In addition, at the second level of this scheme, the activities of a set of hippocampal cells that are activated in sequence during a particular episode are preserved. This may be accomplished by cells whose plasticity properties can incorporate features of two or more sequential events, thus providing a mechanism for tying together the individual representations of multiple events. This combination of a set of sequential individual event codings and the codings that link multiple event sequences constitute the complete representation of a single episodic memory.

Finally, at the third level of this scheme, it is proposed that there are other "nodal" hippocampal cells that encode features that are common across multiple episodes. According to this account, these cells receive strong inputs from some information about specific stimuli, behaviors, or location or other contextual information that is a salient element among otherwise distinct experiences. This feature could include a common critical stimulus to be remembered across different types of training trials, a common response one made to various stimuli in different trials, or a common location where different experiences occurred.

The combination of these three functional prototypes of hippocampal cells provides the fundamental elements of a "memory space" that could support the properties of declarative memory. The event cells would capture unique combinations of behavioral and location information that would mark specific episodes. The cells that encode sequences of multiple events could allow the recovery of entire episodes. The nodal cells could provide a bridge between episodic representations that could support the capacity for flexible and inferential memory expression by linking together indirectly information obtained across distinct episodes. What is the evidence that hippocampal cells have the properties of these prototypical units? A review of the story of efforts to characterize hippocampal neuron activity provides strong support for this model and insights into the workings of memory processing within the hippocampus.

Early observations on the firing patterns of hippocampal neurons

Following on the advent of technologies for recording the extracellular spike activity in behaving animals, several investigators began to explore the firing patterns of the large pyramidal cells in the hippocampus of rats. Electrophysiological techniques allowed these investigators to make the recordings in awake and behaving animals, providing the opportunity to correlate neuronal activations with stimulus events and motor patterns during a broad variety of behaviors, including learning. The expectations of investigators in these explorations were marked by caution. James Ranck, Jr., as he pioneered the earliest recording of hippocampal neurons in behaving animals, worried that cells in a brain structure located so many synapses from sensory input and motor output would have firing activity significant only as part of a large network; he suspected that neural firing patterns in response to external stimuli or behavioral output would be uninterpretable. But this clearly turned out not to be the case. Quite the opposite—hippocampal neuronal activity is well correlated with a very broad variety of stimuli and behavioral events, with the activity of cells "mirroring" virtually all the combinations of stimulus and behavioral events in any situation. Thus, identifying the scope and nature of information processing by hippocampal neurons has proved a formidable challenge, not because of the paucity of responses they might have evoked, but because of their variety, their complexity, and their plasticity in response to change.

In Ranck's landmark 1973 paper, he described a large number of behavioral correlates of hippocampal neuronal activity. His categorization included cells that fired associated with specific orienting behaviors, approach movements, or cessation of movement, and with consummatory behaviors (feeding and drinking) or the mismatch of expected consummatory event (e.g., the absence of water when it is usually found). At the same time, John O'Keefe was also recording from hippocampal cells in rats exploring open environment. His observations on hippocampal cellular activity led him to a different conclusion—rather than neuronal activity reflecting ongoing behaviors, O'Keefe and his colleague John Dostrovsky made the remarkable and historic discovery that hippocampal cells fire associated with locations the animal occupies at least as much as with the ongoing behavioral events. Ranck noted the possibility that his findings might be characterized in terms of the spatial specificity of firing patterns, and for some period the "behavioral" correlates of hippocampal firing patterns were largely overwhelmed with excitement about the spatial coding properties of these cells. This led to a period when considerable attention was given to the spatial properties of hippocampal neuronal activity, within the framework of the cognitive map theory of O'Keefe and Nadel, as introduced in the preceding chapter.

What are place cells? Do they compose a "cognitive map"?

The existence of location-specific neural activity in hippocampal neurons has been confirmed in many systematic studies. The common observation is that pyramidal neurons of the CA1 and CA3 fields of the hippocampus fire at high rates when the animal is in a particular location in the environment and fire little or not at all when the animal is located in other places. This observation led to the conclusion that each hippocampal cell has a distinct "place field," or area of the environment associated with high firing rate. Many current studies of place cells involve computerized tracking of the animal's position continuously in space, and automated means of determining the firing rate of the neuron associated with a matrix of locations. These studies show that many hippocampal cells have spatially specific activity that can be observed in many behavioral situations. A particularly clear example comes from a simple protocol where a rat forages for small food pellets distributed randomly throughout an open field. The rat continuously searches in all directions for extended periods (Fig. 6–3A). In this situation many hippocampal cells fire at a high rate only when the rat crosses a particular area in the environment (the place field), regardless of the rat's orientation within the environment. Once established, place fields can be very stable, and have been observed to show the same spatial firing pattern for months. However, the probability of firing of place cells is highly variable, in that sometimes the rate exceeds 100/sec on a pass through the field. Yet, on other passes, the cell may not fire at all, such that the average firing rate within the place field is typi-

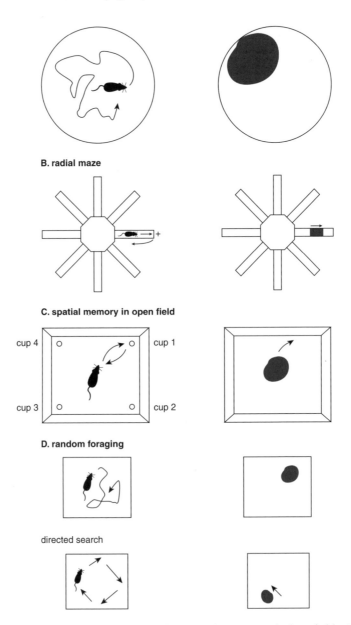

A. random foraging in open field

B. radial maze

C. spatial memory in open field

cup 4   cup 1

cup 3   cup 2

D. random foraging

directed search

Figure 6–3. Four different protocols used to map hippocampal place fields. For each protocol, the task is illustrated on the left. On the right is a mapping of an example place field (filled area), the location in the environment where the cell increased firing rate of the cell. Directional place fields are indicated by an arrow showing the direction of movement associated with increased firing.

cally about 10/sec. This variability portends that factors other than the location of the animal *per se* determine the activity of these cells.

In their initial report, O'Keefe and Dostrovsky realized immediately the potential significance of this neural correlate, and suggested that the hippocampus might subserve the creation and utilization of cognitive maps that animals use to navigate their environment, just as Tolman proposed in his efforts to characterize maze learning capacities in animals. In support of this view, O'Keefe later reviewed the existing findings on hippocampal place cells, focusing on the number and types of stimulus features in the environment that were encoded by place cells. He concluded that "a place cell is a cell which constructs the notion of a place in the environment by connecting together several multisensory inputs each of which can be perceived when the animal is in a particular part of the environment" (O'Keefe, 1979, p. 425). He supported this characterization by showing that the location-specific firing of most hippocampal neurons is controlled by the global configuration of the distant salient stimuli, and that any substantial subset of the spatial cues is sufficient to support spatially specific activity in some cells. More recent studies have shown that while some cells encode all of the available sensory cues, the location-specific activity of most hippocampal neurons is controlled by a subset of the spatial stimuli. Therefore, the overall representation of space is a composite of many partial representations where each cell encodes the spatial relations between a few of the cues.

The view that hippocampal cells encode spatial position is a critical feature of O'Keefe and Nadel's cognitive mapping hypothesis. The concept of hippocampal spatial representation that has emerged from these findings, illustrated in Fig. 6–4, is that the hippocampus contains a map-like representation of space. At a conceptual level, the map constitutes a coordinate grid, instantiated by intrinsic connections among hippocampal neurons. During investigation of a novel environment, representations of the relevant environmental stimuli are associated with appropriate spatial coordinate points. The resulting map is Cartesian in that it provides metric representations of distances and angles between the relevant stimuli. At the physiological level, a place cell reflects the occurrence of the rat at a particular coordinate position within the map. Thus, implicit in this model is the assumption that place fields can be considered "pointers" within a unified map, such that either every cell contains information about all of the cues or that cells representing subsets of the cues are all linked and bound by the global coordinate framework. O'Keefe and Nadel's central notion then is that the hippocampus constructs a facsimile of the environment, including the salient environmental cues.

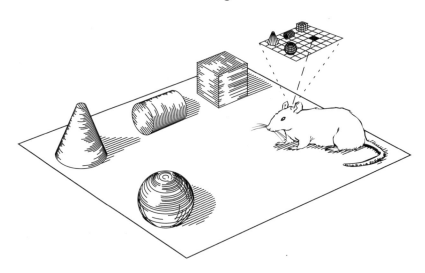

Figure 6–4. A schematic illustration of how an environment is mapped in the hippocampus, according to the cognitive mapping hypothesis (from Eichenbaum et al., 1999).

Despite the attractive features of a cognitive map in the hippocampus, there is little in the way of evidence that hippocampal cells act as elements of a cohesive map of the environment. Indeed, in contrast to this view, there is no topographical relationship between place cells in the hippocampus and locations in space. Furthermore, in many situations individual place cells are simultaneously controlled by different cues in the environment. So, while the existence of place cells as encoding location-specific sensory information is now widely accepted, there is no strong evidence that these place representations are elements of a cohesive map of space. Instead, a strong possibility is that place cells represent familiar places as complex contextual information rather than as coordinates of a map. Additional evidence that place cell activity is strongly influenced by nonspatial factors suggests that location-specific activity may reflect the encoding of the places where important events happen.

Hippocampal cells encode actions in places

Do hippocampal place cells encode only the location of the animal? Even in his earliest description of place cells O'Keefe reported that the spatial activity of hippocampal neurons was influenced by more than just the location of the animal in the environment. Indeed, the preliminary study by O'Keefe and Dostrovsky emphasized that all the place cells fired only when the rat was facing a particular direction. O'Keefe's subsequent full analysis reported several variables in addition to location that determined place cell firing rate, including orientation, how long the rat was in the place field, and the elicitation of particular behaviors such as eating, grooming, and exploratory sniffing. Motion- and behavior-related correlates were the focus of Ranck's analysis of hippocampal firing properties, in which he described cells that fired primarily as a rat was involved in orientation, approach to particular objects or goals, consummatory movements, or cessation of movement.

Several studies have now demonstrated that place cell firing is strongly influenced by movement direction and speed. Indeed, as rats perform in maze tasks, such as the radial maze, the majority of place cells in rats running on a radial maze fired almost entirely when the animal was running outward or returning inward on the maze arms (see Fig. 6–3B), and the firing rate was somewhat higher when the rat was running with greater speed. This finding is not dependent on the structure of the maze itself, but rather on the movement patterrns of the rat in the task. For example, in one study rats were required to begin each trial at the center of the open rectangular environment, and then could approach any of the four corners to obtain a reward. Subsequently they had to return to the center and then approach a different corner to obtain another reward, etc. The majority of place cells fired differentially according to the direction the rat was moving (see Fig. 6–3C). In addition, most place cells were also tuned for the speed of movement, and in many of these cells there was an optimal movement speed such that the cell fired at lower rates for both slower and faster movements through the place field. Also, the majority of the place cells fired differentially depending on the angle of the turn taken during movements. The activity of most cells was best described not so much in terms of spatial parameters but simply as firing at a particular time during the trip to or from a particular goal.

A critical role for the animal's behavior, as much as the nature of cues available or the shape of the apparatus, was most directly demonstrated in a study that involved training rats in two different versions of the same task (see Fig. 6–3D). In one version the rats were initially trained to forage in an open environment for tiny food pellets distributed in random locations, causing the rats to move in all directions throughout the environment. In the second version of the task, the same rats were subsequently trained to find food only at four specific locations in the same open field that were repeatedly baited. Consistent with other descriptions of place cells of rats performing the random foraging task, in this situation the place cells were generally nondirectional, that is, fired similarly regardless of the direction of the animal's movement through the place field. By contrast, when the rats approached a small number of repeated reward locations, most of the cells (even the same cells) were directional, that is, fired only during the approach to, or the departure from, a particular location. These findings are distinct from the conventional characterization of place cells as localized with respect to static cues in the environment, and show that the ongoing behavior, defined as direction of movement, can strongly influence cell activity.

Furthermore, these findings show that, even in the identical apparatus, place cells can exhibit a specific movement correlate depending on whether the task makes particular movement direction patterns significant to the structure of the task. Thus, in this context, the cells are not well characterized as place cells, because their activity does not reliably predict the animal's location. Rather, these cells seem to encode a particular relevant action in a particular place. This conclusion opens up the possibility that hippocampal cells may also encode other variables, including stimuli, behaviors, or other events that have no particular identity in location.

Hippocampal neurons encode nonspatial stimuli and events

As noted previously, even the earliest studies on hippocampal activity in animals exploring open environment included some cells that appeared to have nonspatial firing correlates. Consistent with these early findings, several investigators who have intentionally looked for event-related neural activity have demonstrated firing patterns of hippocampal neurons related to nonspatial stimuli and events. In most of these studies, as in the earliest place cell studies, the relevant stimuli and behaviors were confounded with spatial location in that each event is associated with the animal's presence in one place. Nevertheless, these studies show that nonspatial stimuli and events can be a necessary component of cellular activation, and a recent study provides compelling evidence of nonspatial firing patterns that occur independent of the animal's spatial location.

Among the first findings of nonspatial correlates of hippocampal cellular activity were observations that hippocampal neurons fire associated with the development of a Pavlovian conditioned eyeblink, even when the animal was restrained throughout the training session. In addition, several studies have shown hippocampal neural activity associated with stimulus sampling in rats performing learned sensory discriminations or delayed matching or nonmatching to sample tasks. Notably in all these tasks other individual hippocampal cells exhibited striking responses associated with various behaviors including approach to the relevant discriminative stimuli or the reward. Indeed, the activity of the population of hippocampal cells could be characterized as a set of neurons firing selectively at each phase of the task.

Perhaps the most striking of these studies is a series of experiments by Sam Deadwyler and his colleagues, who have studied the firing properties of single hippocampal neurons and neuronal ensembles in rats performing delayed matching and nonmatching to sample in a discrete trials version of the task where the cues were left and right positions of two response bars. On each trial one bar was extended into the apparatus and pressed by the animal to obtain an initial reward. During the delay period the bar was withdrawn and the animal had to nose poke at a port on the opposite side of the apparatus. Finally both bars were extended into the apparatus and the animal could press the matching or nonmatching bar to obtain a second reward. In Deadwyler's analysis of single hippocampal cells, many of the neurons fired during the sample or match responses or upon the delivery of the reward, or combinations of these events. Many of these cells fired differentially depending on the left–right position of the bar pressed, or whether the response was correct or an error. In addition, many individual cells fired during the delay period, but their activity did not predict the position of the correct response.

Deadwyler and colleagues' characterization of the activity of ensembles of cells recorded at several locations in the hippocampus focused on a statistical analysis that could extract patterns of covariances among the cells associated with different task events. These analyses showed that specific task parameters accounted for most of the overall variance in ensemble activity. The major components corresponded to encoding of the sample versus choice phase of the task regardless of bar position, encoding of the spatial position of the lever independent of task phase, encoding of left versus right error responses, and encoding of the sample position during the sample and choice phase. The encoding of lever position may be regarded as a spatial mapping. However, the coding of task phase cut across locations where the rat was positioned, and the coding of the sample position lingered into the choice phase when the rat was at the opposite bar on correct trials. Thus, while all the correlates of these cells can be considered "spatial" in various ways, a considerable amount of the variance in ensemble activity was not associated strictly with the animal's location but rather with the encoding of task-relevant spatial information.

Analyses of the firing properties of hippocampal neurons have been extended to studies on the primate hippocampal region. In general the evidence for pure place-specific activity is poor, although sensory-evoked neural activity is often modulated by a variety of spatial variables. In humans, visually evoked responses of hippocampal neurons have also been observed, and a substantial fraction of these cells fired on the sight of a particular word or face stimulus or during execution of task-relevant key press responses. In one recent study, Itzak Fried and his colleagues characterized the responses of hippocampal neurons in human subjects performing a recognition memory task with face and visual-object cues. Again a substantial number of cells responded to the stimuli, and individual cells had activity that differentiated faces from objects, or distinguished facial gender or expression, or new versus familiar faces and objects. The largest fraction of cells differentiated combinations of these features. Some of the cells had a specific pattern of responsiveness across all of these parameters.

Some studies have been directly aimed at dissociating spatial and nonspatial firing patterns of hippocampal neurons by requiring animals to perform the same tasks using identical cues located at different locations in the environment. A particularly compelling study involved olfactory cues that were moved systematically among locations within a static environment, and provided unambiguous evidence of place-independent nonspatial hippocampal activity. Rats were trained to perform an odor-guided delayed nonmatch to sample task at multiple locations on a large open field (Fig. 6–5A). The stimuli were plastic cups that contained playground sand scented with one of nine common odors (e.g., coffee, cinnamon, etc.). On each trial one cup was placed randomly at any of nine locations on the open field. Whenever the odor differed from that on the previous trial (i.e., was a nonmatch) a Froot Loop was buried in the sand, and the rat would dig for the reward. Whenever the odor was the same as that on the previous trial (i.e., was a match) no Froot Loop was buried and the rat would turn away. The firing rate of hippocampal cells was assessed during the approach to the cups, focusing on the last second of the approach during which the animal arrived at the cup and generated its response. Firing rates were statistically compared across the set of odors, the set of locations, and match–nonmatch conditions.

About two-thirds of hippocampal cells fired in association with one or more of these variables during the task. About one-third of the active cells' firing was not differentiated by the location of the cup, and about one-third of the active cells demonstrated some spatial component of firing. Some of the nonspatial cells were activated during the approach to any of the odor cups at any of the nine locations. Other cells fired differentially across the odor set (Fig. 6–5B), or between match and nonmatch conditions, or some combination of these variables and the approach. Only a small proportion of the location-selective cells fired associated only with the position of the cup (Fig. 6–5C). For the majority of cells, their activity was conjointly associated with the position where the cup was pre-

A. delayed non-match to sample task

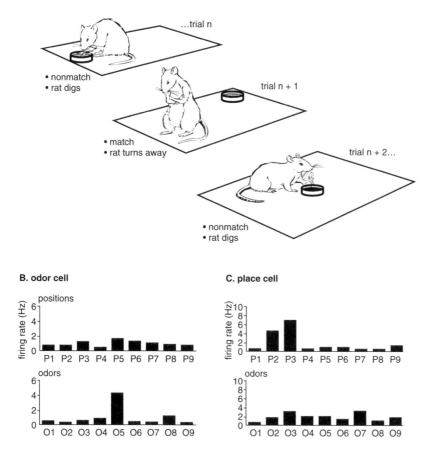

Figure 6–5. Delayed nonmatching to sample test where the location of trials varies randomly. *A:* On those trials when the odor is different from that presented on the preceding trial (i.e., a nonmatch) the rat can dig in the scented food cup for a buried reward. On those trials when the odor is the same as that on the preceding trial (i.e., a match), there is no reward and the rat turns away. *B:* Example of a cell that fires associated with trials when odor 5 (O5) was presented but not when other odors were presented. The activity of this cell did not distinguish the locations where the trial was performed or the match–nonmatch status of the odor. *C:* Example of a cell that fired when trials were performed at adjacent locations P2-P3, but not when the trial was performed at other locations. The activity of this cell did not distinguish between different odors or their match–nonmatch status (data from Wood et al., 1999).

sented, the odor, the status of the odor as a match or nonmatch, and many of the cells fired at some point as the animal approached any cup. These results show that the activity of fully half of the activated cells acted completely independent of location, and most of the location-specific cells involved more than purely spatial features of the task. In addition, while some cells encoded particular odors or places, the activity of most cells was associated with one of the many potential conjunctions of odors, places, approach movements, and match–nonmatch events. These data indicate that, when important stimuli move unpredictably within an environment, a segment of the hippocampal population encodes the regularities of these stimuli without coding of the global topography. Combined with the other findings described before, these data provide compelling evidence that hippocampal cells can encode purely nonspatial information that is relevant at many locations in the environment.

The hippocampal network mediates a "memory space"

The preceding review both confirms the existence of location-specific activity of hippocampal neurons, and suggests that place cells are parts of a neural representation that is both less than, and more than, a map of space. The representation is less than a map because it is clear that place cells individually and independently encode pieces and patches of an environment without acting as part of a full mapping. The representation is also more than a map because spatial codings are modulated by relevant nonspatial task variables and hippocampal cells encode nonspatial stimuli and events. How can the impressive location-specific activity be reconciled within a larger framework of memory representation? The properties of hippocampal firing patterns are entirely consistent with the memory space scheme proposed earlier in this chapter.

To place the properties of hippocampal firing patterns in the context of this scheme, let us review the firing patterns of hippocampal cells in rats performing two prototypical tasks, a spatial task similar to the radial maze task, and an odor-guided memory task. Begin with the data from rats performing the spatial memory task in a large arena (see Fig. 6–3C). Many of the cells can be described as place cells having a place field in a particular portion of the arena, with their activity modulated by several movement parameters such that the cells fire maximally when the rat is moving at a particular speed, in a particular direction, and when the rat is turning in one particular angle. One cell, whose firing patterns are depicted in Fig. 6–3C, can be described as a cell with a place field near the center of the arena, and its activity is modulated by several movement parameters: It fires maximally when the rat is moving at a moderate speed, when the rat is moving "north," and when the rat is turning slightly to the right. Alternatively, however, virtually all of the activity of this cell can be characterized more simply as firing when the rat initiates its approach to cup 1. Most cells recorded as rats performed this task could similarly be described by a complex combination of place, direction, and turning angle, or could be at least as well described by when the cell fired during movements toward, or in return from, a particular reward cup. Furthermore, the population of hippocampal neurons contains cells that fire at virtually every point in the path to and from each of the cups (Fig. 6–6A). So one can best describe the full data set as a network of neurons each of which encodes one fragment of the approach and return from each reward cup. Of course, within the memory space framework outlined previously, the hippocampal network representation contains a subset of cells that represents distinct events, each defined by a specific location and a specific set of movement attributes, linked to encode a particular kind of trial episode, defined as the approach to and return from a particular goal location.

Now let us expand the same kind of characterization to hippocampal cellular activity in rats performing the odor-guided tasks such as those described earlier, with the additional insight into how "secondary" nonspatial firing properties are accommodated into hippocampal spatial activity (Fig. 6–6B). As animals perform these tasks individual cells activate at vir-

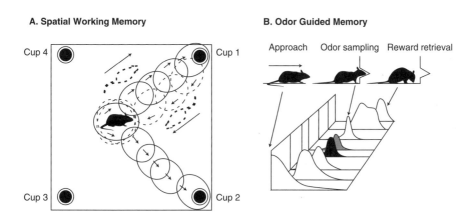

Figure 6–6. Temporal organization of hippocampal neuronal activity. *A:* Schematic illustration of firing patterns of a set of cells as the rat performs a spatial memory test. Different cells fire at each successive moment as the rat approaches each cup and returns. Note that each cell has a place field and directional firing preference associated with a particular segment of a particular outward-bound or inward-bound episode. *B:* Schematic illustration of firing patterns of a set of cells as the rat performs an odor discrimination task. Different cells fire at each successive moment as the rat approaches the odor ports, samples the odors, and retrieves the reward, and other behaviors. Some cells fire on all trials, others fire only if a particular odor is presented (data from Eichenbaum et al., 1999).

tually every instant of the task, defined as time-locked neural activity to identifiable stimulus and behavioral events. Individual cells in animals performing the odor-guided nonmatch to sample task fired at different times associated with the approach to the odor sampling port, during the odor sampling period, and during the discriminative response and reward period. Thus, overall hippocampal activity in this situation, like that in the spatial task described before, can be described as a network of cells that encode each event that characterizes each type of discrimination trial episode.

In addition, in both spatial and odor tasks, some of the hippocampal cells showed considerable specificity for particular locations of approach or odors sampled, whereas other cells fired on every trial for different directions of movement and different types of odor trials. This observation leads to an additional characterization of how hippocampal cells are "tuned" to brief segments of behavioral episodes. Let us first consider the cells that show the greatest specificity for particular conjunctions or relations among stimuli or events. Prominent examples include conjunctions or relations between the places and actions that occur in those places, or between sequences of odors. A similar characterization can be offered to describe the data from the odor-guided delayed nonmatch to sample task where the trials were performed at different locations on an open field. Some cells associated only with particular conjunctions of events, places, or both, and virtually every possible conjunction was represented. These most selective cells might be thought of as reflecting ever more rare variations of events.

Now let us consider the cells that fired consistently on different types of trials in spatial and odor tasks. Indeed, many of these cells fired associated with locations or events that were common across all the different types of trials within a task. In the spatial task, some cells fired whenever the animal's path crossed a particular place regardless of what cup was being approached or left behind. In the odor tasks, some cells fired during a particular common behavioral event, for example, during the approach movement regardless of spatial location, and others fired on all match or nonmatch trials. In the task where the odor test was performed at multiple locations some cells fired on all trials at a particular location regardless of the current odor or type of trial. These cells might be thought of as the "nodal" cells introduced in the scheme presented in Figure 6–2, the cells that encode intersections among the episodes that have in common a particular place or a particular stimulus or behavior. Of course, the full range of cells extends continuously from the most common nodal point cells to the most highly specific cells. From this perspective, "pure" place cells (ones that are location specific and have no other quality) are one of the more common nodal correlates, whereas the highly combinatorial cells represent events that occurred only a few times in a session.

Evidence of episodic-like representations in the hippocampus

More direct evidence of coding for information specific to particular types of episodes comes from another experiment where hippocampal cells fire differentially even in situations where the overt behavioral events and the locations in which they occur are identical between multiple types of experience. In this experiment rats performed a spatial alternation task, a simple version of one of Olton's episodic memory tasks, performed in a T-maze. Each trial commenced when the rat traversed the stem of the T and then selected either the left- or the right-choice arm (Fig. 6–7A). To alternate successfully the rats were required to distinguish between their left-turn and right-turn experiences and to use their memory for the most recent previous experience to guide the current choice. Different hippocampal cells fired as the rats passed through the sequence of locations within the maze during each trial. Most important, the firing patterns of many of the cells depended on whether the rat was in the midst of a left- or right-turn episode, even when the rat was on the stem of the T and running similarly on both types of trials—minor variations in the animal's speed, direction of movement, or position within areas on the stem did not account for the different firing patterns on left-turn and right-turn trials (Fig. 6–7B). Other cells fired when the rat was at the same point in the stem on either trial type. Thus, the hippocampus encoded both the left-turn and right-turn experiences using distinct representations, and included elements that could link them by their common features. In each of these experiments, the representations of event sequences, linked by codings of their common events and places, could constitute the substrate of a network of episodic memories.

Elaboration of a general scheme for memory representation by the hippocampus

There are three central aspects of this novel characterization of the firing properties of hippocampal neurons in animals performing a broad range of learning and memory tasks. First, cellular activity can be described as a sequence of temporally and spatially defined events that constitute each trial. Second, some cells show a very high degree of specialization, such as the approach to a particular odor at a particular place only when it is

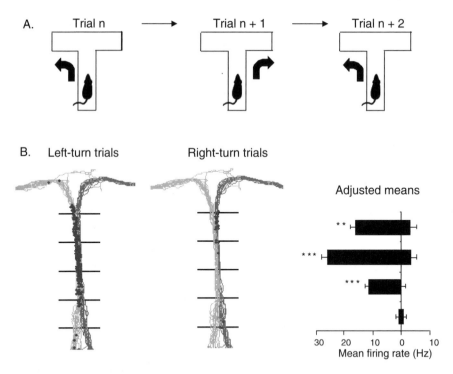

Figure 6–7. T-maze alternation. A: Illustration of trials in this task. On each trial the rat must remember the previous episode and then turn in the opposite direction. B: Example of a hippocampal cell that was active when the rat is traversing the stem section of a T-maze while performing the spatial alternation task. This cell fired almost exclusively during left-turn trials. In the left and middle panels, the paths taken by the animals on the central stem are plotted for left-turn trials (light gray) and for right-turn trials (dark gray). The locations of the rat when individual spikes occurred are indicated by dots for left-turn trials (left panel), and then right-turn trials (middle panel). In the right panel, the mean firing rate of the cell for each of four sectors of the maze, adjusted for variations in firing associated with other behavioral factors, is shown separately for left-turn trials (left bars) and right-turn trials (right bars). (significant differences: ** $p<.01$, *** $p<.001$) (data from Wood et al., 2000).

on a nonmatch trial. Third, other cells are activated on different kinds of trials, and the activity of some reflects the common places animals pass through and behavioral actions they take on all such trials. One hypothesis that may account for these three aspects of the firing patterns is that, when the animal enters a novel situation, the activity of the hippocampal neural network reflects specific ongoing behavioral episodes. As more and more experiences are accumulated within that overall situation, common locations, stimuli, and actions are reflected in enhanced firing by cells that initially are active during the relevant parts of episodes. Eventually the hippocampal network encodes the organization of related episodes, including both the frequent elements common across many similar events, and rare conjunctions of elements that define infrequent episodes in the task. This view of hippocampal representation puts the hippocampus squarely as central to episodic memory but also assigns its purpose in identifying and organizing events into a general memory organization that relates events to one another.

How might such hippocampal episodic codings and organizational processing serve the global declarative memory function of the hippocampus? The present considerations provide support for a working hypothesis about a common organization of spatial and nonspatial memories in the hippocampus. According to this view, individual hippocampal neurons encode all manner of conjunctions and relations among combinations of perceptually independent cues. The domain of relations captured within hippocampal codings is broad, indeed may involve virtually any conceivable dimension by which stimuli can be related through experience. Furthermore, hippocampal representations include behavioral actions as well as stimuli, internal stimuli (e.g., hunger, fear) as well as exteroceptive stimuli.

Consider the example of T-maze performance. In this situation distinct subsets of hippocampal neurons are active during either of the two trial types (left-turn and right-turn), and some cells are active at least to some extent on both. Thus, a way to view these findings is that specific networks of cells encode the sequence of places passed through, as well as the direction of running, motivation, etc., for each trial type, as if the composite of these firings were a videoclip of that type of trial. In addition, the cells that fire similarly on both trial types contribute representations of the "overlap" in the different codings, presumably by sharing subsets of the overall set of relevant cues. This creates a framework that extends the set of stimuli and actions represented in the network, and it constrains the nature of the network organization by the accommodation of both types of trial representations into a single larger framework for the entire task (Fig. 6–8).

The same scheme can be extended to account for the development of spatial memory representations for an environment. The findings just summarized, and other studies, indicate that hippocampal place cells encode small portions of space, or, more specifically, the spatial relations among subsets of the environmental cues. How can one build a representation of the environment that would support the important spatial navigation functions of the hippocampus? Suppose the environment as a whole is not rep-

T-maze Alternation

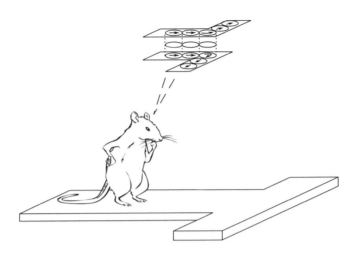

Figure 6–8. Idealized firing patterns of sets of hippocampal neurons that form separate network representations of left-turn and right-turn trials, and cells that represent the overlapping spatial information that links the two representations into a larger "memory space."

resented explicitly by a "map" in the hippocampus. Rather, spatial memory could be mediated as the byproduct of a large set of overlapping representations of specific subsets of the environmental stimuli. Within this view, during a sequence of episodes in which the animal explores the environment, individual hippocampal cells encode relative distances between small sets of cues, as well as the distance from the subject to those cues as they were experienced from a particular perspective or set of perspectives during different paths taken through the environment. Furthermore, each cell encodes only a subset of the available cues, and different cells encode overlapping combinations of those cues. The "map" of space, then, is constituted as a large collection of cue conjunctions that overlap so as to constrain the spatial relations among all the cues, and to provide a framework for moving among the cues.

A simplified version of this model is illustrated in Figure 6–9A. In this illustration, each cell is conceived as encoding only two cues in terms of their spatial separation and the distance of the animal from each of them as experienced in a separate episode. Furthermore, different cells encode overlapping pairs of cues, such that an organization of the cues emerges within the hippocampal population. To the extent that these overlapping codings constrain the overall population code, the network hippocampal

A. Representation of space

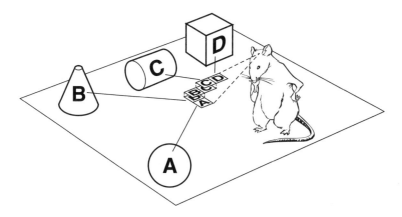

B. Representation of paired associates

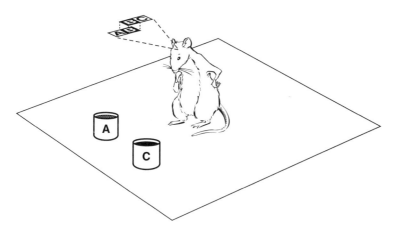

Figure 6–9. Memory space models: *A:* For the representation of space, separate "episodes" composed of distinct views of AB, then BC, then CD, are linked. *B:* For the representation of the paired associates task, separate episodes composed of each stimulus pairing (AB and BC) are linked to support inferential memory expression of B versus C.

representation crudely approximates the relative topography among all the codings. In this example, the topography of the network representation of stimuli A–D is constrained to form an L-shape, like the topography of the actual stimuli. Furthermore, this model can be envisioned as sufficient to support "navigation" among the cues in the sense that it can begin with any particular cue and know how to proceed to any other one by generating the entire set of representations. In the example, one can conceive of activation of each pair-wise coding as also exciting adjacent copings that share overlapping elements. We will call this conception the "memory space" model because it describes a network of associative connections among related stimuli. The model is "spatial" only in the sense that the specific representations are based on spatial relations. However, the links between representational elements are based on associative strengths, not on metric distance or angle representations.

Now imagine that precisely the same kind of hippocampal representation supports entirely nonspatial learning dependent on the hippocampus. A particularly good example of this learning that involves overlapping representations of nonspatial stimulus items comes from the study of transitivity in paired associate learning in rats. In the study described in Chapter 5, intact rats were trained on sets of overlapping odor associations, and demonstrated the capacity to infer relations among indirectly related items. For example, after they had learned that stimulus A was associated with stimulus B, and B was associated with C, they could infer that A was associated with C. This task directly demonstrates that rats can represent overlapping stimulus associations, and that these associations become linked to support inferential judgments. Furthermore, the capacity to build the overlapping associations into a network representation that supports inferential judgments depends on the hippocampus. In our conceptual model of the "memory space" for this task, distinct sets of hippocampal neurons might encode each pairwise trained cue relationship (Fig. 6–9B). Because of the structure of the learning task, these codings would necessarily provide a set of overlapping representations. Assuming the different representations that contain the shared item C are each activated by presentation of C in any one of them, it would be expected that the representation of the entire odor series (A–C) would be activated to support the inferential choice among nonadjacent items B and C.

Within this overall conceptual framework, three guiding principles can account for both spatial and nonspatial memory dependent on the hippocampus: (1) discrete subsets of cues and actions are encoded by hippocampal cells in terms of appropriate relations among the items; (2) the contents of these representations overlap to generate a higher-order framework or "memory space"; (3) animals can conceptually "navigate" this memory space stepping across learned associations to make indirect novel associations or other inferential judgments among items in the memory space. From this view, the key properties of spatial memory performance are particularly powerful examples of a memory space in operation. For example, the capabilities for taking "shortcuts" and "roundabout routes," types of spatial inference outlined by Tolman as defining properties of a cognitive map, can be accomplished within such a memory space without performing metric calculations of exact distances or angles. Rather, they are reflections of inferential memory expression within a constrained framework of associations.

These considerations serve to show how the spatial and nonspatial firing properties of hippocampal neurons might be reconciled. Furthermore, the "memory space" model offers insights into how the hippocampus serves its global role in declarative memory, by mediating the establishment of a relational representation among items in memory. Finally, this model shows how such a relational representation can mediate the capacity for flexible, inferential expression of memory from nonspatial as well as spatial organizations. These considerations provide a preliminary, yet clear, view of how "cognitive" memory is accomplished by the brain.

Summing up

Studies using brain imaging techniques complement the findings on human amnesia showing a critical role for the medial temporal lobe in declarative memory. These studies have shown that the medial temporal region is activated for a broad range of materials, and shows the laterality of hemispheric differences in verbal versus nonverbal information processing observed throughout the cortex. In addition, the medial temporal area is activated when a large amount of novel information is being processed, by the processing of new stimulus associations, and associated with explicit, conscious recollection.

In addition, further insights into the neural coding mechanisms of declarative memory have been made through observations on the firing properties of hippocampal neurons in behaving animals. Many cells fire selectively when an animal is in a familiar location in its environment, showing that remembered locations are an important component of the information coded by hippocampal neurons. In addition, hippocampal neurons are activated by nonspatial stimuli and their activity is associated with behavioral events. Some cells fire only when the animal is in a particular place and is engaged in a particular behavior or is presented with a particular stimulus. These cells encode combinations of places and behaviors that define specific events within learning episodes. Furthermore, the sequential activations of sets of these cells could be used to represent the sequences of events in episodic memories.

Other hippocampal cells fire associated with a spatial or nonspatial feature that is common across multiple related learning episodes. These cells could be used to link the representations of distinct experiences together within a larger organization of memories, called a "memory space." This perspective on observations on hippocampal neuron firing patterns offers clear insights into the structure of relational representations that support the properties of declarative memory.

READINGS

Amaral, D.G., and Petersen, S., Eds. 1999. Functional imaging of the human hippocampus. A special issue of *Hippocampus* 9(1).

Eichenbaum, H., Dudchencko, P., Wood, E., Shapiro, M., and Tanila, H. 1999. The hippocampus, memory, and place cells: Is it spatial memory or a memory space? *Neuron* 23: 209–226.

Henke, K., Buck, A., Weber, B., and Wieser, H.G. 1997. Human hippocampus establishes associations in memory. *Hippocampus* 7:249–256.

Muller, R.U. 1996. A quarter of a century of place cells. *Neuron*, 17: 813–822.

O'Keefe, J.A. 1979. A review of hippocampal place cells. *Prog. Neurobiol.* 13:419–439.

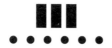

COMPARTMENTALIZATION: CORTICAL MODULES AND MULTIPLE MEMORY SYSTEMS

There are two parts to the story on the compartmentalization of memory in the brain. The first part is a continuation on the theme of cortical localization, with regard to both its information processing functions and memory *per se*. Enormous progress has been made in identifying functional modules within the cerebral cortex, and in showing how memory is compartmentalized within the same cortical areas that subserve specific perceptual, motor, or cognitive functions. The second story is a continuation of the revelations about different kinds of memory introduced in the last section of this book. That review focused on distinctions between "cognitive" memory and other noncognitive forms of memory, and characterized some fundamental aspects of the mechanisms and neural coding scheme that subserve cognitive memory. This part expands the notion of multiple memory systems and considers compartmentalization both within the cognitive memory system and other memory systems.

Localization of memory in the cerebral cortex

The early neurologists and physiologists characterized the cerebral cortex into a large set of sensory processing areas, identified with regions within the posterior cortex, and motor processing areas, mainly in the anterior cortex. Pavlov had just succeeded famously in identifying a conditioned reflex, showing that a very simple kind of memory could be reduced to the association between an arbitrary stimulus and a similarly arbitrary response. Combining these findings, a prevalent view was that associations were instantiated within specific circuits that connected sensory and/or motor representations in the cortex.

Guided by this view, Karl Lashley pioneered the effort to localize stimulus–response associations to specific sensory–motor connections. He surveyed the entire cerebral cortex, attempting quite directly to disconnect the critical sensory-to-motor connections by knife cuts between posterior sensory and anterior motor cortical areas (Fig. III–1). In later studies the damage went further, and involved removing portions of the cortex from virtually all areas and to varying extent in different animals. He then trained rats on a set of maze problems that were progressively more difficult and compared the severity of subsequent learning deficits with the location and extent of cortical damage. In other studies he examined the effect of the disconnections or lesions on retention of previously learned maze problems.

Lashley found that maze performance was not affected, and therefore that maze memories were not stored in any single location or in any particular pathway within or between sensory and motor areas. While not rejecting the idea of cortical localization of function in general, Lashley concluded that one also cannot view memories as stored in switchboard-like fashion within specific circuits or locations; instead he argued that memories were diffusely distributed in the brain.

At about the same time that Lashley left the field with the issue of localization unresolved, the Canadian psychologist Donald Hebb provided a possible reconciliation of the stimulus–response (S-R) and antilocalization views. In his classic 1949 monograph, Hebb recognized both the "switchboard" and cognitive theories, and argued that the eventual explanation of mental phenomena would have to incorporate plasticity of neural transmission mechanisms that lead from sensory excitation to motor responses. But to expand beyond a simple "habit" mechanism, Hebb proposed the notion of "cell assemblies," diffuse circuits of connected neurons that develop to represent specific percepts and concepts. These as-

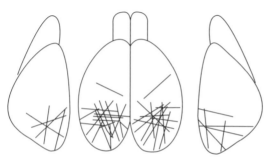

Figure III-1. Composite diagram showing top and lateral views of the rat brain indicating long axes of lesions that separated cortical areas. None of these lesions produced a substantial effect on learning ability (from Lashley, 1929).

semblies could involve diffuse circuits within a brain area, and indeed might involve sets of cell assemblies across multiple areas. His proposal retained the idea that structural changes in specific synapses would make lasting memory possible. But rather than relying on a single stimulus-to-response circuit to mediate any memory, Hebb emphasized some kind of reverberatory activity among a network of many cells, outlasting the learning event and leading to a stabilization of the cooperative activity of cells in that cell assembly. He suggested that short-term memory could be maintained within the reverberatory activity of such circuits, but long-term memory would require the ability to reinstantiate the activity within cell assemblies through changes in the connectivity of the elements and the particular pathways among them excited during learning. This view incorporated both the specificity of functions of connections in the cortex, and the distribution of global functions across cortical areas. This part reviews further advances in our understanding of how memory is compartmentalized in cell assemblies throughout the cortex.

Multiple memory systems

The findings on H.M. and other amnesic patients made it clear that structures in the medial temporal lobe including the hippocampus mediate one type of memory function, declarative memory. Conversely, these findings showed that other brain areas are sufficient to mediate other nondeclarative memory functions. What is the full extent of the declarative memory system? What are the types of nondeclarative memory and what brain systems support them? It turns out the story on the declarative and nondeclarative memory systems focuses not on the issue of cortical localization previously discussed. Rather, the story on multiple memory systems involves brain systems in which widespread areas of the cortex feed into, and are influenced by, different subcortical areas. Thus, the multiple memory systems story should be viewed as a set of parallel, functionally dedicated memory systems each of which stems from and involves cortical processing plus a separate stream of subcortical processing. After a consideration of the modular organization of the cortex, this part of the book also considers the number and nature of memory systems in the brain. I expand on the considerations of the medial temporal lobe system, to outline the entire brain system in which the hippocampus operates to support declarative memory. A review of other memory systems follows, outlining both the brain pathways and characteristics of the different forms of nondeclarative memory.

READINGS

Hebb, D.O. 1949. *The Organization of Behavior*. New York: Wiley.

Lashley, K.S. 1929. *Brain Mechanisms and Intelligence: A Quantitative Study of Injuries to the Brain*. New York: Dover (1963 edition).

7
• • • • • •

The Cerebral Cortex and Memory

STUDY QUESTIONS

What is the functional organization of the cerebral cortex?

Is the organization of the cortex fixed during the course of development?

Is the organization of the cortex fixed in adulthood?

How are ordinary memories encoded by neurons in the cerebral cortex?

Franz Joseph Gall was the first to propose a detailed formulation of cortical specialization in which distinct types of memory are imbedded within the functional domains of different cortical areas (see Chapter 1). Although Gall's phrenology was justifiably discredited (for reasons described in Chapter 1), it turns out that the notion that cerebral cortex is made up of multiple, functionally distinct processing regions has proven correct. Also correct is Gall's notion that memory is integrally tied to these various processing systems. As will become apparent, memory is both a necessary part and an obligatory product of the ongoing processing activities of areas of the cerebral cortex.

This chapter begins with a brief summary of the evidence regarding functional specialization of the cortex. Then the role of experience in shaping the responses of neurons in various cortical areas is reviewed. There are striking commonalities in the forms of plasticity observed across cortical areas and among different types of experiential modifications. These commonalities provide the basis for the subsequent outline of general rules for how memories are represented in the cortex and, more specifically, how memory is embedded in the various networks, a fundamental part of these networks in operation.

Cortical localization

Parallel with the discoveries on functional distinctions in cortical areas, in 1909 Korbinian Brodman provided the first architectonic map of the cerebral cortex, a parcellation in which cortical areas were subdivided based on cell types and their laminar organization (Fig. 7–1). Several subsequent mappings of the human and animal cortex followed, and there was (and still is) disagreement about the number and types of areas, and about their evolutionary origins. From the outset, it was expected that the micro-anatomical differences among these areas would provide the substrate for, and therefore have been seen as reflecting, functional differences. These original observations have been extensively supplemented by further anatomical techniques, including histochemistry and connectional studies, as well as by physiological techniques, including recording and stimulation studies. The latter have provided substantially greater resolution of the anatomical divisions and, perhaps more important, given us a greater understanding of the functional distinctions among these areas in a number of species. In addition, functional neuroimaging, using positron emis-

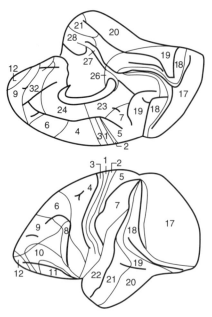

Figure 7–1. Brodman's (1909) cytoarchitectonic map of the macaque monkey cortex.

sion tomography (PET) and functional magnetic resonance imaging (fMRI), has provided strong confirmation of the functional specialization of different cortical regions. These techniques have permitted detailed mapping of the functionally distinct cortical areas specialized from processing highly specific types of information processing.

Summarizing this still unfolding story about the functional specializations of cortex is well beyond the scope of this book. Indeed, it is the subject of various books or texts in cognitive neuroscience and cognitive neuropsychology. However, a few very general principles should be committed to mind for the present purposes. First, the cortex can roughly be divided into posterior fields that are involved in perceptual processing and anterior areas that are involved in motor processing (Fig. 7–2). Second, in the posterior cortex, most of the fields are divided by sensory modality. Third, the fields in both the anterior and posterior cortex involve processing hierarchies. In the anterior cortex, there is the primary motor area just in front of the central sulcus, where the muscles of the body are mapped out in a topographic organization, with adjacent areas of cortex representing muscle groups in adjacent areas of the body. The primary motor cortex is the origin of a progression of projections to higher-order processing areas that are involved in the sequencing and organization of response output and, more generally, in the planning, executing, and withholding of goal-directed behaviors.

In the posterior cortex there are distinct primary areas for each sensory modality. Each of these is characterized by cells that respond to stimulation within a small circumscribed spatial region of the sensory field, known as a receptive field, and respond preferentially to other specific trigger features of the stimulus. The receptive fields and other trigger features

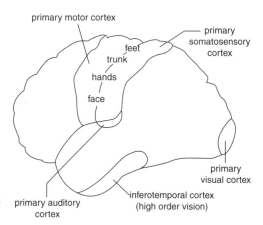

Figure 7–2. Some of the functional areas of the human cerebral cortex.

are organized in a topographic map of the sensory field and of other relevant sensory dimensions, such that adjacent neurons represent contiguous parts of the field and closely related dimensions of the trigger features. For each sensory modality these primary areas are the origins of a hierarchy of specialized processing regions leading to more and more complex perceptual areas. Eventually, some of these streams of sensory processing are combined in multimodal cortical areas, which in turn project to the supramodal processing areas in frontal, temporal, and parietal cortices.

The intertwining of information processing and memory storage in the visual cortex

To appreciate how memory is integrally related to specific cortical processors a specific example of functional specialization and memory representation in cortex will be considered in some detail. The obvious choice for this example is vision, because its functional properties and its cortical substrates have been so extensively studied. There exist more than 30 functionally distinct visual fields that encompass a large proportion of the primate brain. These different visual areas follow a complicated combination of parallel and sequential pathways that are organized hierarchically into several stages of processing. At the earliest processing stages, distinct areas are involved in identification of basic properties of visual stimuli such as their orientation, spatial frequency, speed, color, and location in the visual world. At the highest levels of visual cortex, distinct areas are responsible for localization of salient stimuli in visual space and categorization of visual stimuli according to their meaning. An example from the lowest and highest levels, and the characteristics of memory representation at both levels, are discussed next.

The primary visual cortex can alter its functional organization in response to the competition of input activities

The early visual cortical areas are particularly well characterized. The first stage of visual cortical processing involves a "topographic" representation of simple visual features. In this representational scheme small groups of neighboring cells have the same receptive fields, or areas of the visual world in which they are responsive to visual stimuli. The best understood of these areas is primary visual cortex, where cells of the input layer respond to small spots of light in highly restricted receptive fields. Neighboring principal cells in other layers respond to stable or moving contrast edges with similarly small receptive fields. Furthermore, cells with these response properties are organized topographically along two dimensions. One dimension corresponds to a preference for activation by the ipsilateral (same side of the head) or contralateral (opposite side) eye—this is called the ocular dominance property of these cells. The other dimension, which applies to cells that respond to edges of light, corresponds to preferences for an optimal orientation of the contrasting edge (Fig. 7–3). The cells are arranged in columns, such that through the depths of the cortical layers, neurons have very similar properties in ocular dominance and orientation selectivity. Ipsilateral and contralateral ocular dominance columns alternate, and orientation columns are arranged in a systematic sequence. The combination of a full set of ocular dominance and orientation columns that represent the same small receptive field area is known as a "hypercolumn." Sets of such modules are organized systematically to provide a full representation of the contralateral visual field for each hemisphere.

The linkage between memory and perceptual processing involves the experience-driven tuning and modification of the cells in this organized network—a rewiring of the cells in the network and of the maps they form. The tuning and modification of cortical processing networks by experience was first observed in the primary visual cortex associated with development in young animals. The classic studies by David Hubel and Torsten Wiesel showed that response properties of primary visual cortex neurons are plastic, that is, modifiable by experience, during a "critical period" of the first 4 weeks of life. They found that closure of one eye during this period in kittens resulted in a shift in ocular dominance of all

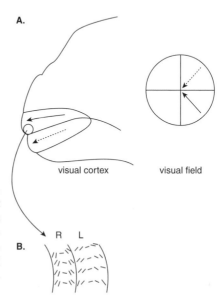

Figure 7–3. Map of primary visual cortex. A: Areas on the medial surface of the left visual cortex sensitive to parts of the arrows designated in the right visual vield. B: Expansion of the circled area in A showing orientation selectivities indicated by slanted lines and right (R) and left (L) ocular dominance stripes.

cells toward a preference for the active eye. Similarly, restricting exposure in kittens to stimuli with only certain orientations of visual contrast (e.g., only vertical or only horizontal) during the critical period resulted in a shift of all cells toward selectivity for the trained orientation. Such manipulations are not nearly so effective in producing tuning of visual cortex after this early critical period ends, a finding that led most investigators to conclude that cortical organization becomes fixed in adulthood.

There are indications that the reorganization of sensory maps, as well as the normal initial organizing of sensory maps, arises from a competition of activity among different inputs to each cell. Some of the earliest and most impressive evidence for competitive mechanisms underlying cortical organization, and reorganization, came from studies of the optic tectum in frogs. In frogs, the major projection of the retina arrives in the part of the midbrain known as the optic tectum, the highest visual area of the frog brain. This projection is entirely crossed such that all of the fibers from the left eye arrive in the right tectum and *vice versa* (Fig. 7–4A). This pattern of connections can be visualized by injecting a radioactively labeled amino acid into one eye and then observing the transport of radioactivity into the synapses of the optic tectum.

Studies of plasticity in this system exploited the regenerative capacities of the frog nervous system to examine the effects of additional abnormal inputs to the optic tectum. The manipulation in this study was to add a third eye to the head of the frog embryo. At this time the partially developed eyes are only protruding bulges on the head. But, as the animals mature, the retinal elements develop optic nerves that innervate one or the other optic tectum of the host brain. Amazingly, in each of these animals, the topographic pattern of the synapses making these connections was dramatically altered from the normal monocular input pattern, such that in three-eyed frogs there were periodic bands of input from the two eyes innervating half of one tectum (Fig. 7–4B). Thus, inputs from the additional eye mapped onto one or the other tectum along with those from the natural eye. Moreover, in each case, the competition of inputs from two eyes elicited a pattern of ocular dominance stripes essentially the same as that observed in mammals with naturally occurring binocular inputs to each side of the cortex.

Is this peculiar phenomenon restricted to the lowly frog? Not at all. In mammals, normally the retina sends inputs to major targets in the brain stem areas known as the superior colliculus and the lateral geniculate nucleus of the thalamus. Concurrently, the cochlea normally sends auditory inputs to the medial geniculate nucleus of the thalamus. In a landmark experiment on newborn ferrets, the retina of one eye was prevented from

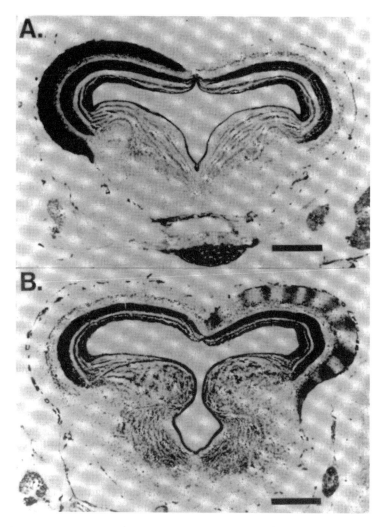

Figure 7–4. Reorganization of the frog optic tectum (top layers in frontal section of the frog brain) *A:* Black area on left side (right hemisphere) indicates deposition of radioactive amino acids transported following an injection into the right eye. This shows that the normal projection is entirely contralateral. *B:* Pattern of transport in a frog with a third eye transplanted near the normal right eye. The left optic tectum (on right) receives alternating zones of input from both eyes (from Constantine-Paton and Law, 1982).

sending its normal inputs to the brain stem by transecting the optic nerve, and the normal inputs to the medial geniculate were severed. Subsequently, the retinal projections innervated the disconnected medial geniculate nucleus, resulting in visual responses being observed in normally auditory parts of the thalamus and the auditory cortex. Furthermore, a visual map developed in auditory cortex and it involved an organized topographic map in which the two-dimensional visual fields were mapped precisely onto the cortical area that normally holds a one-dimensional representation of auditory frequencies. These findings indicate that the competitive activities of inputs are sufficient to determine the general aspects of cortical organization. Thus, the pattern of cortical reorganization after sensory deprivation is no different from that by which the processing system becomes organized during development.

The adult cortex also shows plastic changes in response to altered input activity

Is this kind of plasticity observed only in the developing brain? Or is plasticity associated with a competition among inputs a property of the mature brain as well? One way in which the plasticity of the adult cortex has been explored is by creating small and selective damage to a part of the normal inputs to the cortex and subsequently examining the effects of this deprivation of input on the area of cortex that had previously received those inputs.

There is now considerable evidence that such selective deprivation of inputs produces a reorganization in the adult visual cortex. In the most sophisticated of these experiments, a laser light was used to produce a very small lesion of the retina that deprives animals of a small area of the visual field. This lesion initially produces a correspondingly small area of silent primary visual cortex. However, after a 2-month recovery period, the topography of the cortex is reorganized such that the formerly disconnected zone becomes responsive to neighboring parts of the visual field (Fig. 7–5). Also, whereas *complete* recovery requires a prolonged period, some cells at the border of the deafferented area become responsive to stimulation of intact visual field areas within hours of the lesion.

A parallel pattern of reorganization follows selective deafferentation of other primary cortical areas in the adult cerebral cortex. For example, in the monkey primary somatosensory (touch) cortex, the normal representation of the hand is extremely orderly, involving a systematic mapping of sequential finger surfaces. When the nerve innervating the surface of some of the fingers was cut, the cortical region normally representing these areas was initially unresponsive. However, after several months this cortical area became responsive to stimulation of neighboring regions of the palm and to intact portions of remaining fingers. In other studies where the input from one finger was eliminated, the area that had been disconnected became responsive to stimulation of the neighboring fingers and the palm.

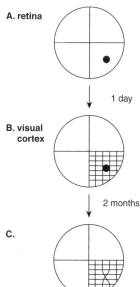

Figure 7–5. Reorganization of visual cortex after a small retinal lesion. *A:* Initially a very small area of damage is created in a spot on the retina. *B:* This results in loss of responsiveness in the corresponding area of the primary visual cortex, determined the next day. *C:* After 2 months of recovery, that region of cortex becomes responsive to visual stimulation in the adjacent areas of the retina.

A similar pattern of results in seen in the reorganization of rat motor cortex representation when a single whisker is eliminated—the disconnected area becomes responsive to stimulation of the neighboring intact whiskers.

Similar results have been obtained in studies on the primary auditory cortex. In this system the cochlea, or inner ear, is normally organized such that successive parts of its surface area are responsive to sequential frequencies of sound. Furthermore, the auditory cortex is topographically organized in a sequence of frequency bands that receive inputs from adjacent areas of the cochlea, similar to the topographic organization in the visual cortex. In these studies a restricted area of the cochlea was lesioned, such that a single frequency band of the auditory cortex representation was deprived of its normal input. Initially, cells in this band became silent to normal levels of stimulation, although they were responsive to louder stimuli. After a month of recovery, these cells became fully responsive to tones in the frequencies neighboring that lost after the lesion.

All of these phenomena speak to the integral role of real-world experience in the basic processing functions of these various cortical systems. Experience shapes the operation of these systems, altering the mapping of the sensory and motor world by primary sensory and motor cortices. Thus, a record of experience is embedded in these networks. A fundamental aspect of these networks in operation involves the competition among inputs to dominate the activity of, and representation in, cortical areas.

Cortical reorganization also occurs as a result of learning

Are these dramatic changes in cortical organization limited to drastic alterations or disconnection of inputs? Do similar changes occur during "real" learning, and, if so, are such changes of sufficient magnitude to be observable after the typically brief and subtle experiences of real-life learning? It is now clear that reorganizations of primary cortical areas indeed do occur as a consequence of conventional learning experiences.

An early report of learning-related reorganization in the visual cortex came from an experiment where young kittens were outfitted with special goggles that could be used to present each eye separately with a vertically or horizontally oriented set of lines. The kittens were trained to avoid a forearm shock by moving the arm to a particular position when signaled by an oriented visual grating presented to one eye. A visual grating of the opposite orientation was presented to the other eye, and its presentation was not associated with shock. Following several weeks of training, recordings were made in the forearm area of the somatosensory cortex, and cells were examined for both tactile and visual responsiveness. In trained animals a large number of cells showed selective visual responses to the training cues. Presentations of the oriented visual stimuli in the correspondingly stimulated eyes produced robust responses in the forelimb area of the somatosensory cortex that represented the shocked arm, whereas presentation of other line orientations were relatively ineffective. These studies showed that cortical areas that are normally responsive only to tactile stimulation could, through training, become activated by visual stimuli. Furthermore, the acquired visual responsiveness is closely related to the significance of the association between an arbitrary visual stimulus and tactile stimulation.

Since that time, a number of studies have now shown changes in cortical responses following Pavlovian conditioning. Among the most elegant of these demonstrations come from experiments by Norman Weinberger and his colleagues, showing shifts in the tuning curves of auditory cortical cells following training in tone-cued classical conditioning. Initially, recordings were taken from a single auditory cortex neuron of an anesthetized guinea pig, and its frequency tuning curve fully characterized (Fig. 7–6). Then a nonoptimal frequency was selected as the conditioning stimulus and its presentation was paired repeatedly with foot shocks, which typically produce unconditioned pupillary dilation responses. Following several pairings of the tone and shock, presentation of the tone alone produced a pupillary conditioned response that reflects an expectancy of the shock.

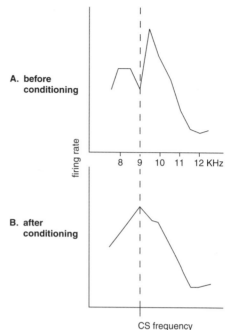

A. before
conditioning

firing rate

8　9　10　11　12 KHz

B. after
conditioning

CS frequency

Figure 7–6. Learning related firing pattern in an auditory cortex neuron. *A:* The tuning curve for an auditory cortex neuron before classical conditioning indicates an optimal response at about 9.5 KHz. *B:* After conditioning with a 9 Khz tone as the conditioning stimulus (CS), the cell shifts its tuning curve to be most responsive at the CS frequency and less responsive at the preconditioning optimum (data from Weinberger, 1993).

After this training the frequency tuning curve of the cell was again characterized. The typical finding was that auditory cortex neurons showed enhanced responses to the initially nonoptimal tone frequency, and reduced responses to other frequencies including the former best frequency of the cell. When the training involved a discrimination between one tone associated with shock and another not paired with shock, responses to the tone associated with shock increased, whereas those to the other tone decreased, as did the responses to other frequencies including the cell's former best frequency. These effects developed in just a few conditioning trials and were long-lasting. Indeed, the magnitude of the novel response grew over the hour after training and was maintained at least 24 hours, for as long as observations could be made. Overall, these changes in the response distribution across the population of auditory cells indicate a general shift in the topographic map. The map would shift strongly toward greater representation of the task-relevant frequency at the expense of other frequencies in the audible spectrum—a pattern of results markedly similar to results from the sensory deprivation experiments in various developing and adult cortical areas.

Similar enhancements of tuning of auditory cortical cells toward relevant conditioning frequencies have also been observed in monkeys. In monkeys who were trained to discriminate small frequency differences, it was found that the monkeys' performance improved progressively over a period of several weeks. In subsequent recordings, changes were found in the size of the auditory cortex representation of the task-relevant frequencies, the sharpness of tuning to these frequencies, and the latencies of cellular responses—all were greater than those of untrained frequencies or of all frequencies in untrained animals. Furthermore, the changes in area of the cortical representation were correlated with the improvement in task performance.

In parallel studies on tactile discrimination learning, monkeys were trained to hold a joystick while a 20 Hz vibration was applied to a small area of a single finger. To obtain rewards the monkey had to release the stick whenever the stimulations were presented at any of several higher frequencies. After months of training the animals, the investigators recorded cellular responses in the primary somatosensory cortex and found that the hand representation in the stimulated finger area was more complex, and had increased in size severalfold, and receptive fields were substantially increased in overlap (Fig. 7–7). These expansions of the stimulated area occurred at the expense of other parts of the finger representation, similar to the findings on auditory responses after training. Using a different task that required monkeys to discriminate the roughness of tactile stimuli presented to varying loci on the finger, the receptive fields in the somatosensory cortex were *reduced*, unlike the preceding findings, although the overall area of the finger representation was, as in the preceding study, increased greatly to take over regions previously unresponsive to these stimuli. Thus, the overall size of the network of neu-

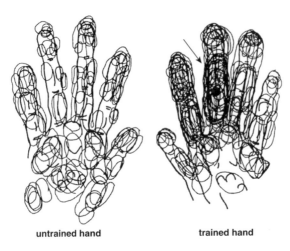

untrained hand　　　　**trained hand**

Figure 7–7. Receptive fields of somatosensory neurons in a monkey's hand before training, and then after training where tactile stimulation was presented in the area indicated by the black circle. Note the large number of overlapping receptive fields after training (arrow) (from Recanzone and Merzenich, 1991).

rons was increased, as was the resolution for detection of fine differences in somatosensory input.

How do higher areas of cortex respond to learning?

At higher levels of sensory processing, the relevant cortical areas are involved in more complex distinctions, and, accordingly, the cells in these areas have more complex response properties that appear to arise from combinations of inputs from the lower levels. One of these areas that has been extensively studied is the inferotemporal cortex (IT). IT is the highest-order cortical visual processing area, whose function is the identification of objects by their visual qualities—and this area is thought to be the site of long-term storage of memory about visual objects. This section reviews the role of IT as indicated mainly by studies of the effects of damage to this area, then describes the normal sensory response properties of IT cells. A discussion of the nature of memory coding by IT cells follows.

Damage to inferotemporal cortex in humans results in visual agnosia, a selective deficit in visual object recognition, and this area has been observed to be activated in various PET or fMRI studies of neurologically intact individuals performing tasks requiring visual object recognition. Damage to inferotemporal cortex in monkeys produces a complex visual impairment. Unlike damage to early visual cortical areas, there is no blindness as a result of IT damage—monkeys with damage to this area have normal thresholds and acuity of visual detection. However, their capacity for visual discrimination is impaired whether the discriminative stimuli involve color, brightness, two-dimensional patterns, or three-dimensional objects, and the deficit is exacerbated when the stimuli are perceptually similar or the number of stimuli to discriminate is large. The deficit in monkeys with IT damage may result from the loss of "perceptual constancy," that is, loss of the ability to recognize a target stimulus across changes in many perceptual qualities including retinal location, rotation, size, color, or contrast, as revealed in studies showing an exception to the generality of an impairment on difficult discrimination problems. Monkeys with inferotemporal lesions perform surprisingly well on mirror-image or inverted stimulus problems, which normal monkeys find rather difficult because of their tendency to see the stimuli as identical in form. It appears that the lesion of the inferotemporal cortex eliminates the appearance of similiarity among mirror-image and inverted stimuli, making this aspect of discrimination less of a problem for monkeys with such lesions.

IT cortex receives information from earlier stages in the ventral visual stream that, when combined, permit it to compute the three-dimensional form of objects. Accordingly, neurons in inferotemporal cortex respond exclusively to visual stimuli and are responsive to whole objects positioned almost anywhere within the visual fields. These cells respond best to the presentation of two- and three-dimensional objects, or to some aspect of visual color or form. Many of these cells respond similarly to a particular stimulus regardless of its size, degree of contrast from the background, or details of its form, location in the visual field, or motion.

The selectivity of IT cells is sometimes highly specific. For example, the first explorations of IT described a cell that responded best to the silhouette of a monkey's hand. Other cells responded to the shape of a banana or a toilet brush (used to clean monkey cages). Studies have concluded that some of these responses to complex stimuli can be reduced to more elemental, albeit still somewhat complicated, forms. Perhaps most widely studied are IT cells that respond best to faces, a finding that has been replicated and studied extensively in a number of laboratories. The responses of these cells are relatively invariant to size, color, contrast, and position. Some cells respond to particular features of faces, but others respond selectively to a particular face orientation, or decrease firing rate when parts of the face are eliminated or scrambled. Some of these cells have selective responses to face identity, that is, to a particular person, and the selectivity of these responses is maintained across a variety of stimulus transformations.

Neurons in inferotemporal cortex change their firing patterns in accordance with their recent past history. The initial evidence for this came from studies of short-term or working memory. In the standard delayed match to sample task typically used to study short-term memory, an animal is presented with a sample cue, followed by a memory delay during which that sample has to be remembered. Then one or more choice stimuli are presented and the animal is required to respond depending on whether the choice cue is the same as the sample (a match) or not (a nonmatch). Joaquin Fuster and his colleagues performed the first studies in which cortical neurons were recorded in monkeys performing this task. They characterized the responses of cells in the inferotemporal cortex following presentations of the sample and choice cues, and during the delay period. In one version of their task the monkey was presented with a color cue and was required to retain it for up to 20 seconds prior to the choice. They identified cells that fired differentially to specific colors of the sample and choice. Some of these cells maintained high levels of activity during the memory delay, and this activity was specific to the sample cue.

In another version of the task, compound stimuli with both color and pattern information were presented as samples. When one particular pattern was presented, the color dimension had to be remembered. When other patterns were presented, the pattern information had to be remembered. Some inferotemporal cells responded selectively to a color or pattern, and the activity of many of these responses was strongly modulated by the relevant memory dimension. In a subsequent study, Fuster found that the magnitude of the enhancing effect was correlated with the animal's response latency.

Other studies have revealed that many inferotemporal cells show suppressed responses to repeated stimuli, and suggested that this phenomenon may provide signals for short-term memory. In the earliest observations of this phenomenon, Malcolm Brown and his colleagues found that inferotemporal cells showed suppressed stimulus-selective responses to stimulus repetition in monkeys performing a delayed matching task where stimuli were reused repeatedly across trials. More recently, Earl Miller and his colleagues have reported multiple correlates of short-term memory in the inferotemporal cortex. They elaborated the delayed match to sample task to include multiple choice cues, and the monkey was required to restrain from making a behavioral response until the matching choice appeared. Their initial main finding was that inferotemporal cells showed suppressed responses on repetition of the sample cue as choice. These responses were maintained across intervening items, but were reset between trials, except for a general decrement in responses across the entire session. A few cells showed the opposite response, an enhancement for matching choice stimuli. In addition, delay firing was observed in some cells, but this activity ceased upon presentation of any subsequent stimulus.

In subsequent studies, the task was changed so that the intervening nonmatch choice stimuli repeated prior to representation of the sample as a choice. In this situation the proportions of inferotemporal responses changed such that many cells showed suppression for any repeated stimulus, whether it was a repetition of the sample or of a nonmatching intervening stimulus. However, now a much larger proportion of cells showed match enhancement responses, and these were observed only for repetition of the sample cue. This pattern of findings was interpreted as evidence for a combination of memory mechanisms within the inferotemporal cortex. Match suppression was viewed as a passive consequence of stimulus repetition such that it occurs whether or not the stimulus had to be remembered. On the other hand, match enhancement was viewed as reflecting the continued processing of a stimulus to maintain a memory. Sustained firing could also be used to bridge a memory delay, but it appears this mechanism cannot be maintained through interfering stimuli by the inferotemporal cortex.

Other studies on inferotemporal cortex have revealed activity patterns that reflect long-lasting stimulus associations. An early study inadvertently found a capacity for cross-modal associations in IT neurons of animals performing a visual discrimination task. In this experiment, monkeys were trained to discriminate four different visual patterns, including a plus sign, a triangle, a square, and a circle. Before presentation of each of those stimuli, a brief tone signaled the monkey to fixate its eyes on the central position of the visual display in anticipation of the visual stimulus onset. To the surprise of the investigators, a third of the visually responsive inferotemporal neurons fired after the onset of the tone at long latencies, and continued to fire after the onset of the visual stimulus. At that point the cells either increased firing rate if the optimal cue was presented, or ceased firing if a different stimulus was presented.

In a study explicitly designed to evaluate such "associative" neuronal responses, Miyashita and his colleagues examined responses of inferotemporal neurons to 24 fractal stimulus patterns. These stimuli were arbitrarily paired such that on each trial one stimulus of a pair was presented as a sample cue, and after a delay period was followed by a choice between the assigned paired cue and one of the other stimuli. After acquisition of this paired associate task over a series of training sessions, two different associative correlates were observed in the firing of these neurons. "Pair-coding" neurons fired maximally for the two cues that were paired associates, more so than for any other cues (Fig. 7–8 top). "Pair-recall" neurons increased firing rate during the delay period following presentation of the associate of the optimal cue (Fig. 7–8 bottom). This study made clear that the preferences of inferotemporal neurons for specific objects can be permanently modified to incorporate a preference for the objects associated with them during learning.

Taken together, these findings suggest that in the course of processing, cortical neurons are sensitive to both short-term and long-term contingencies of the items they are called upon to handle. Here too, then, memory becomes an integral part of the normal operation of these cortical processing systems, as experience continues to shape the nature of processing that is performed.

Summing up

The cerebral cortex is subdivided first into major zones called the frontal, parietal, occipital, and temporal lobes. Within these are a multitude of functionally specific areas segregated into motor, specific sensory modal-

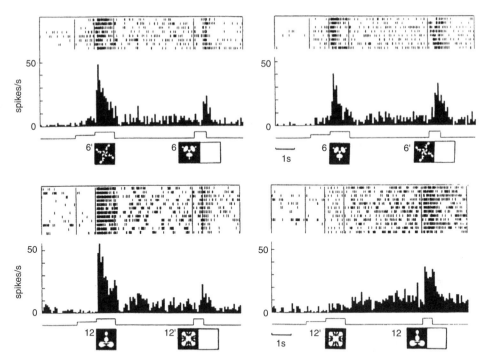

Figure 7–8. Two types of firing patterns that reflect the paired association. *Top:* A "pair-coding" neuron that fired for both associated stimuli. *Bottom:* A "pair-recall neuron" that fired when one of the cues was presented, or in anticipation of that cue predicted by its associated stimulus (from Sakai et al., 1994).

ities, and "association areas" that mediate higher-order functions that often involve a combination of modalities. The general organization of early stages of cortical processing involve systematic topographies of specific sensory or motor features onto the cortical surface. In higher stages of processing these systematic topographies are lost. All cortical areas, both in development and in adulthood, demonstrate considerable plasticity in the form of alterations in the size and topographic organization of cortical areas corresponding to increases or decreases in the activity of inputs to these areas.

The cortical code for memory involves the plasticity of the inherent information processing attributes of the cortex. Sometimes the broad variety of cellular memory correlates in the cortex seems almost as large as the number of studies that report them. However, these diverse findings can be consolidated by thinking about memory as encoded within the cortex in two general ways, each of which involves a modification of the normal sensory processing function of the cells in these areas. First, memory is reflected in the capacity of cortical cells to shift or modulate the responses evoked by the stimuli that drive them. This kind of memory coding is observed as an increment (or enhancement) or as a decrement (or suppression) of sensory responsiveness. A combination of incremental and decremental changes could be integrated to shift a tuning curve, and many of such coordinated tuning-curve shifts could account for the expansion or shrinkage of parts of the overall sensory representation within a cortical area. These response biases can be held briefly, as observed in working memory tasks, or permanently, as observed in an increased resolution within the cortical maps for a relevant stimulus dimension. In working memory tasks, enhanced responses could amount to an attentional "filter" that generates a bias in signals that generate the selection of choice stimuli. Suppressed responses could reflect a kind of subthreshold sustained activation, that is, "primed" neural activity that subsequently requires less processing to identify the familiar stimulus, and this would appear as less activation of the cells required to reidentify a familiar stimulus.

Second, memory is encoded in the capacity of cortical cells to sustain or reactivate their normal sensory responses in the absence of the stimulus ordinarily required to evoke the representation. This type of coding can be observed in firing patterns maintained during the delay in working memory tasks, providing a confirmation of Hebb's "reverberating circuit" notion. In addition, the capacity of cortical cells to regenerate item-specific firing patterns when cued by an associated event seems to confirm Hebb's model of complex memories as "phase sequences" involving replays of linked stimulus representations.

These observations serve to emphasize a fundamental theme, that memory should be conceived as intimately intertwined with information processing in the cortex, indeed so much so that the "memory" and "information processing" are inherently indistinguishable. One understanding of this view holds that memory is nothing more or less than the plastic properties of specific cortical information processings. Another equally valid point of view holds that all cortical information processing inherently involves adaptations to stimulus regularities and contingencies, and/or storage of the information processed. By either view, the mechanisms of the cerebral cortex involve a combination of information processing and memory to constitute neural networks that contain the structure of our knowledge about the world. The memory code is thus both constrained by and revealed in acquired biases in evoked activity patterns and in the ability to recreate those knowledge representations.

READINGS

Constantine-Paton, M., and Law, M.I. 1982. The development of maps and stripes in the brain. *Sci. Am.* 247: 62–70.

Fuster, J.M. 1995. *Memory in the Cerebral Cortex: An Empirical Approach to Neural Networks in the Human and Nonhuman Primate.* Cambridge: MIT Press.

Gilbert, C.D. 1992. Horizontal integration and cortical dynamics. *Neuron* 9: 1–13.

Gross, C.G. 1992. Representation of visual stimuli in inferior temporal cortex. *Phil. Trans. R. Soc. Lond. B* 335: 3–10.

Kaas, J.H. 1995. The reorganization of sensory and motor maps in adult mammals. In *The Cognitive Neurosciences*, M.S. Gazzaniga (Ed.). Cambridge: MIT Press, pp. 51–71.

Kandel, E.R., and Schwartz, J.H. 1985. *Principles of Neural Science,* 2nd edition. New York: Elsevier.

Merznich, M.M., Recanzone, G.H., Jenkins, W.M., and Grajski, K.A. 1990. Adaptive mechanisms in cortical networks underlying cortical contributions to learning and nondeclarative memory. In *The Brain,* Cold Spring Harbor Press: Cold Spring Harbor Symposium LV, pp. 873–887.

Miyashita, Y. 1993. Inferior temporal cortex: Where visual perception meets memory. *Annu. Rev. Neurosci.* 16:245–263.

Perrett, D.I., Mistlin, A.J., and Chitty, A.J. 1987. Visual neurones responsive to faces. *T.I.N.S.* 10: 358–364.

Tanaka, K. 1993. Neuronal mechanisms of object recognition. *Science* 262: 685–688.

Weinberger, N.M. 1995. Retuning the brain by fear conditioning. In *The Cognitive Neurosciences*, M.S. Gazzaniga (Ed.). Cambridge: MIT Press, pp. 1071–1089.

8

• • • • • •

Multiple Memory Systems in the Brain

STUDY QUESTIONS

What are "behaviorism" and "cognitivism"?

What strategies do rats use in maze learning?

What is a double dissociation, and why does it allow powerful conclusions about functional assignments of brain areas?

What functional dissociations characterize the existence of multiple independent memory systems in both rats and humans?

Much of the thinking and research about the nature of cognitive processes in memory, specifically the "behaviorist" versus "cognitivist" debate, proceeded independently of the explorations on cortical localization. Picking up from where we left off in Part II, the evidence from Tolman's work showing capacities that exceeded the predictions of the behaviorist position did not end the debate. Rather, the evidence simply inspired more sophisticated additions to the behaviorists' construction of the internal representation of habit. The debate became focused on the central issue of whether rats acquire maze problems by learning specific turning "responses" or by developing an expectancy of the "place" of reward.

The issue was addressed using a simple T-maze apparatus where "response" versus "place" strategies could be directly compared by operational definitions (Fig. 8–1A). The basic task involves the rat beginning each trial at the base of the T and being rewarded at the end of only one

• 195

A.

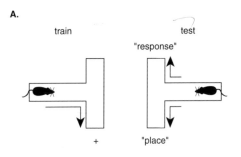

train   test

"response"

+   "place"

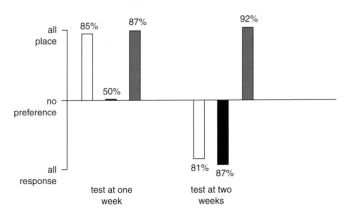

B. proportion of subjects selecting "place" or "response"

Figure 8–1. Place versus response learning. *A:* Initially rats were trained in the T-maze to turn right in order to obtain a food reward in a particular place. In a subsequent probe test the maze was rotated 180 degrees and then rats were run a single trial to determine if they chose the same right turn "response" or instead chose to go to the same "place." *B:* Probe test performance when given a placebo or lidocaine in the hippocampus or striatum. When tested after 1 week of training most normal control rats chose the "place" strategy, whereas after 2 weeks of training most chose the response strategy. Inactivation of the hippocampus abolished the place strategy at 1 week, but had no effect on selection of the response strategy at 2 weeks. Inactivation of the striatum did not affect selection of the place strategy at 1 week, but at 2 weeks abolished the response strategy and returned the rats to the place strategy. Open bars = placebo; black bars = hippocampus; shaded bars = striatum (data from Packard and McGaugh, 1996).

arm, for example, the one reached by a right turn. The accountings of what was learned in this situation differ strongly by the two theoretical approaches. According to behaviorist theory, learning involves acquisition of the reinforced right-turn response. By contrast, according to Tolman's account, learning involves the acquisition of a cognitive map of the environment and the expectancy that food was to be found at a particular location in the test room. The critical test involved effectively rotating the T by exactly 180 degrees, so that the choice arms still end at the same two loci (albeit which arms reach those loci are now exchanged), and the start point would now be at the opposite end of the room. Behaviorists would predict that a rat would continue to make the previously reinforced right-turn response at the choice point, leading it to a different goal location than that where the food was provided during training. By contrast, Tolman's account predicts that the rat would switch to a left-turn in order to arrive at the expected location of food in the same place in the room where it was originally rewarded.

Many experiments ensued, with mixed results indicating that place learning was more often favored but that there were conditions under which response learning was preferred, and the nature of the available cues was the primary determining factor for the differences in the results. In general, whenever there was salient extramaze visual stimulation that differentiated one goal location from the other, a place representation predominated; and whenever such differential extramaze cues were absent, the response strategy would predominate. Such a pattern of results did not, of course, declare a "winner" in the place-versus-response debate. Instead, these results suggested that both types of representation are available to the rat, and that it might use either one under conditions of different salient cues or response demands.

Tolman himself was conciliatory in his explicit suggestion that "there is more than one kind of learning." He offered that different theories and laws might all have some validity for some types of learning. He suggested the possibility of both stimulus-response and cognitive map representations, and elaborated variations on each. He also suggested a distinct form of learning for emotional dispositions for stimuli, calling these *cathexes*, similar to Main de Biran's sensitive memory. Tolman did not consider whether these different types of learning were mediated by different brain pathways. But it turns out that different types of learning do exist, that they follow different rules, and that they are supported by different brain mechanisms.

A most elegant demonstration of such a conclusion was recently provided by Mark Packard and James McGaugh, 50 years after the classic Tolman studies. In Packard and McGaugh's experiment, rats were trained for a week on the T-maze task, then given the rotated-maze probe trial. Then they were trained for another week with the maze in its original orientation, and then finally presented with an additional probe trial. Packard and McGaugh found that normal rats initially adopted a place representation, as reflected in their strong preference for the place of the previous goal during the first probe trial. However, after the additional week of overtraining, normal rats switched, now adopting a response strategy on the final probe test. So, under these training circumstances, rats developed both strategies successively. Their initial acquisition was guided by the development of a cognitive map, but subsequent overtraining led to development of the response "habit."

But Packard and McGaugh's experiment went beyond merely showing that the same rats can use both learning strategies. In addition to the behavioral testing, Packard and McGaugh also examined whether different brain systems supported these different types of representation. Prior to training, all animals had been implanted with indwelling needles that allowed injection on the probe tests of a local anesthetic, which would silence all the cells in a local area for several minutes, or saline placebo directly and locally into one of two brain structures, the hippocampus or the striatum. The choice of these particular brain structures follows from work conducted in the 50 years intervening between Tolman's and Packard and McGaugh's work, particularly the work on human amnesia that so conclusively ties the hippocampus to certain aspects of memory, to be described in subsequent sections of this chapter.

The results on normal animals described previously were from those subjects that were injected with placebo on both probe tests (Fig. 8–1B). The effects of the anesthetic were striking and different depending on when and where the drug was infused. On the first probe trial after only 1 week of training, animals that were injected with anesthetic into the striatum behaved just as control subjects had—they were predominantly "place" learners, indicating the place representation did not depend on the striatum. In striking contrast, the animals that had been injected with anesthetic into the hippocampus showed no preference at all, indicating that they relied on their hippocampus for the place representation, and that this was the only representation normally available at that stage of learning. On the second probe test after 2 weeks of training, a different pattern emerged. Whereas control subjects had by now acquired the response strategy, animals given an anesthetic in the striatum lost the turning response and instead showed a striking opposite preference for the place strategy. Animals given an injection of anesthetic into the hippocampus maintained their response strategy.

A clear picture of the evolution of multiple memory representations emerges when these data are combined. Animals normally develop an initial place representation that is mediated by the hippocampus, and no turning-response representation has developed in this initial period. With over-training, a turning-response representation that is mediated by the striatum is acquired, and indeed predominates over the hippocampal place representation. The latter is not, however, lost—it can be "uncovered" by inactivating the striatum and suppressing the turning-response strategy. Why in particular the hippocampus and striatum might serve these particular roles in memory is discussed extensively later. For now, these findings offer compelling evidence that elements of both the behaviorist and the cognitive map views were right: There are distinct types of memory for place and response, and they are distinguished by their performance characteristics as well as by the brain pathways that support them.

The power of "double dissociation"

The Packard and McGaugh experiment demonstrates the power of the neuropsychological approach in providing compelling evidence both for the existence of two different kinds of learning and for the mediation of different forms of memory by distinct memory systems. Of course, the existence of the hippocampal memory system, and many of its characteristics, was well known long before the Packard and McGaugh study, as outlined in detail in Chapters 4 and 5. And the Packard and McGaugh study was not the first to reveal a role for the caudate nucleus and other parts of the striatum in response learning. But most of the experiments that preceded Packard and McGaugh were based on investigations of only one brain structure in a particular experiment. Although many of these studies, as outlined in the previous chapters, have provided compelling evidence of high specificity in the functional contribution of one brain structure, it is generally agreed that the strongest evidence of differential roles of particular brain structures comes from a design called "double dissociation." In this experimental design, the object is to demonstrate that damage to brain structure A, but not structure B, results in impairment on task X, but not task Y, while damage to brain structure B and not structure A results in impairment on task Y and not task X. Such a design shows, at the same time, that both loci of damage are effective in altering behavior, and both structures play a selective role. The Packard and McGaugh study is a particularly good example of the success of the strategy of double dissociation. This strategy has been extended in several other studies on memory, and the results reveal the existence of and some of the critical brain structures participating in, distinct memory systems.

An anatomical framework for parallel memory systems in the brain

The studies to be described in the remainder of this chapter are examples of research guided by the view that distinct types of memory processing are mediated by distinct functional systems of the brain. A general, anatomically based framework for some of the major memory systems has emerged from this research. A preliminary outline is presented here to provide a framework for discussing the hypotheses and results of the dissociation experiments that follow. In subsequent chapters, greater detail on the anatomical circuits of each pathway is provided.

An outline of some of the most prominent memory pathways currently under investigation is provided in Fig. 8–2. In this scheme, the origin of each of the memory systems is the vast expanse of the cerebral cortex, focusing in particular on the highest stages of the several distinct sensory and motor processing hierarchies, the cortical association areas. As discussed in Chapter 7, each of these areas is responsible for both perceptual, motor, or cognitive processing and for memory of the same domain of information. The cerebral cortex then provides major inputs to each of three main pathways of processing related to distinct memory functions. One pathway, already discussed in part in Chapters 4 and 5, is to the hippocampus via the parahippocampal region. In addition, the main output of hippocampal and parahippocampal processing is back to the cortical areas, the sites of storage and consolidation of long-term declarative memories. As we have seen, this pathway supports the relational organization

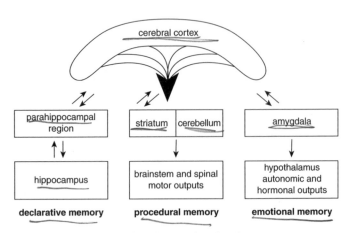

Figure 8–2. Schematic diagram of pathways for the three major "memory systems" discussed in this chapter plus other pathways and modules that are introduced later.

of cortical representations and representational flexibility in declarative memory expression. Further details on the operation of this entire system are discussed in detail in Chapter 9, and its contribution to memory consolidation is considered in Chapter 12.

Two other main pathways highlighted here involve cortical inputs to specific subcortical targets as critical nodal points in processing leading to direct output effectors. One of these systems involves the striatum as a nodal stage in the association of sensory and motor cortical information with voluntary behavioral responses via the brain stem motor system. Another component of this system involves the cerebellum. The putative involvement of these pathways in the acquisition of specific behavioral responses has led many researchers to consider this system as specialized for habit or skill memory, examples of "procedural memory." This hypothesis is tested in the experiment described below in this chapter, and is considered in more detail in Chapter 10.

The other system involves the amygdala as a nodal stage in the association of exteroceptive sensory inputs to emotional outputs effected via the hypothalamic–pituitary axis and autonomic nervous system. The putative involvement of this pathway in such processing functions has led many investigators to consider this system as specialized for "emotional memory." This hypothesis is treated in experiments described below in this chapter and in Chapter 11.

The goal of the remainder of this chapter is to provide a preliminary characterization of the roles of these systems, and in particular to show how they operate differently in the acquisition of different types of memory for the same materials. The comparisons I describe are some of the most striking examples of the success of the double dissociation approach in demonstrating and defining distinct memory systems. The first experiment described involves a "triple dissociation" of memory functions in rats. This study reveals three different patterns of sparing and impairment of memory following damage to three different brain structures. Then two studies are described that involve double dissociations of memory functions in humans with specific types of brain damage. Taken together, the findings suggest a similar set of memory functions supported by homologous brain areas in animals and humans.

Distinct memory functions and brain areas supporting radial maze performance in rats

One of the most striking dissociations among memory functions supported by separate brain structures comes from studies by Normal White and his colleagues. These studies involved multiple experiments in which separate groups of rats were trained on three different versions of the spatial radial maze task. Each version of the task used the same maze, the same general spatial cues and approach responses, and the same food rewards. But the stimulus and reward contingencies of each task differed, each focusing on a different kind of memory processing demand. For each task, performance was compared across three separate groups of rats operated to disrupt the hippocampal system, the amygdala, or the striatum. In addition, different methods of brain damage were compared. Hippocampal system disruption was accomplished by either a fornix transection, which disconnects the hippocampus from important subcortical areas, or by direct lesion of the hippocampus. The effects of these kinds of damage were compared to different methods for direct damage to the amygdala and the striatum.

One test was the conventional version of the radial maze task (Fig. 8–3A). In this version of the task, an eight-arm maze was placed in the midst of a variety of stimuli around the testing room, providing animals with the opportunity to encode the spatial relations among these stimuli as spatial cues. On every daily trial, a food reward was placed at the end of each of the eight maze arms, and the animal was released from the center and was allowed to retrieve the rewards. Optimal performance would entail entering each arm only once, and subsequently avoiding already visited arms in favor of the remaining unvisited arms. The central memory demand of this task was characterized as a "win–shift" rule; such a rule emphasizes memory for each particular daily episode with specific maze arms. Also, the task requires "flexible" use of memory by using the approach into previously rewarded locations to guide the selection of other new arms to visit (see Chapter 5). Accordingly, it was expected that performance on this task would require the hippocampal system.

It was found that normal animals learned the task readily, improving from nearly chance performance (four errors out of their first eight arm choices) on the initial training trial to an average of fewer than half an error by the end of training. Consistent with expectations, damage to the hippocampus resulted in an impairment on this version of the radial maze task. Compared to normal animals, rats with hippocampal damage made more errors by entering previously visited maze arms. Even after extended training, hippocampal-damaged rats continued to make substantially more errors than controls. By contrast, amygdala and striatum lesions had no effect on task performance. Indeed, the group of animals with amygdala lesions performed at least as well as the controls.

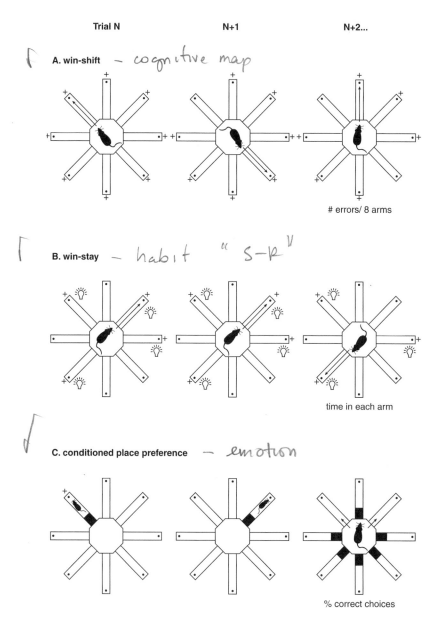

Figure 8–3. Illustrations of example trials in different variants of the radial arm maze task. For each, the measure of performance is indicated below the N + 2 trial. + = rewarded arm (from descriptions in McDonald and White, 1993).

The second test involved a variant of the same radial maze task (Fig. 8–3B). In this version, the maze was surrounded by a curtain, and lamps were used to cue particular maze arms. On the first trial of each daily training session, four arbitrarily selected arms were illuminated and baited with food, whereas the other four arms were dark and had no food. When a lit arm was entered for the first time, that arm was rebaited, so the animal could return to the arm for a second reward. Subsequently that lamp in that particular arm was turned off and no more food was provided at that arm. Thus, here the task was characterized by a "win–stay" rule in which animals could approach any lit arm at any time and could even re-execute the approach to a particular arm for reward one time in each daily trial. This version of the task minimized the availability of spatial cues, and indeed associated rewards with different sets of locations across days. Thus, the task emphasized the approach to a specific cue (a light) across all trials and made no demand to remember particular trial episodes. Also, this version of the task did not require flexible expression of memory under conditions different than original learning—memory was expressed in choice selections during repetitions of the learning trials. Therefore, performance was not expected to rely upon the hippocampus. Furthermore, following learning, the expression of the acquired approach responses is not sensitive to manipulations of the reward level, indicating the task is mediated by stimulus–response habits, rather than by the stimulus–reward association. For these and additional reasons to be made clearer later, performance on the win–stay task was expected to rely on the striatum.

Results showed that normal control subjects learned the appropriate behavioral response to approach the lit arms gradually over several training sessions. In the first few sessions they selected lit arms on only 50% of the trials, but, by the end of 24 sessions, they performed at about 80% correct. Consistent with expectations, animals with striatal damage were impaired, barely exceeding chance performance even with extended training. By contrast, animals with hippocampal damage succeeded in learning and even outperformed the control subjects in learning rate. Animals with amygdala lesions were unimpaired, learning the task at a normal rate.

The third test involved yet another variant of the radial maze task in which animals were separately conditioned to be attracted to one maze arm and habituated to another arm (Fig. 8–3C). In this version, the maze was surrounded by a curtain to diminish the salience of spatial cues. Six of the maze arms were blocked off to make them inaccessible, and one of the remaining two arms was illuminated by proximal lamps, whereas the other was only dimly illuminated. After a preliminary session in which rats could explore both available arms, conditioning proceeded with daily exposures to one of the two arms. For each rat, either the lit or the dark arm was associated with food by confining the animal in that arm for 30 minutes with a large amount of food on four separate trials. On another four trials, the same animal was confined for the same period of time to the other arm, but with no food. Thus, in half of the rats, the lit arm was associated with food availability and the dark arm was not; for the other half of the rats the opposite association was conditioned. In a final test session, no food was placed in the maze and access to both the lit and dark arms was allowed. The amount of time spent in each arm for a 20-minute session was recorded to measure the preference for each of the two arms. This version of the radial maze task emphasized the strong and separate associations between food reward or absence of reward with a particular maze arm defined by a salient nonspatial cue. This task minimized the availability of spatial relations among stimuli. Also, because the same lit and dark arms used during training were re-presented in testing, the task did not require flexible expression of memory under conditions substantially different than original conditioning. Thus, it was not expected that the hippocampal system would be critical to learning. Also, no overt approach response was required during initial learning, minimizing the involvement of learning specific behavioral responses. For these and additional reasons to be discussed later, learning would seem to depend on memory processes associated with emotional conditioning that is expected to depend upon the amygdala.

It was found that normal animals showed a strong preference for the arm associated with food, typically spending 50%–100% more time in the maze arm in which they had been fed compared to the arm where no food was previously provided. Consistent with expectations, rats with amygdala damage showed no conditioned preference for the cue arm associated with food. By contrast, rats with hippocampal or striatal damage showed robust conditioned cue preferences. Despite their lesions, they performed at least as well as intact animals.

The results of this study confirmed all of the findings described earlier, showing that selective ablation of the hippocampus disturbs a form of episodic memory, that selective ablation of the striatum disturbs response or habit learning, and that selective ablation of the amygdala disturbs a conditioned emotional preference.

Double dissociation of memory systems in humans

Studies on human patients provide another potential source for the possibility of double dissociations among the functional memory systems. Studies on humans can extend the dissociations described so far to the distinction between declarative memory, as it is defined in humans, and different forms of nondeclarative or implicit memory, and can reveal significant similarities in the memory dissociations across species. The following sections summarize the findings of two recent studies that have compared different patient populations on a variety of learning and memory paradigms. Despite some potentially important differences across studies in the nature of the disorders represented in these patients, there are strong similarities across studies in the overall pattern of findings. In each study, the learning and memory capacities of amnesic patients with damage to the medial temporal lobe were compared with the capacities of "nonamnesic" patients, that is, humans with brain pathologies not producing the classic amnesic syndrome discussed in Chapter 4. Also, in each study, the performance of these patient groups was compared on standard tests of declarative memory for the learning materials used in each of the tests. The resulting double dissociations in human patients with various memory disorders provide especially compelling evidence for the existence of multiple parallel memory systems in the brain.

There have been no fully parallel triple dissociation experiments performed on humans. However, in the next sections of this chapter, two double dissociation experiments are described—one study compares the abilities of amnesic subjects to the performance of patients with damage to the striatum, and the other study compares the abilities of amnesics to those of patients with damage to the amygdala.

Procedural (habit) learning and declarative memory

One example of a double dissociation involves the analysis of an unusual form of habit learning. Barbara Knowlton and her colleagues studied patients in the early stages of Parkinson's disease, associated with degeneration of neurons in a part of the brain stem (the substantia nigra) resulting in a major loss of input to the striatum, and a set of amnesic patients with hippocampal damage or damage elsewhere in that memory system. Subjects were trained in a probabilistic classification learning task formatted as a "weather prediction" game. The task involved predicting one of two outcomes (rain or shine) based on cues from a set of cards. On each trial, one to three cards from a deck of four were presented. Each card was associated with the sunshine outcome only probabilistically (Fig. 8–4A) and the outcome with multiple cards was associated with the conjoint probabilities of the cards presented in any configuration. After presentation of the cards for each trial, the subject was forced to choose be-

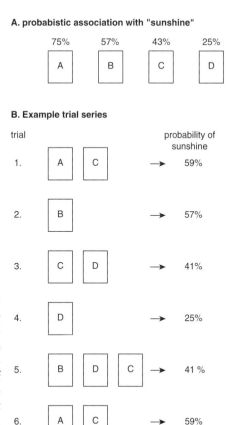

Figure 8–4. The "weather prediction" probabalistic learning task. *A:* The four stimulus cards and their individual assigned associations with the outcome "sunshine." A–D stand for distinct complex stimulus patterns. *B:* An example of a series of trials and the average probability of sunshine for each. Note a repeat of the same stimulus pair on trials 1 and 6.

tween rain and shine, and was then given feedback as to the outcome. The probabilistic nature of the task made it largely counterproductive for subjects to attempt to recall specific previous trials, because repetition of any particular configuration of the cues could lead to different outcomes. In the example set of trials shown in Fig. 8–4B, when presented with the pattern shown on trial 6, subjects might remember their response to the same pattern on trial 1—but the outcome on the current trial need not be the same as on that first trial, leading to confusion. Instead, the most useful information to be learned concerned the probability associated with particular cues and combinations of cues, acquired gradually across trials much as conventional motor habits or skills are acquired.

Over the initial block of 50 trials, normal subjects gradually improved from pure guessing (50% correct) to about 70% correct, a level consistent with the optimal probability of accuracy in this task. However, the patients with Parkinson's disease failed to show significant learning, and the failure was particularly evident in those patients with more severe Parkinsonian symptoms. By contrast, amnesic patients were successful in learning the task, achieving levels of accuracy not different from those of controls by the end of the 50-trial block.

Subsequent to training on the weather prediction task, these subjects were debriefed with a set of multiple-choice questions about the types of stimulus materials and nature of the task. Normal subjects and those with Parkinson's disease performed very well in recalling the task events. But the amnesic subjects were severely impaired, performing near the chance level of 25% correct. These findings demonstrate a clear double dissociation, with habit learning disrupted by striatal damage and declarative memory for the learning events impaired in amnesia, providing further evidence for the view that different forms of memory are represented for the identical learning materials within parallel and separable brain systems.

Declarative memory and emotional memory

Another double dissociation in the literature on amnesia involves the analysis of a type of emotional conditioning. Antonio Damasio and his colleagues studied three patients with selective damage to the hippocampus or amygdala. One patient suffered from Urbach-Wiethe disease, a rare disorder resulting in selective bilateral calcification of the tissue of the amygdala, sparing the adjacent hippocampus. Another patient experienced multiple cardiac arrests and associated transient hypoxia and ischemia that resulted in selective bilateral hippocampal atrophy, sparing the neighboring amygdala. The third patient suffered herpes simplex encephalitis resulting in bilateral damage to both the amygdala and hippocampus.

This study focused on a form of classical conditioning involving an association between a neutral stimulus and a loud sound that produces a set of autonomic nervous system responses (Fig. 8–5A). All subjects were conditioned twice, once in the visual modality where the conditioning stimulus (CS+) was a simple colored slide, and then again in the auditory modality where the CS+ was a pure tone. Subjects were initially habituated to the CS+ as well as to several other stimuli in the same modality (different colors or different tones) that would be presented as CS− stimuli. Subsequently, during conditioning, the CSs were presented in random order for 2 seconds each. Each presentation of the CS+ was terminated with the unconditioned stimulus (US), a loud boat horn that was sounded briefly. The loud horn produced a set of involuntary emotional responses, including sweating that was measured through electrical recordings of skin conductance.

Normal control subjects showed skin conductance changes to the US, and robust conditioning to the CS+, with smaller responses to the CS−

A. conditioning protocol

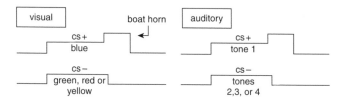

B. declarative memory questions

1. How many colors?
2. Name the colors.
3. How many colors were followed by the horn?
4. Name the colors followed by the horn.

Figure 8–5. Protocols for emotional conditioning and declarative memory. *A:* The protocols for visual and auditory classical conditioning. *B:* The questions asked in the post-training interview.

stimuli (Fig. 8–6). The patient with selective amygdala damage showed normal unconditioned skin conductance responses to the US, but failed to develop conditioned responses to the CS+ stimuli. By contrast, the patient with selective hippocampal damage showed robust skin conductance changes to the US and normal conditioning to the CS+ stimuli. This pa-

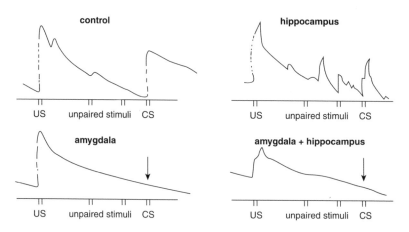

Figure 8–6. Skin conductance responses to the boat horn unconditioned stimulus (US) followed by responses to the unpaired stimuli and the conditioning stimulus (CS). Note that all subjects show strong unconditioned responses to the US. Controls also show a strong conditioned skin conductance response to the CS but not to the unpaired stimuli. The subject with hippocampus damage only shows a strong response to the CS and some generalization to the unpaired stimuli. Subjects with amygdala damage did not acquire a response to the CS (from Bechera et al., 1995).

tient also showed responsiveness to the CS− stimuli, but clearly differentiated these from the CS+ stimuli. The subject with combined amygdala and hippocampal damage failed to condition, even though he responded to the US.

After the conditioning sessions, the subjects were debriefed with several questions about the stimuli and their relationships (see Fig. 8–5B). Control subjects and the patient with selective amygdala damage answered most of these questions correctly, but both patients with hippocampal damage were severely impaired in recollecting the task events. These findings demonstrate a clear double dissociation, with a form of emotional conditioning disrupted by amygdala damage and declarative memory for the learning situation impaired by hippocampal damage. The finding that these different forms of memory for the identical stimuli and associations are differentially affected by localized brain damage further supports the notion of multiple memory systems.

Summing up

Combining the results of the studies presented in this chapter permits some critical nodal points for memory processing to be identified, and these functional assignments are similar across species. These multiple dissociations show that the hippocampal region mediates memory for adoption of the "place" strategy in a T-maze and expression of episodic memories in rats, and memory for facts and events in humans. These dissociation studies show additionally that the striatum plays a critical role in the learning of habitual behavioral responses as reflected in the "response" strategy in a T-maze and stimulus–approach learning in the radial maze by rats and in probabilistic cue–response associations in humans. Furthermore, these studies have provided compelling evidence that the amygdala is critical to emotional learning, as reflected in the acquisition of cue preferences in rats and conditioned emotional responses in humans. Across all these experiments, a salient theme is that these different forms of memory, even for the identical learning materials, are mediated largely independently and in parallel.

Note that although particular nodal brain loci are claimed critical to particular forms of memory, we should not think of these particular brain structures as "black boxes" that contain and perform different types of memory in isolation. Specific brain structures, including (but not restricted to) the hippocampus, the striatum, and the amygdala, are key centers for processing one of the many streams of the flow of cortical information outward to other brain systems. Because these particular structures are central "bottlenecks" for particular pathways, and because each is part of only one of the main functional pathways, these structures become loci of critical and selective processing for that type of memory. Thus, one should be wary of viewing the hippocampus as "the" center for relational or declarative memory. Rather, it is only one (albeit crucial) part of that memory system, but perhaps the only part that is not shared in the pathways for other memory systems. A similar characterization fits for the striatum and for the amygdala. Further details on the circuitry and functional properties of those two memory systems follow in the next three chapters.

READINGS

Bechera, A., Tranel, D., Hanna, D., Adolphs, R., Rockland, C., and Damasio, A.R. 1995. Double dissociation of conditioning and declarative knowledge relative to the amygdala and hippocampus in humans. *Science*, 269: 1115–1118.

Knowlton, B.J., Mangels, J.A., and Squire, L.R. 1996. A neostriatal habit learning system in humans. *Science*, 273: 1399–1401.

McDonald, R.J., and White, N.M. 1993. A triple dissociation of memory systems: Hippocampus, amygdala, and dorsal striatum. *Behav. Neurosci.*, 107: 3–22.

Packard, M.G., Hirsh, R., and White, N.M. 1989. Differential effects of fornix and caudate nucleus lesions on two radial maze tasks: Evidence for multiple memory systems. *Neurosci* 9: 1465–1472.

Packard, M.G., and McGaugh, J.L. 1996. Inactivation of hippocampus or caudate nucleus with lidocaine differentially affects expression of place and response learning. *Neurobiol. Learn. Mem.* 65: 65–72.

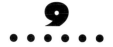

A Brain System for
Declarative Memory

STUDY QUESTIONS

What are the main components of the declarative memory system, and what are the subcomponents of each of them?

What is the general pattern of connectivity among the main components of the system and within each of the main components?

What is the evidence for a selective and independent role for the parahippocampal region in the persistence of representations in intermediate-term memory?

What is the evidence for a separate and selective role for the hippocampus itself in the organization of memories into a relational representation?

How is information differentially encoded in the parahippocampal region versus the hippocampus?

So far the discussion of declarative memory has considered the role of the entire medial temporal lobe region, or the hippocampus specifically, making little distinction between anatomically separate components of this area of the brain. However, the hippocampus is many synapses from sensory inputs and motor outputs, and so its contribution must be considered in the context of how the hippocampus performs its functions within the larger system of brain structures of which it is a part. Indeed, the hippocampus is only one of several structures that compose the full brain system that mediates declarative memory. The aims of this chapter are to identify the main components of this system, to outline the anatomical pathways by which information flows through the system, and to characterize the functional contributions of its different components.

Anatomical characterization of the hippocampal memory system

The *declarative memory system* is composed of three major components: the cerebral cortex; the parahippocampal region, which serves as a convergence center for neocortical inputs and mediates two-way communication between cortical association areas and the hippocampus; and the hippocampus itself. Figure 9–1 illustrates the multiple areas of the cerebral cortex that are involved in this system, and shows the basic anatomical connections between the several neocortical areas that provide specific per-

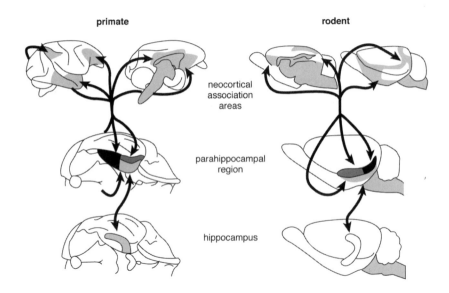

primate   rodent

neocortical
association
areas

parahippocampal
region

hippocampus

Figure 9–1. The anatomy of the hippocampal memory system. In both monkeys and rats the origins of specific information to the hippocampus include virtually every neocortical association area. Each of these neocortical areas projects to one or more subdivisions of the parahippocampal region, which includes the perirhinal cortex, the parahippocampal (or postrhinal) cortex, and the entorhinal cortex. The subdivisions of the parahippocampal region are interconnected and send major projections to multiple subdivisions of the hippocampus itself. Thus, the parahippocampal region serves as a convergence site for cortical input and mediates the distribution of cortical afferents to the hippocampus. The outcomes of hippocampal processing are directed back to the parahippocampal region, and the outputs of that region are directed in turn back to the same areas of the cerebral cortex that were the source of inputs to this region (from Eichenbaum, 2000).

ceptual and motor information to the relevant medial temporal lobe areas, and are the main recipients of the outputs of processing by structures within the medial temporal area. The diagram also shows the location of the components of this system that lie within the medial temporal area. In the terminology suggested by Menno Witter and his colleagues, the large collection of structures within the medial temporal lobe that participate in this system are consolidated into two functional components, the *hippocampus* and the *parahippocampal region*. This diagram also indicates the flow of information among the three major components of the system, highlighting the similarity of the main pathways in monkeys and rats.

The flow of information within the hippocampal memory system

The major pathways of the hippocampal memory system connect the system's three main components, with one set of bidirectional connections between the cortex and the parahippocampal region and another set of bidirectional connections between the parahippocampal region and the hippocampus. This three-stage, two-way communication scheme provides both the basic framework of information flow through the system and strong limitations on how the system works. In this anatomical scheme the cortex provides specific information to the medial temporal lobe structures, this information is manipulated in two stages, and the product of these manipulations is targeted to influence the same cortical areas that provided the original inputs. The message one should take from these anatomical facts is that the role of the medial temporal lobe is to enhance the storage of, change the organization of, or otherwise modify the nature of cortical representations. The next sections provide an overview of the anatomy of each of the main components of the system and outline the main pathways of communication between them.

Areas of the cerebral cortex that interact with the medial temporal lobe

Only highly preprocessed sensory information reaches the medial temporal lobe structures, but these inputs come from virtually all higher-order cortical processing areas. Thus, the larger scheme in which perceptual information reaches the medial temporal lobe is as follows: Sensory information enters the primary cortical areas, then passes through multiple secondary and tertiary stages of sensory processing that are segregated for each sensory modality, as discussed in Chapter 7. The highest areas for each sensory modality then project to the association areas, multimodal areas in the prefrontal parietal, and temporal lobes, as well as the cortex on the midline called the cingulate area. A somewhat similar hierarchy exists for stages of processing in the motor cortical areas, which also ultimately project to association areas in the cingulate and prefrontal cortex. The functional role of these areas differs, but for each that role involves a very high order form of sensory, motor, emotional, or cognitive processing that includes and supersedes specific sensory modalities of the information these areas receive. For example, the association areas of the parietal lobe process spatial information about visual and other sensory inputs, and association areas of the temporal lobe process are involved in object identification from information from multiple sensory modalities. The precise function of prefrontal and cingulate areas is less well understood, but may involve a combination of information about the significance of stimuli, the rules of tasks, and plans for task solutions. The outputs of these areas are the source of inputs to the parahippocampal region.

The parahippocampal region

The parahippocampal region comprises three distinct and adjacent cortical zones, the entorhinal cortex, the perirhinal cortex, and the parahippocampal cortex (as it is called in monkeys, or postrhinal cortex as it is called in rats; (see Fig. 9–1)). Each of these areas can be characterized as receiving input from multiple neocortical association areas and thus constitutes an important convergence site for neocortical input to the hippocampus.

The input connections to the parahippocampal region arise in virtually all the higher-order association areas, including several parts of the prefrontal cortex, parietal cortex, temporal cortex, as well as olfactory cortex in both monkeys and rats. A major similarity of the perirhinal and parahippocampal (postrhinal) areas is that both heavily project to parts of the entorhinal cortex. These areas connect with subdivisions of the hippocampus and also have major projections back to the same neocortical areas that provided the major inputs.

The cortical inputs to the parahippocampal region demonstrate a systematic organization, but one that is unlike the precise topographies that characterize the primary sensory and motor cortical areas (see Chapter 7). Instead, these projections involve large and overlapping zones of projection, an organization of "topographical gradients." Individual cortical association and olfactory areas project differentially along the parahippocampal region. Generally, inputs from more anterior cortical areas, the ones from olfactory, anterior cingulate, and frontal areas, terminate within anterior parts of the perirhinal and lateral part of the entorhinal cortex.

Conversely, inputs from more posterior cortical areas, the ones from parietal and temporal areas, terminate in more posterior parts of the perirhinal, parahippocampal (postrhinal), and lateral entorhinal cortex. In monkeys, the overwhelming input to perirhinal cortex is from visual association areas, whereas in rats there is a more even distribution of inputs from all the ventral temporal association areas. Olfactory inputs to all areas of the parahippocampal region are more prominent in rats than monkeys. These differences largely reflect species differences in the distribution of cortical specializations, for example, differences across species in the amount of cortical area devoted to vision. The perirhinal and parahippocampal (postrhinal) areas, in turn, project heavily onto entorhinal cortex, providing about two-thirds of their cortical input, and contribute to the inputs to the hippocampus itself. There are also major connections between the perirhinal and parahippocampal (postrhinal) cortex. Therefore, these three areas are viewed as highly interconnected cortical zones that, as a whole, accumulate and send cortical information to the hippocampus.

The hippocampus

The hippocampus is composed of several subfields that are distinguished according to the types and layout of cells, and the anatomical connections of these cells. These subfields include an area called Ammon's horn (composed of two main subdivisions called CA1 and CA3), the dentate gyrus, and the subiculum (Fig. 9–2A). The hippocampus is connected to other brain areas via two main bidirectional routes. One of these routes is via a major axon bundle called the fornix, which carries input and output connections with the hippocampus and several subcortical areas. This connection pathway supports multiple modulatory influences on the hippocampus, including attentional controls that tell the hippocampus when to become activated and rhythmic controls that pace its processing cycles. The other route of communication for the hippocampus is via the parahippocampal region. This route, by contrast to the fornix pathway, supports specific informational inputs to the hippocampus from a variety of cortical areas as well as outputs from the hippocampus to these same cortical areas.

There are two main routes by which the parahippocampal area projects into the hippocampus; these are characterized here as the "long" and "short" routes (see Fig. 9–2B). The long route is the so-called trisynaptic circuit, which begins with the perforant path, composed of axons of the entorhinal cortex that penetrate the hippocampal fissure to invade the dentate gyrus. The perforant path originates in superficial cells of the entorhinal and perirhinal cortices, and the projection into the dentate gyrus

A.

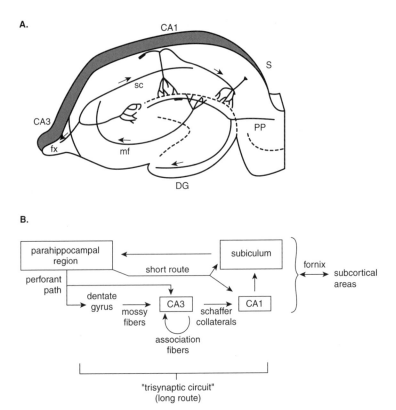

B.

Figure 9–2. Pathways within the hippocampus. *A:* A hippocampal slice indicating the anatomical positions of the major areas and pathways. DG = dentate gyrus; fx = fornix; mf = mossy fibers; sc = Schaffer collaterals; pp = perforant path; S = subiculum. *B:* A flow diagram of the major pathways through subdivisions of the hippocampus, including the several known "loops" between these areas. The traditional "trisynaptic circuit" is the lower "loop" proceeding successively from the parahippocampal region, to the dentate gyrus, to CA3, to CA1, to the subiculum, and then back to the parahippocampal region. The short route involves direct connections between the parahippocampal region and CA1 plus subiculum.

involves well-organized but coarse topographic gradients. These projections pervade the superficial layer of granule cells in the dentate gyrus and on the apical dendrites of pyramidal cells in CA3. Then the dentate granule cells, via the mossy fibers, project to the proximal dendrites of CA3 cells in Ammon's horn. Next, the CA3 pyramids give rise to a large number of collateral outputs: First, some of these axons terminate on other CA3 cells broadly in the hippocampus, via the so-called association fibers.

Second, the CA3 pyramidal cells give rise to the earliest projection out of the hippocampus via the fornix to subcortical areas. Third, CA3 pyramids also give rise to the Schaffer collateral system that provides the major long-route input to the pyramidal cells of CA1. CA1 pyramidal cells project broadly onto cells in the subiculum. The short route of communication involves direct input from the deep layer cells of the parahippocampal cortex to the subiculum and to CA1. The organization of these inputs is essentially the same as that of the entorhinal–dentate inputs.

The return circuit out of the hippocampus begins with the subiculum giving rise to major subcortical and cortical outputs of the hippocampus. The subcortical projection is through the fornix and into multiple subcortical areas (other fibers of the fornix carry subcortical inputs into all the subfields of the hippocampus). The cortical projections, involving outputs of both CA1 and the subiculum, project primarily to deep layers of the entorhinal cortex, completing the parahippocampal–hippocampal loops. These projections follow the same topographic arrangement as the input connections.

Next, the deep pyramidal cells of entorhinal and perirhinal cortex project to the same cortical areas from which inputs originated. In addition, part of the prefrontal cortex receives a direct projection from the CA1. Thus, the cortical recipients of parahippocampal output include the polymodal association areas of the frontal, cingulate, and temporal areas, and the unimodal higher cortical areas in the piriform (olfactory) cortex and neocortex. The organization of these projections follows that of the input organization: More anterior parts of the parahippocampal region project to anterior cortical areas and more posterior parahippocampal areas to more posterior cortical sites.

These anatomical details provide the framework for understanding the functional roles of each of the major components of the system. The cortical association areas provide specific information to the parahippocampal region and hippocampus and in turn are influenced by the outputs of processing in these areas. Notably, in this scheme the parahippocampal region has prominent bidirectional connections with the cortex, and so could support some aspects of memory function on its own even without the contribution of the hippocampus—this possibility is explored in the next section. In addition, the hippocampus depends on two kinds of connections, the general modulatory connections with subcortical areas through the fornix and the specific informational connections with cortical areas. As you will see, both kinds of connections are important to its contribution.

Functional distinctions between the components of the medial temporal lobe

There is now substantial evidence that the major components of the hippocampal memory system contribute differentially to overall memory functions of the system. Here evidence is presented indicating two sequential functions corresponding to the parahippocampal region and the hippocampus. First, it is argued that the parahippocampal region by itself mediates the representation of isolated items and can hold these representations in a memory "buffer" for periods of at least several minutes. This "intermediate-term memory" function bridges the gap between the very brief period of immediate (or short-term) memory and the potentially permanent (or long-term) memory store. Second, it is argued that during this intermediate period, the hippocampus itself mediates comparing and relating these individual representations to other memory representations, creating or modifying the overall memory organization according to the relevant relations between the items and the structure of any already established memory organization that involves those items. The combination of these two processing functions constitutes *declarative memory* as it has been characterized in previous chapters.

Although these two processing functions are seen as supported independently, they normally function interactively, with relational memory processing by the hippocampus operating on new items being held in the intermediate-term store in the parahippocampal region. The intermediate storage function is accomplished at the earlier stage of parahippocampal processing, which contains a full set of input and output connections with neocortical areas, as described earlier. Thus, even without a functional hippocampus, one might expect that the parahippocampal region may be able to support intermediate-term memory for individual items. By contrast, the hippocampus itself interacts with the neocortex only via the parahippocampal region, so one might expect that damage to the parahippocampal region would eliminate any relational processing contribution of the hippocampus. Thus, the intermediate-term storage of single items does not require the relational memory processing function, but relational memory processing depends on the intermediate-term store. This sequential stage model is entirely consistent with the known anatomy of the system.

Further supporting evidence comes from observations concerning the behavioral physiology of the parahippocampal region and the hippocampus. Consistent with the functional distinction proposed earlier, neural activity within the parahippocampal region reflects encoding of individual items and intermediate-term storage for specific items, whereas activity in the hippocampus involves highly specific conjunctions of behavioral events and place where they occur, sequences of information in episodic memories, and extraction of information that is common across episodes, as described in Chapter 6.

In the following sections of this chapter other relevant findings are presented, offering specific comparisons between the parahippocampal region and hippocampus both in their critical functional roles and in their information coding properties. The memory functions assigned to these two regions are seen as reflecting the separation between two general aspects of memory dependent on the medial temporal lobe. First, there is an aspect of this function in which information is held for some period of time that outlasts a single experience. This aspect of medial temporal function is reflected by evidence showing that this region is critical in very rapid acquisition of information and in persistence of memory representations bridging the gap between short-term and long-term memory. Capacities for rapid acquisition and intermediate-term memory persistence are evident in a broad range of human memory tasks and are particularly prominent in the studies on simple recognition in monkeys and rats. Second, there is an aspect of medial temporal function by which this region is involved in aspects of memory organization and expression that mediate the fundamental properties of declarative memory in humans and that are particularly evident in studies on relational learning in rats. In the next sections, it is argued that the parahippocampal region is more critical to the persistence functions of the medial temporal region, whereas the hippocampus is more critical to the organizational functions of this region.

The parahippocampal region and intermediate-term memory

The persistence properties of declarative memory have been studied extensively in animals using the simple recognition memory test known as delayed nonmatch to sample (DNMS), introduced in Chapter 5 (see Fig. 5–1C). Reiterating briefly here, in the original development of this task for monkeys, the subject is presented with a novel "sample" object and rewarded for displacing it. Then, after a variable memory delay, two objects are presented, one identical to the sample and the other a novel one. In this choice phase, the monkey is rewarded for selecting the novel, nonmatching object. The nonmatching rule is easily learned because monkeys are naturally attracted to novel objects. More to the point, the delayed nonmatch to sample task is ideal for measuring the persistence of memory representations for single, isolated stimuli. Indeed, to the extent that memory performance can be related specifically to variations in the length of the memory delay, it would seem that this task selectively assesses the persistence of memories as supported by medial temporal lobe structures.

Following on the initial successful studies showing that large medial temporal lobe ablations produce severe deficits on long delay performance in DNMS, this assay was used to determine which specific structures within the temporal lobe are critical. In H.M. the entire medial temporal lobe region was removed, including the amygdala, the hippocampus, and the immediately surrounding cortex. The ability to produce selective ablations of each of these structures within the monkey allowed the investigation of the role of each of these structures individually.

One part of the story about which there is general agreement is that the amygdala is not critical to the kind of memory modeled by these tasks. A surgical method was developed that allowed selective ablation of the amygdala, including virtually all of its nuclei, without damaging the surrounding cortical areas. Circumscribed lesions of the amygdala had no effect on performance on tasks for which larger medial temporal ablation produces a deficit, specifically DNMS (Fig. 9–3A), as well as retention of object discriminations and concurrent object discrimination.

The other obvious structure that was implicated in the early neuropsychological studies of human amnesia was the hippocampus. Its specific role, independent of the surrounding cortex, has been examined in several ways, including different means for ablating the hippocampus itself and transecting the fornix, the major fiber bundle connecting the hippocampus with subcortical areas. Given the focus on the hippocampus in studies on human amnesia, it came as somewhat of a surprise that the deficit following hippocampal damage or fornix transection is modest compared to that of medial temporal lobe ablation. Monkeys with damage to the hippocampus involving less damage to the surrounding parahippocampal cortical region were less severely impaired than those with full medial temporal ablations (see Fig. 9–3A). Moreover, monkeys with selective hippocampal ablations or fornix transections either show a reliable but small deficit, or perform fully normally (Fig. 9–3A,B) on the conventional DNMS task with delays as long as 2 minutes or sample lists as long as 10 items. In perhaps the most challenging version of the DNMS task, Elizabeth Murray and Mortimer Mishkin presented monkeys with a list of 40 sample objects at 30-second intervals. Subsequently, choice tests were presented in the reverse order at 30-second intervals, so that the effective memory delays spanned from 30 seconds to 40 minutes, and the longest delay was filled with all of the other testing. Under these difficult conditions normal monkeys showed very good performance up to 5 minute delays, with a smooth dropping in performance to about 60% correct at de-

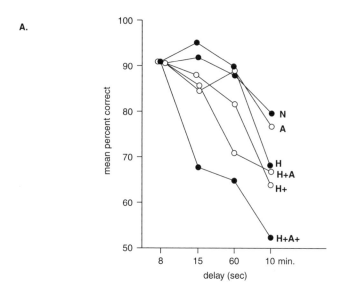

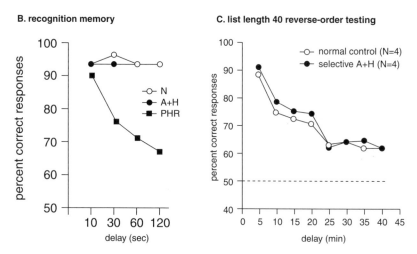

Figure 9–3. Performance of monkeys with different medial temporal lesions on delayed nonmatch to sample (DNMS). *A:* Comparison of the effects of different lesions from one series of studies. N = normal controls; A = amygdala; H = hippocampus; H+ = hippocampus plus a part of the surrounding parahippocampal region; H + A = hippocampus plus part of surrounding cortex and amygdala; H+A+ includes the hippocampus, amygdala, and most of the parahippocampal region (data from Alvarez et al., 1995; Zola-Morgan et al., 1989). *B:* Comparison of the performance on DNMS in another series of studies in normal monkeys (N) with that of monkeys with lesions of the amygdala plus hippocampus and no cortical damage (A + H) or of the parahippocampal region (PHR). *C:* Performance on a variant in which a list of 40 items is tested in the reverse order of their presentation (data from Murray and Mishkin, 1998).

lays over 20 minutes (Fig. 9–3C). Monkeys with ablations of the hippocampus (as well as the amygdala) showed a virtually identical pattern of performance.

These findings of modest or no effect of selective hippocampal damage contrasted sharply with data from contemporaneous studies that examined the role of the cortical areas immediately surrounding the hippocampus and amygdala. Damage to the combined perirhinal, parahippocampal, and entorhinal cortex produces a very severe deficit on the acquisition, long delay, and sample-list performance of DNMS (Fig. 9–3B, see also Fig. 9–3A H+A+), as well as on retention of object discriminations and concurrent object discrimination, and on the acquisition and long delay performance of the tactual version of DNMS. Furthermore, there was no impairment on pattern discrimination. The severity of the impairment was at least as much as that of the original combined medial temporal lobe ablation that involved the hippocampus, amygdala, and surrounding cortex. Indeed, to achieve the learning criterion with short delays on DNMS, monkeys with damage to the perirhinal and entorhinal cortex required remedial training with repetition of the sample trial. Finally, there appears to be a hierarchy of importance of distinct areas within this region. Perirhinal damage produces the greatest deficit, parahippocampal lesions less effect, and entorhinal lesions produce a significant, yet lesser effect.

The evidence from studies on rats supports this basic pattern of findings. In one series of studies on rats, a variant of the delayed nonmatch to sample task, called continuous delayed nonmatch to sample (cDNM), was developed (Fig. 9–4A). This task employed odor cues and involved a stimulus presentation protocol suitable for characterizing neural firing patterns to single memory stimuli as well as behavioral responses in accordance with the nonmatch memory contingency. On each trial, one of a large set of odors was presented with the contingency that a response to the odor was rewarded only if that odor was different from (i.e., a nonmatch with) the immediately preceding one. Rats were trained initially with a very brief interval between odor presentations. Subsequently, the interstimulus interval was manipulated to vary the retention delay, allowing an assessment of the persistence of memory as in the earlier studies on monkeys.

An initial experiment compared the effects of selective ablation of the parahippocampal region versus a fornix transection that selectively disrupted hippocampal function. Normal rats acquired the task within approximately 150 trials and neither of the lesion groups was impaired on

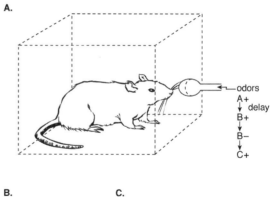

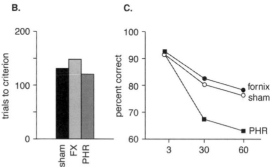

Figure 9–4. The continuous delayed nonmatch to sample (cDNM) task. *A:* A single odor is presented on each trial when the rat inserts its snout into a port on the wall. The sequence of odors (A, B, C) is random, and each is associated with reward if it is different from (a nonmatch with) the one that precedes it. *B:* Acquisition of the cDNM task with short delays by SHAM rats (that is, with surgeries involving no brain damage), rats with fornix transections (FX), and rats with lesions of the perirhinal and entorhinal cortex (PHR). *C:* Performance on short and long delays (data from Otto and Eichenbaum, 1992).

acquisition (Fig. 9–4B). Subsequent testing of memory across various delays showed that intact rats performed at a level of 90% or better at the shortest delay, with performance gradually declining as the retention interval was increased (Fig. 9–4C). Rats with damage to the parahippocampal region also showed good retention at the shortest delay, but their performance declined abnormally rapidly across delays, showing a severe deficit within 1 min. By contrast, rats with fornix lesions performed identically to normal rats across delays, showing intact performance at the short delay and the normal gradual memory decay as a function of increasing delay. These findings indicated that neither the parahippocampal region nor hippocampus is critical for perception of the odor cues, for acquisition of the nonmatch rule, or for short-term retention of odors. However, the parahippocampal region was shown to be critical for mediating a memory representation that persists beyond immediate memory in rats, as it is in monkeys. Furthermore, we may infer from these results that through its direct, reciprocal connections with the cortex, the parahippocampal region is sufficient to mediate the persistence of single-item memories independent of hippocampal processing.

Electrophysiological studies of the parahippocampal region

Using the odor-guided cDNM task in electrophysiological studies of rats, the response properties of neurons in the parahippocampal region and in the hippocampus have been examined. In the studies of the parahippocampal region, the firing patterns of cells were examined associated with three critical aspects of odor coding (Fig. 9–5). First, firing during the period when rats were sampling the odor cues was compared across all the odors presented in order to assess the extent to which odors were selectively encoded. Second, firing during the memory delay was assessed to determine the capacity of these areas for maintaining an odor memory representation in the absence of the stimulus. The focus on delay activity was particularly for the end of the delay period, immediately preceding the initiation of the subsequent odor presentation. At this time, the overt behavior of the animal is consistent across trials—the rat is approaching the stimulus port, in the absence of an odor cue—allowing one to determine if neural activity varies as a function of the memory for the identity of the preceding sample cue just before the recognition judgment must be made. Third, firing during odor sampling was also examined comparing activity

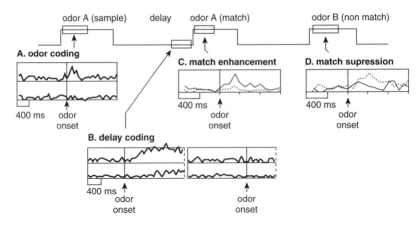

Figure 9–5. Firing patterns of cells in the parahippocampal region during analysis periods in the continuous delayed nonmatch to sample (cDNM) task. *A:* A cell in the entorhinal cortex that shows odor selective responses in the sensory period of the cDNM task. Top panel: strongest response to an odor; bottom panel: weakest response. *B:* A cell in the entorhinal cortex that showed a selective response and sustained selective firing during the delay. Top panel: strongest response to an odor; bottom panel: weakest response. *C:* A "match enhancement" cell that showed a greater response when the odor was a match (solid line) than when it was a nonmatch (dotted line). *D:* A "match suppression" cell that showed a greater response when the odor was a nonmatch (dotted line) than when it was a match (solid line) (data from Young et al., 1997).

levels when a stimulus was a match and when the same stimulus was a nonmatch, to determine the capacity of cells to signal the outcome of the comparison of the preceding and current odor.

A substantial proportion of cells in each of the subdivisions of the parahippocampal region fired during the odor sampling or delay periods. Many cells encoded the identity of the odor cues during the odor sampling period (Fig. 9–5A). Some of these cells fired selectively or differentially to odors at odor onset and ceased firing when odor sampling was concluded, much as one would expect of a sensory neuron. Other cells showed striking odor-specific activity at the end of the memory delay period, indicating some form of intermediate-term storage that was still available just before the choice phase of the trials regardless of the length of the delay. Some of these cells fired during odor sampling and then throughout the delay period, such as the example shown in Figure 9–5B.

Another set of cells showed selective activity that reflected the match and nonmatch qualities of the odor cues during the choice phase. Some of these cells, called "match enhancement cells," fired at a higher rate when the rat was sampling a repeated (matching) odor, and this differential response was largest for the most preferred odor for that cell (Fig. 9–5C). Other cells, called "match suppression cells," fired at a higher rate when the rat was sampling a different odor than the one on the previous trial (i.e., a nonmatch), and this differential response was largest for the most preferred odor for that cell (Fig. 9–5D).

Taken together, neurons in the parahippocampal region have all the properties required to support recognition performance. They encode specific odors, hold these representations (either by maintaining their activity or by regenerating activity) during an extended delay period during which an intact parahippocampal region is required, and they detect match versus nonmatch qualities of the presented choice odors.

In the studies of hippocampus itself, CA1 pyramidal neurons of rats were recorded in animals performing the same cDNM task. A large proportion of hippocampal cells could be activated in association with virtually every identifiable behavioral event in the task. A substantial subset of CA1 cells was selectively active during the odor sampling period, and the activity of some of these hippocampal cells reflected the "match" or "nonmatch" relationship critical to performance in this task. By contrast with the cells in the parahippocampal region, however, no hippocampal cells fired in association with the sampling of a particular odor or with particular combinations of odors that composed specific matching comparisons. Rather, hippocampal cellular activity reflected all comparisons with the same outcome. This finding is entirely consistent with the results of the lesion studies. It appears that the hippocampus itself is *not* involved in the encoding and storage of representations for *specific items* in this task.

Findings from recording studies of monkeys are entirely consistent with the observations of hippocampal system activity in rats. Malcolm Brown and his colleagues first compared the firing properties of neurons in the cortical area surrounding the hippocampus versus the hippocampus itself in monkeys performing a delayed matching task guided by complex visual pattern cues. The cortical cells showed stimulus-specific decrements in response (match suppression) when the choice stimulus was a repetition of the sample, but no such responses were observed in the hippocampus itself. In subsequent studies, Brown and colleagues confirmed that a large percentage of cells in the perirhinal cortex demonstrated match suppression responses. They showed evidence of three different types of recognition-related decremental responses in those cells. Some cells, called "novelty neurons," fired only on the first presentation of a novel visual pattern, and did not recover for at least 24 hours. Other cells, called "familiarity neurons," did not decrement on the choice phase of the first trial in which the stimulus appeared, but showed reduced responses on all subsequent presentations. Yet other cells, called "recency neurons," showed match suppression only on the choice phase of each trial when a particular stimulus appeared, but recovered fully when the same cue was presented as a sample on a subsequent trial. Brown has argued that all of these recognition-related firing patterns coexist, and may serve different roles in visual recognition. Importantly, no stimulus-specific match suppression responses were observed in the hippocampus in any of his studies.

Other recent studies have provided evidence of intermediate-term memory processing by the parahippocampal region in monkeys performing a more complex delayed matching to sample task. Earl Miller, Robert Desimone and their colleagues trained monkeys to perform a variant of delayed matching to sample, where a pattern cue was presented as the "sample," and, followed by several choice stimuli, the monkey had to respond only to the matching choice stimulus. In these studies, cells in the perirhinal cortex of monkeys showed selective responses to the visual cues. Some cells fired persistently during the initial part of the delay, but ceased firing when the first choice item was presented. In a version of the task where each choice stimulus was presented only once per trial, the predominant observation was "match suppression," where many cells fired less to the matching choice item. In another version of the task, where incorrect (nonmatching) choice items were presented repeatedly, forcing the animal to attend to the designated sample cue, a substantial number of "match enhancement" cells were also observed.

Wendy Suzuki and her colleagues employed the same task to study the firing properties of neurons in the entorhinal cortex of monkeys. They found a fraction of entorhinal cells that fired selectively to specific visual cues. In addition, unlike perirhinal cells in the monkey but like cells throughout the parahippocampal region in the rat, neurons in the entorhinal cortex fired throughout each of the delay periods between the sample stimulus and each of the choice items. Finally, entorhinal neuronal activity also reflected the match and nonmatch qualities of the choice stimulus, by showing match suppression and match enhancement responses.

The role of the hippocampus and parahippocampal region in relational memory

The parahippocampal region plays a more critical role in some forms of simple recognition memory than the hippocampus itself. Indeed, some researchers have suggested that the parahippocampal region plays a more critical role than the hippocampus for a broad range of memory tasks, at least as tested in monkeys. However, as seen in Chapters 4 and 5, studies of memory in humans and animals indicate that the hippocampus itself does play a critical role in some types of memory, and recent studies have extended this role even to other forms of recognition memory. The role of the hippocampus is seen most clearly in tasks that emphasize the representational properties of declarative memory rather than the temporal properties. It turns out that the heavy reliance of primate work on the DNMS task has led to emphasis in that literature on the temporal characteristics of the hippocampal memory system and has therefore focused attention on the role of the parahippocampal region, which has the ability to maintain a persistent intermediate-term memory representation. Work on amnesia in humans and rats, by contrast, has explored a variety of tasks that call upon the special representational characteristics of the hippocampal memory system, namely the ability to perform relational memory processing, which depends critically on the hippocampus itself. To clarify this point, we turn now to one further set of results in which the ability to learn the relations among items is challenged in rats with selective damage either to the parahippocampal region or to hippocampus (following transection of the fornix).

In Chapter 5, evidence was presented that the hippocampus plays a critical role in transitive associations in the representation of multiple paired associates. A more ambitious test of the role of the hippocampus was provided in an experiment that examined the capacity for learning and remembering large and structured odor memory organizations and the ability for representational flexibility. This experiment involved the development of a task that required animals to learn an orderly hierarchy of odor representations, and then tested their ability to make transitive inference judgments. The task was based on a test Piaget pioneered to assess human cognitive development. In tests of this type in human children, subjects are initially presented with a set of *premises*, such as "the blue rod is longer than the red rod" and "the red rod is longer than the green rod." Then the children are asked whether they can make an inference that the blue rod is longer than the green rod. The capacity for inferential judgment in this test is interpreted as prima facie evidence of the representation of orderly relations; moreover, it is the kind of relational representation structure that we attribute to the hippocampal memory system.

In the study on rats, the stimuli were different scents added to sand-filled cups in which the animals dug to find buried rewards (Fig. 9–6A), similar to the paired associates task described in Chapter 5. Initially the animals were trained on a series of two-item odor discriminations called premise pairs that collectively included five different odors (e.g., A+ versus B−, B+ versus C−, C+ versus D−, D+ versus E−, where + or − refers to which item is rewarded; see Figure 9–6B). Animals were initially trained on the series of premise pairs using a trial-blocking method that introduced the pairs and their correct responses gradually. Ultimately, however, they were presented with premise pairs in random order. Learning could occur by representing each of the discriminations individually or they could instead be represented within an orderly hierarchy that includes all five items.

To examine which of the representations was actually employed by the animals, they were given probe tests derived from two pairs of nonadjacent elements (Fig. 9–6B). When presented with the probe pair B versus D, two nonadjacent and non-end elements, consistently choosing B provides unambiguous evidence for transitive inference. B and D have never been presented together, and judging between them requires knowledge about their indirect relations via a representation of the missing item C. The other probe involved items A and E. Note that in this pairing correct choices could be entirely guided by the independent reinforcement histories of these elements individually, because choices of A during premise training were always rewarded and choices of E were never rewarded. Thus, the combination of the probe tests B versus D and A versus E provided a powerful assessment of capacities for making novel judgments guided by inferential expression of the orderly organization or by reward history of the individual elements, respectively.

After achieving solid performance on the premise pairs, probe trials containing the critical B versus D problem and the control A versus E prob-

A. Testing method

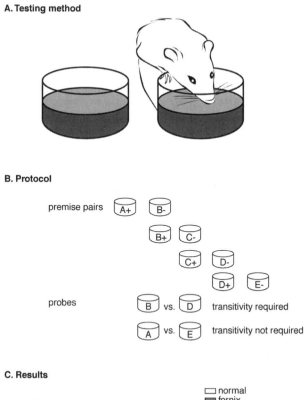

B. Protocol

premise pairs

probes

B vs. D   transitivity required

A vs. E   transitivity not required

C. Results

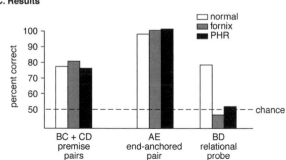

Figure 9–6. The transitive inference task. *A:* Illustration of a rat and the odor stimuli presented on a trial. *B:* Odor pairs presented on training (premise pairs) and transitive inference on control testing (probes). *C:* Average performance on inner premise pairs, on the control probe AE, and on the transitive inference test BD (data from Dusek and Eichenbaum, 1997).

lem were presented intermingled with repetitions of the premise pairs. On these probe trials, animals were rewarded for the "correct" (transitive) selection, in order to avoid dissuading them from making transitive choices and to maintain performance on the probe trials. To minimize new learning of the B versus D problem, probes were presented only twice per test session and were widely spaced among repetitions of premise pairs. In addition, to test for possible contamination by new learning of the B versus D problem, all animals were subsequently tested for their ability to learn about new odor cues presented in the probe test format.

The performance of normal rats was compared to that of rats with fornix transection, preventing the normal operation of the hippocampus, and rats with ablation of perirhinal and entorhinal cortices. Both normal rats and rats with fornix transections or parahippocampal ablation achieved criterion performance on each training phase very rapidly. In addition, all rats readily reached criterion with randomly presented premise pairs in an equivalent number of trials. In probe testing, all rats continued to perform well on the premise pairs during the test sessions, and in particular performed at about 80% correct on the "inner" pairs BC and CD (Fig. 9–6C). Also, all rats performed extremely well on the A versus E trials, which can be solved without a transitive judgment.

On the critical B versus D probe test, normal subjects demonstrated robust transitive inference. Their performance on B versus D trials significantly exceeded chance level and was not different from their performance on premise pairs that included items B and D (the B versus C and C versus D pairs; see Fig. 9–6C). In striking contrast, the rats with either type of hippocampal damage performed no better than chance on the BD probe—their performance on the B versus D problem was much lower than that on the premise pairs that included B and D, and on the other novel probe (AE), and much worse than the performance of normal animals on this test of transitivity.

A further analysis of transitivity examined performance on the very first presentation of the B versus D pair, which may be considered a "pure" test of inferential responding uncontaminated by food reinforcements given on repeated probe trials. Of the normal subjects, 88% chose correctly on the first B versus D probe, whereas only 50% of the rats with either type of hippocampal damage were successful on the initial B versus D judgment. Thus, by several measures, the data strongly indicate that rats with hippocampal damage have no capacity for transitive inference, despite their having learned each of the premise problems as well as normal subjects.

Most important for our considerations of anatomical distinctions within the hippocampal region, in this challenging test of relational memory, transection of the fornix and ablation of the parahippocampal region produced equivalent full-blown impairments. These findings strongly implicate the common structure compromised by these disconnections, the hippocampus itself, as playing the critical role in the representational properties of declarative memory. Furthermore, this pattern of findings is quite different than the selective effect of parahippocampal damage, and not hippocampal damage or fornix transection, on delayed nonmatch to sample. Thus, whereas the parahippocampal region can mediate sustained representations for single items without hippocampal involvement, the hippocampus itself is required for the organization of memories required to perform the relational task.

Differential activation of the parahippocampal region and hippocampus

Two recent studies, one in rats and the other in humans, provide further evidence consistent with the notion that the parahippocampal region and hippocampus are differentially activated in different types of memory processing. One study involved an extension of Brown and colleagues' examination of *c-fos* (a marker for gene expression) activation in the hippocampal region. In this study they presented rats with computer images of novel and familiar object stimuli, and compared responses to changes in the familiarity of particular stimuli or the familiarity of stimulus arrangements. To initiate each trial the rat placed its nose into an observing hole that stabilized the position of its eyes. Then two images were presented in the extreme left and right visual fields; because the visual circuitry of the rat involves a nearly complete hemispheric crossing of the most lateral parts of the visual fields, these images would be expected to drive neurons primarily in the opposite hemisphere. In each case a familiar image was presented to one visual field and a novel image was presented to the other— the key variable in this study was the nature of the images. For some animals the images involved pictures of single objects, whereas in other animals the images involved novel and familiar spatial arrangements of the same three objects. When the images involved single stimuli, the perirhinal cortex showed greater *c-fos* activation in the perirhinal cortex on the side that viewed novel as compared to familiar pictures. No differential activation was observed for single stimuli in the hippocampus. By contrast, when the images involved arrangements of multiple stimuli, hippocampal subdivisions (as well as the postrhinal cortex) showed greater *c-fos* activation for novel as compared to familiar stimulus arrangements. In this condition, no differential activation was observed in the perirhinal cortex.

The other recent study, performed by John Gabrieli and his colleagues, involved an examination of human brain activation using fMRI associated with the presentation of novel pictures. This study also involved two conditions. In one condition, subjects were presented with a series of novel pictures of indoor and outdoor scenes or line drawings. In this condition, the parahippocampal region was activated but the hippocampus itself was not. In the other condition, prior to scanning, subjects were presented with, and asked to remember, a set of line drawings of common objects and animals, or the names of these items. Then, during scanning, the subjects were presented with the names of the drawings they had seen, or with the drawings of the items whose names they had previously seen, respectively. In this condition, a subdivision of the hippocampus (specifically, the subiculum) was activated when the items were accurately remembered, whereas no activation was observed in the parahippocampal region. This study provided evidence in human subjects of a dissociation of memory processing functions in the hippocampal region.

Furthermore, the evidence from both of these studies can be viewed within the framework outlined here based on single neuron recordings and lesion experiments in animals. In both rats and humans, the parahippocampal region is activated during the perception and encoding of novel pictures. This could reflect the activity of neurons in the parahippocampal region associated with recognition of specific single items, as observed in rats and monkeys. These activation findings complement the observations of selective deficits in recognition memory for single items in rats and monkeys with parahippocampal damage. Furthermore, in rats the hippocampus itself is activated when memory processing involves the identification of novel arrangements of multiple items. In humans the hippocampus is activated when memory processing involves the identification of a word from a picture or vice versa. Both of these types of processing are likely to invoke the processing of relationships between items in memory, consistent with the role of the hippocampus in relational processing.

Summing up

The findings we have discussed speak to the roles of the parahippocampal region and the hippocampus in realizing the persistence and organizational properties, respectively, of hippocampal-dependent memory processing. But how do these components provide their separate functions within the declarative memory system, and how do they interact to produce declarative memory? To address this question, this chapter concludes with a model for successive stages of memory processing within the entire declarative memory system.

Prior to processing by the medial temporal lobe, neocortical areas create specific perceptual representations that can be sustained briefly within those processing areas. Such memory traces are able to support perceptual matchings between current and stored representations, and can support performance in short-term recognition, consistent with the observed sparing of working memory even in severe amnesia.

At the first stage of processing within the medial temporal lobe, perceptual codings from the neocortical processors reach the parahippocampal region, where functionally distinct representations of the to-be-remembered events converge prior to processing in the hippocampal formation itself. In the parahippocampal region, specific information is encoded, and neural activity representing that information is sustained, persisting through considerable interference and intervening processing. Furthermore, the parahippocampal region is capable of processing the matchings between current representations and the contents of the intermediate-term store. This processing appears to be sufficient to support delayed nonmatch to sample performance in the absence of normal function of the hippocampus.

At the final stage of declarative processing, the hippocampus enters the picture, *not* to maintain a memory representation of single sensory cues, but rather to process comparisons among the various current stimuli and events and between current stimuli and representations of previous stimuli and events, presumably those maintained at earlier levels of this system. Hippocampal processing appears to be quite different from the perceptual matching taking place in cortical areas. Thus, hippocampal processing relies on cortical inputs and presumably will exert its effects by modifying those inputs or by making connections among those cortical areas. In recognition memory, the hippocampus processes comparisons between current and previous stimuli as well as rich episodic and contextual information that goes beyond the strict perceptual properties on which cortical matchings are based; this may in some cases make a distinctive contribution to intermediate-term memory. Moreover, when the requirements of the task go beyond what can be accomplished by sensory matching processes, requiring comparisons among experiences with items and the flexible expression of memories, the entire system contributes critically to a distinctly new capacity for declarative memory representation.

Putting together the results of the studies presented here, a preliminary picture of the processes that mediate declarative memory emerges. It appears that the parahippocampal region contributes to declarative memory by "buffering" specific representations that can be accessed and manipulated by the hippocampus. Then the hippocampus represents the critical relations among the items and other event information held by the parahippocampal region, and indeed has access to the much larger organization of item representations in cortical association areas via the parahippocampal region. We presume the full relational memory organization comes about through multiple iterations of cortical input to the parahippocampal region and temporary storage there. This might be followed by hippocampus-mediated relational processing that adds to, or restructures, interconnections among parahippocampal and cortical representations. Over extended time periods, new experiences that bear on the established organization reactivate established representations as well as add new ones, and these are processed together by this hippocampal circuit to weave the new information into the established relational network. Precisely because this network is so extensive and systematically interconnected, access to items via novel routes and in novel experiences is not only possible but also occurs continuously as we express memories to guide almost every aspect of daily life. These interactions, by feeding back and forth, can go on for a significant period, and may be reinstated repeatedly by experiences that bear partial similarity to the learning event. This repetitive processing could contribute to the consolidation of memories over very long periods. The larger issue of memory consolidation itself is considered in Chapter 12.

READINGS

Amaral, D.G., and Witter, M.P. 1995. Hippocampal formation. In *The Rat Nervous System*, 2nd edition. G. Pacinos, (Ed.). San Diego: Academic Press, pp. 443–493.

Brown, M.W., and Xiang, J.Z. 1998. Recognition memory: Neuronal substrates of the judgement of prior occurrence. *Prog. Neurobiol.* 55:149–189.

Burwell, R.D., Witter, M.P., and Amaral, D.G. 1995. Perirhinal and postrhinal cortices in the rat: A review of the neuroanatomical literature and comparison with findings from the monkey brain. *Hippocampus* 5:390–408.

Dusek J.A., and Eichenbaum, H. 1997. The hippocampus and memory for orderly stimulus relations. *Proc. Nat. Acad. Sci. U.S.A.* 94:7109–7114.

Eichenbaum, H., Otto, T., and Cohen, N.J. 1994. Two functional components of the hippocampal memory system. *Brain Behav. Sci.* 17:449–518.

Miller, E.K., Li, L., and Desimone, R. 1991. A neural mechanism for working and recognition memory in inferior temporal cortex. *Science* 254: 1377–1379.

Suzuki, W.A., Miller. E.A., and Desimone, R. 1997. Object and place memory in the macaque entorhinal cortex. *J. Neurophysiol.* 78: 1062–1081.

Witter, M.P., Groenewegen, J.J., Lopes da Silva, F.H., and Lohman, A.H.M. 1989. Functional organization of the extrinsic and intrinsic circuitry of the parahippocampal region. *Prog. Neurobiol.* 33:162–243.

Young, B.J., Otto, T., Fox, G.D., and Eichenbaum, H. 1997. Memory representation within the parahippocampal region. *J. Neurosc.* 17: 5183–5195.

..10..
• • • • • •

A Brain System for Procedural Memory

STUDY QUESTIONS

What are the basic types of procedural memory?

What are the major anatomical subsystems involved in procedural memory?

What is the role of the striatum in habit learning?

What is the role of the cerebellum in conditioning?

What is the role of the motor cortex in learning?

Procedural memory. It's a term I use when I coach baseball to 10-year olds. I tell them each time they use the correct form in throwing a ball, and in swinging a bat, they strengthen the program for that correct movement. And, conversely, each time they do it wrong, they strengthen that incorrect style to the detriment of their overall performance. Some coaches call it "muscle memory." But while that term gets closer to the observable behavioral output, we know the memory for such complicated coordination is not stored in the muscles. It is stored in the nervous system, and in particular in a complicated brain system that plans and executes coordinated motor programs or procedures. From playing a sport to the act of reading aloud this manuscript and writing notes on its content, an endless array of coordinated behaviors we execute in everyday life are the product of *procedural memory,* the habits and skills that our motor system has acquired and built into its very circuitry. Other than in such painful circumstances as trying to learn a new skill in adulthood, we typically take procedural memory for granted. It goes on seamlessly and unconsciously. Yet, while development of these procedural memories is a prominent part of our childhood—as we learn to write and to ride a bicycle—they are never fully complete. Instead, procedural memories are continuously modified by experience and tuned by repeated practice throughout life.

From the perspective of the study of motor systems, a number of investigators have separated procedural memory into two general types. One type involves the acquisition of habits and skills, the capacity for a very broad variety of stereotyped and unconscious behavioral repertoires. These can involve a simple refinement of particular repeated motor patterns and extend to the learning of long action sequences in response to highly complex stimuli. These abilities reflect both the acquisition of general skills (writing, piano playing, etc.) and the unique elements of personal style and tempo in the expression of these behaviors.

The other type of procedural memory involves specific sensory-to-motor adaptations, that is, adjustments of reflexes, such as changing the force exerted to compensate for a new load, or acquisition of conditioned reflexes that involve novel motor responses to a new sensory contingency, as characterize many instances of Pavlovian conditioning described earlier. An analysis of the brain systems that support these two types of unconscious learning is the focus of this chapter.

Overview of brain anatomy relevant to procedural memory

The anatomy of brain systems that mediate procedural memory is highly complex and only partly understood, so only a few parts of these pathways that support different aspects of procedural memory are sketched here. At the top level of these various circuits is the primary motor cortex, a cortical area that is critically involved in directing the force and flow of muscle contractions generated by neural controls at the level of the spinal cord. An additional neighboring critical structure is the premotor cortex, which plays a central role in the preparation for movement and in the coordination of movements on the two sides of the body, as well as the sequencing of motor coordination over time. These cortical motor areas work in close concert with two major subcortical structures, the *striatum* and the *cerebellum* (Fig. 10–1). Each of these subcortical structures forms the nodal point in a major circuit "loop" that begins with downward projections from the cortex and ends in a route from the thalamus back to the cortex. However, there are important differences between these two subsystems with regard to the specific sources of cortical input and output, and the connections with the brain stem and the spinal cord.

A. striatal subsystem

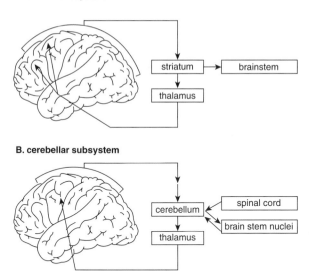

B. cerebellar subsystem

Figure 10–1. Two major motor system pathways. *A:* Connections from virtually every cortical area are sent to the basal ganglia. The major output of this subsystem is through the thalamus back to the frontal cortex. *B:* Connections from frontal and parietal cortical areas indirectly reach the cerebellum, which interacts directly with the spinal cord and brain stem motor and sensory nuclei. This system also has outputs via the thalamus back to parts of the frontal cortex.

The striatum is the combination of the anatomically distinct caudate nucleus and putamen. It works together with other components of the so-called basal ganglia, and is the focus of most of the recording and lesion studies on procedural memory in this subsystem. The striatum receives its cortical inputs from the entire cerebral cortex, and these projections are capable of activity-dependent changes in responsiveness. These projections are topographically organized into divergent and convergent projections into modules within the striatum that could sort and associate somatosensory and motor representations. The striatum projects mainly to other components of the basal ganglia and to the thalamus, which project back to both the premotor and motor cortex, and the prefrontal association cortex. Notably, there are minimal projections of this circuit to the brain stem motor nuclei and none to the spinal motor apparatus.

This pattern of anatomical connectivity suggests that the striatum is not involved directly in controlling the details of motor output. Instead, the connections to premotor and prefrontal cortex suggest that the cortical–striatal loop contributes to higher motor functions including, many researchers believe, the planning and execution of complex motor sequences. When the striatum is considered together with the anatomical connections between parts of the striatum and the brain structures involved in motivation and emotion, the suggestion has arisen that the striatum may be involved more generally in the planning and execution of goal-oriented behavior.

The cerebellum is a distinctive structure, remarkable particularly for the regularities of its internal circuitry. It has several subdivisions associated with different sensory and motor functions. The cerebellum receives cortical input from a much more restricted cortical area than the striatum, including only the strictly sensory and motor areas projecting via brain stem nuclei into the lateral part of the cerebellar cortex. Like the striatal subsystem, the cerebellum has a thalamic output route to the cerebral cortex, although the cortical target is also more restricted than that of the striatum, limited to motor and premotor cortex. In addition, the cerebellum receives somatic sensory inputs directly from the spinal cord and has major bidirectional connections with brain stem nuclei associated with spinal cord functions. Based on these connections, and on behavioral and electrophysiological data to be discussed later in this chapter, the cerebellum is believed to more directly contribute to the execution of movement details, and to the acquisition of conditioned reflexes and body adjustments to changing environmental inputs.

The striatal habit subsystem

In the preceding chapter, the striatal habit system was introduced via experiments that dissociated this system from the hippocampal and amygdala memory systems. Those experiments provided evidence indicating a role for the striatum in the acquisition of specific stimulus–response associations, as contrasted with declarative memory and emotional memory functions of the hippocampal and amygdala systems, respectively. Here the role of the striatum in habit acquisition is further elaborated, considering further the nature and scope of learning mediated by this system.

One early study illustrates the scope of memory mediated by this system and shows a particularly striking dissociation between regions within the striatum that control approach behavior conditioned by different cues. In this study, thirsty rats with lesions of the posterior-ventral or ventral-lateral regions of the striatum were trained to approach a water spout over several days. Subsequently, they were given foot shocks in the same chamber in the presence of a conditioning cue, which was either a light or an odor. The animals were tested later for their latency to approach the water spout when the conditioning cue was present versus when it was absent. Animals with lesions of the posterior-ventral striatum failed to show discriminative avoidance of the light cue, but showed good avoidance of the olfactory cue. Conversely, animals with ventral-lateral striatal lesions failed to show discriminative avoidance of the olfactory cue, but showed good avoidance of the light cue.

It was clear from the early studies, taken together, that the scope of striatal involvement is not limited to a particular sensory or motivational modality, or to a particular type of response output. The studies by Packard, McDonald, and their colleagues outlined in Chapter 8 indicate that the striatum is also essential for learning that involves acquisition of a consistent approach response to a specific stimulus. How broadly does this characterization apply to the larger body of data on lesions of the striatum in animals? In addition to the dissociation of hippocampal and striatal involvement in radial maze learning described Chapter 8, other studies by the same investigators have provided parallel data on versions of the aversively motivated water maze task. For example, in one study rats with hippocampal or striatal damage were trained on two variants of the Morris water maze task (see Chapter 5) that used the same stimuli but involved different stimulus–response demands. In both tasks, the animals were always presented with two rubber balls distinguished by different visual patterns as the learning cues. One of the cues was attached to a stable submerged platform on which the animals could climb in order to escape swimming, and the other cue was anchored to a thin pedestal that could not be mounted.

In the "visual discrimination" task variant, the positions of the cues varied, but the cue with a particular visual pattern was always mounted to the escape platform (Fig. 10–2A); here, the animal had to ignore the locations of previous escapes and consistently approach a particular visual pattern. Conversely, in the "place learning" task variant, the escape platform was always located in the same place in the maze, but the visual pattern on the cue above it varied randomly (Fig. 10–2B). In this version of the task, the animal had to ignore the visual pattern and swim consistently to a particular location defined by extramaze stimuli.

The results of this study indicated a clear double dissociation of hippocampal and striatal memory functions. Animals with hippocampal damage failed to acquire the place learning variant of the task (Fig. 10–2A), performing hardly better than chance (four correct choices out of each block of eight trials) over several training sessions. By contrast, rats with lesions of the striatum succeeded in learning to approach the correct location of the escape platform by the fourth training block, just like nor-

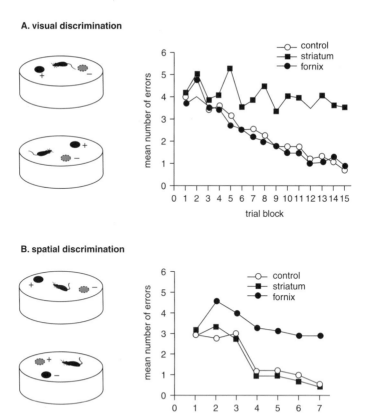

Figure 10–2. Visual or spatial discrimination in the water maze. *A:* In the visual discrimination version, the stimuli varied in location, and the escape platform was always identified by one visual cue (+) and not the other (−). *B:* In the spatial discrimination version, the same two stimuli were employed, but the escape platform was always in the same location regardless of which stimulus was nearby (data from Packard and McGaugh, 1992).

mal rats. The results were precisely the opposite on the visual discrimination task variant. Animals with striatal lesions performed at chance levels over many training blocks, whereas rats with hippocampal damage, like normal rats, gradually acquired the pattern discrimination over the course of training (Fig. 10–2B).

In another study, rats with hippocampal or striatal damage were trained on the visible platform version of the water maze task in which, from multiple starting points, they were to approach a platform that was visible above the surface of the water, always at the same location (Fig. 10–3A). Subsequently, the visible platform was replaced with a submerged plat-

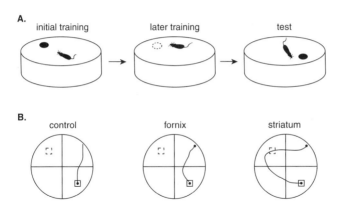

Figure 10–3. Visual versus spatial learning in the water maze. *A:* Stages of training, involving initial training with a fixed visible platform, continued training with a submerged platform at the same location (as well as further training with the visible platform at that locus), and finally testing with the visible platform moved to a new location. *B:* Examples of swim paths on the first test trial in which the escape platform was moved from its original location (dotted square) to a new locus and made visible (filled circle in square) (data from McDonald and White, 1994).

form in the same location for a single block of trials. Then, training continued with repetitions of multiple trial blocks with the visible platform, and a single trial block with the submerged platform. Finally, the visible platform was moved to a new location, and the rats were tested in a single block of trials.

All rats quickly learned to swim to the visible platform. On the first test with the submerged platform after initial training, escape latencies were elevated for all groups. On subsequent trials with the submerged platform, normal rats and rats with striatum lesions quickly learned to approach the correct escape location with shorter latencies, approximating the performance level they had achieved with the visible platform. By contrast, rats with hippocampal damage failed to improve on the submerged platform trials, consistent with their well-described deficits in place learning in the water maze. When the visible platform was moved to a new location, normal rats followed the obvious visible cue and swam to it despite its novel location (Fig. 10–3B). Rats with hippocampal damage behaved similarly, swimming directly to the visible platform as well. By contrast, rats with lesions of the striatum did not swim immediately to the visible platform, but instead swam directly to its previous location and only subsequently to the visible platform at its new site. This finding indicates that the initial successful performance in rats with striatal damage was guided primarily by learning the location of escape. Normal rats demonstrated they were capable of either learning strategy, whereas rats with hippocampal damage were guided primarily by the visual cues. This pattern of results is entirely consistent with the earlier described comparisons of hippocampal and striatal lesions. Furthermore, these data parallel those from the T-maze place-versus-response study of Packard and McGaugh. They reveal that in water maze learning too, even when initial learning performance is equivalent among animals with distinct brain damage, the representational strategies may differ qualitatively as revealed in subsequent probe tests.

These double dissociations of striatal versus hippocampal function followed on earlier studies showing a special role for the striatum in "egocentric" localization, the kind of representation that would mediate learning left or right turns in a T-maze, as illustrated in the Packard and McGaugh experiment described in Chapter 8. Raymond Kesner and his colleagues performed a study that shows compellingly the striatum's role in egocentric as opposed to "allocentric" localization, the ability to locate items in space regardless of the positions relative to the subject, exemplified in water maze learning.

In one of their experiments, a group of rats was trained on the standard eight-arm radial maze task, in which they were required to remember each of the arms they had visited based on their allocentric location in the room. The same rats were also trained in a different maze on a variant of the task in which they began each trial on an arbitrarily selected arm and were required to subsequently select an egocentrically defined adjacent arm. Rats with striatal lesions performed well on the standard radial maze (allocentric) task, but they could not learn the adjacent arm (egocentric) task (Fig. 10–4). In a second experiment, rats were trained on two tasks on different radial mazes. In a place learning (allocentric) task, only one arm of an eight-arm maze was consistently baited, and the rat began each trial from any of the remaining arms chosen at random. In a right–left discrimination (egocentric) task, the animal began each trial in the central area of the maze and two randomly chosen adjacent arms were indicated for a choice. The rat had to choose only the left (or, for other rats, the right) of the two arms regardless of its absolute location. Here, too, rats with striatal lesions performed well on the place learning task but did not learn the right–left discrimination task (Fig. 10–4).

These findings, combined with those of several other similar studies, suggest that the deficit following striatal damage can be characterized as an impairment in generating behavioral responses toward important environmental stimuli. The deficit extends to both approach and avoid-

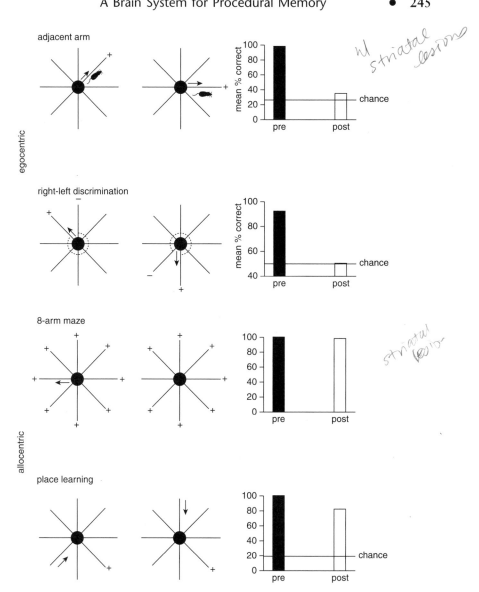

Figure 10–4. Pre- and postoperative performance of rats with striatal lesions on egocentric and allocentric spatial tasks. For each task two successive example trials are illustrated. + = rewarded arm;− = nonrewarded arm; arrow indicates beginning of run on a trial.

ance responses and to both egocentric spatial and nonspatial stimuli. However, it is likely that the deficits in egocentric localization and stimulus–response learning in animals with striatal damage may reflect only a subset of the forms of behavioral sequence acquisition mediated by the striatum.

The striatal habit subsystem: studies on human patients with striatal damage

In Chapter 8, it was shown that patients with striatal dysfunction associated with Parkinson's disease are impaired in probabilistic learning in a weather prediction task. This deficit is just one aspect of the deficit in habit learning in patients with striatal damage. Indeed, the deficit in probabilistic learning is among a number of findings in the clinical literature that raise questions about the scope of learning and memory impairments following striatal damage; more specifically, about whether deficits are limited to habit or motor skill learning or whether, instead, they extend to all domains of skill learning. The weather prediction results can be seen as entirely consistent with the findings in animals with striatal damage indicating an impairment in learning to generate one particular response among many to a complex stimulus, except that here patients were impaired in learning to generate a variety of specific responses to the appropriate sets of complex stimuli. This section considers other findings from the clinical literature. The findings described here demonstrate that this correspondence between the animal and human clinical literatures is strong and extensive.

Patients who have been studied in order to examine the role of the striatum in learning and memory come mainly from two etiologies, Parkinson's disease and Huntington's disease. Both disorders lead to profound motor deficits. In Parkinson's disease, patients suffer from tremor, rigidity, and akinesia (inability to move) following substantial cell death in other parts of the basal ganglia and the resultant depletion of dopamine, a major neurotransmitter in the striatum. Huntington's disease is characterized by primary degeneration of the striatum, and these patients exhibit irregularities in their movement patterns (athetosis and chorea). In addition to the motor deficits, some patients with Parkinson's disease also suffer from depression or dementia, and patients with Huntington's disease always progressively develop dementia. Furthermore, drug treatments administered to these patients, such as L-dopa for Parkinson's disease, have cognitive consequences. Thus, work with such patients aimed at characterizing the role of the striatum in memory is somewhat more complicated than the animal work.

Notwithstanding those limitations, both types of patients exhibit deficits on motor skill learning tasks. In one experiment, subjects were required to maintain contact of a handheld stylus with a target metal disk revolving on a turntable—this task is called rotary pursuit. Normal subjects showed robust learning over repeated practice sessions on this often-studied task, increasing the amount of time they maintained contact with the target. However, patients with Huntington's disease showed virtually no learning. To control for the possible effects on learning of differences in baseline motor performance due to the motor deficits associated with Huntington's disease, the speed of the turntable rotation was manipulated to equate the patients' initial performance to that of control subjects. Equating initial levels did not reduce the learning deficit; indeed, even when initial performance was adjusted to be better than that of normal subjects, the patients with Huntington's disease still failed to show learning.

The motor learning deficit in patients with Huntington's disease and patients with Parkinson's disease extends to unconscious learning in a task called the serial reaction time test. In this task, one of a number of different locations on a computer screen is flashed on each trial and the subject is to press the button corresponding to that location. Unbeknownst to the subject, the locations are flashed in a particular repeating order. For example, in one such item a 12-item fixed sequence involves each of the four locations flashed three times in a particular order. During the course of repetitions, implicit learning of the sequence is revealed in reductions in the subjects' average reaction time to respond to a given item within repeating sequences. Conversely, their reaction times are slower in a transfer test where subjects are presented with randomly ordered items. Several reports have indicated deficits in learning on this task in patients with Parkinson's disease or Huntington's disease, suggesting that tasks requiring memory for and sequencing of responses tap into the selective functions of the human striatum.

Functional brain imaging studies have provided another way to explore the role of the striatum in learning and memory in humans, with results paralleling closely the results of the patient studies just described. Increases in striatal activation have been seen in association with learning of finger movement sequences and with learning in the serial reaction time tasks. More recently, activation has been documented in the striatum in the more perceptual and cognitively based skill learning tasks used in other patient studies of striatal function, including probabilistic classification in the weather prediction task and other skill learning tasks. Taken together, these results indicate that the role of the striatum in habit or skill learning extends beyond the motor domain, encompassing a variety of performances that all involve multiple input or response options and that all show gradual, incremental learning across trials. The number of neuropsychological and functional imaging studies of striatal function is growing very rapidly, offering promise of clarifying the striatum's contribution to human learning and memory.

Learning-related neural activity in the striatum

Recent neurophysiological studies have provided converging evidence for the involvement of the striatum in programming stimulus–response sequences. These studies have characterized striatal neurons as anticipating movements, and have suggested that striatal activity might be associated with the relation between behavioral contexts and responses. Work by Wolfram Schultz and his colleagues has revealed striatal neural activity associated with the expectation of predictable environmental events in monkeys performing conditional responses. In one experiment, such activity was found using a variant of the delayed response task where delayed go and no-go responses were conditioned by visual stimuli. Neuronal activity sustained during the delay period reflected anticipation of either the active arm movement or of withholding that movement. A variety of cellular responses has been seen, including task-dependent anticipatory activity and activity related to the expectation and reception of reward. These findings have led Schultz to suggest that the striatum incorporates knowledge about the behavioral context of the task to plan behavioral responses.

Other studies, focusing on striatal interneurons that are tonically active, have led to a similar conclusion. Ann Graybiel and her colleagues identified a substantial population of tonically active neurons in the striatum that became responsive to an auditory cue only when the cue acquired predictive value for subsequent delivery of a reward. These cells did not respond to primary rewards, but did establish cued responses in expectation of a reward and maintained those conditioned responses for weeks. The conditioned responses were entirely dependent on dopamine inputs from the substantia nigra. Selective depletion of dopamine cells in the substantia nigra, another major part of this system that sends inputs to the striatum, resulted in a reduction of the cued responses of tonically active striatal neurons, to the same level as observed prior to conditioning. Subsequent systemic administration of a dopamine receptor agonist reinstated conditioned responses of these striatal cells. Based on these findings, Graybiel emphasized the role of limbic reward-related inputs via the substantia nigra in mediating the establishment of context-dependent striatal activity participating in the selection and execution of learned behavioral repertoires.

In addition to these observations on simple and conditional motor responses, there are data indicating a prominent role for the striatum during spatial sequencing behavior. In one study monkeys were trained to fixate a central location and encode a sequence of spatial target illuminations, then visually orient to and subsequently reach toward each target in order (Fig. 10–5A). Many striatal neurons responded to the visual instruction stimuli during central fixation or during the saccade or arm move-

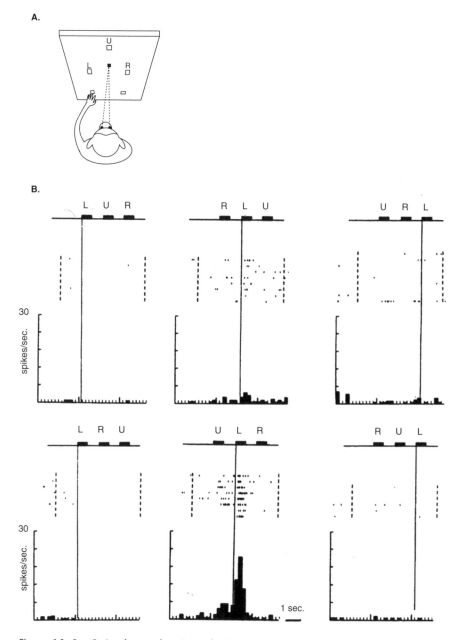

Figure 10–5. Striatal neural activity during sequence memory. *A:* Task protocol. On each trial the animal begins the trial by fixating its eyes at the fixation point (FP). This results in a sequence of brief illuminations of targets at right (R), left (L), and upward (U) positions in a particular order that is reproduced in eye and arm movements. *B:* Example of a striatal neuron that fired upon presentation of the L cue, only when in the ULR sequence (data from Kermadi and Joseph, 1995).

ment. Furthermore, the responses of a substantial proportion of these cells were highly dependent on the sequential order of the targets, responding only to a particular visual cue if it was in a particular position in the three-item sequence (Fig. 10–5B). None of the cells showed sustained activity after the target instructions, but rather the cells fired in anticipation of each item in the sequence, consistent with the view that the striatum participates with other structures in the anticipation of sequential behaviors to be performed.

Summarizing the role of the striatum in habit learning

The findings from different approaches to understanding the role of the striatum converge well, leading to the suggestion that the striatum plays a critical role in habit learning, particularly in tasks involving the learning of response sequences to specific stimuli. The necessary circuitry exists in the striatum for cortical sensory input and direct motor outputs to mediate the association of both simple and highly complex stimuli with specific behavioral outputs. Furthermore, there are clear striatal pathways for, and well-documented influences of, reward signals capable of enhancing the associations of stimuli and responses. The striatum represents a broad variety of cues, motor responses, and rewards, although in the spatial domain its role is limited to egocentric knowledge. There are both direct output pathways for control of voluntary behavior and feedback pathways to the cerebral cortex, particularly the prefrontal cortex, that could mediate complex sequencing and planning. Current research seeks to determine whether the system works to resolve competition among competing input or response options, or to permit manipulation of or shifting among representations of these input/response options, or to learn and execute the desired input–output mappings. It is clear that the striatum is a key element in a pathway for sequence learning and other aspects of habit learning involving the acquisition of stereotyped and unconscious behavioral repertoires. This procedural learning pathway is independent of the earlier described circuits for declarative memory and for emotional memory.

The cerebellum and motor conditioning

The cerebellum has long been considered a brain structure closely involved in motor control and motor learning. Experimental investigations into the role of the cerebellum in motor learning have focused on its highly organized circuitry and emphasized its mechanisms for reflex adaptations. The circuitry involves a complex set of connections among several nuclei in the brain stem. Here some of the details of that circuitry are introduced, allowing insights into the precise mechanisms of plasticity that underlie procedural memory supported within this system.

This relevant circuitry involves both the cerebellar cortex and underlying deep nuclei, plus several other specific nuclei in the brain stem (Fig. 10–6A). The principal cells of the cerebellar cortex are the Purkinje cells, which send entirely inhibitory inputs to the deep nuclei. These cells receive

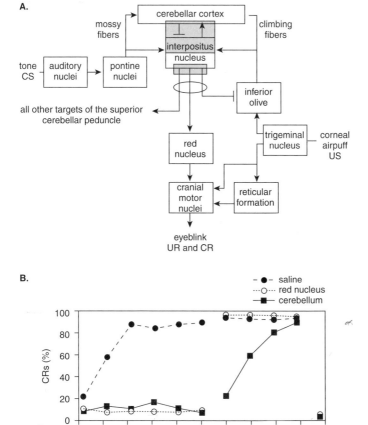

Figure 10–6. A: Schematic diagram of the essential brain circuitry that mediates classical conditioning of the eyeblink response. B: Effects of muscimol on conditioned reflex eyeblinks (CR). All groups received injections prior to training on sessions 1–6, not on sessions 7–10, and all groups received muscimol on session 11 (data from Krupa et al., 1993).

two excitatory inputs, from the mossy fibers and the climbing fibers. The mossy fibers constitute the major afferent input. They originate from several brain stem nuclei that represent the spinocerebellar inputs, and they influence Purkinje cells indirectly through clusters of cerebellar granule cells that lie beneath. The granule cells originate the parallel fibers, the set of axons that run several millimeters along the long axis of the cerebellar folia. The parallel fibers make their excitatory connections onto the dendrites of a row of Purkinje cells, all oriented perpendicular to the parallel fibers.

There is considerable convergence of sensory inputs both at the level of the granule cells and onto Purkinkje cells. The other excitatory input, the climbing fibers, originates in the inferior olivary nucleus of the medulla. These axons rise within the cerebellar cortex and wrap around the Purkinje cell soma and dendrites, making numerous excitatory synaptic contacts. Each Purkinje cell receives input from only one climbing fiber, but these inputs have a powerful influence over the Purkinje cells, resulting in an all-or-none influence over the activity of Purkinje cells. Furthermore, coactivity of mossy and climbing fibers results in a long-term depression (LTD) of the mossy fiber synapse that is thought to play a central role in mediating the cerebellum contribution to motor learning. The cerebellum receives input from, and forms topographic representations of, the entire body surface. In addition, inputs from the vestibular, visual, and auditory areas are conveyed through other deep nuclei. The main outputs of the cerebellum to spinal motor mechanisms are through areas of the brain stem including the red nucleus and reticular formation, in addition to the upward going outputs to the premotor and motor cortex.

Eyeblink conditioning as an example of motor learning supported by the cerebellum

Considerable recent attention has focused on Pavlovian eyeblink conditioning as a model learning paradigm in which to study the role of the cerebellum. In this paradigm, rabbits are placed in restraining chambers where they can be presented with a well-controlled tone or light as the conditioning stimulus (CS), and a photoelectric device records eyeblinks. In classic *delay conditioning*, this stimulus lasts 250–1000 ms and coterminates with an airpuff or mild electrical shock to the eyelid (the unconditioned stimulus, or US) that produces the reflexive, unconditioned eyeblink (the UR). After several pairings of the CS and US, the rabbit begins to produce the eyeblink after onset of the CS and prior to presentation of the US. With more training, this conditioned response (CR) occurs somewhat earlier, and its timing becomes optimized so as to be maximal at the US onset, showing that not only is a CR acquired but also a timing of the CR is established.

Permanent lesions or reversible inactivation of one particular cerebellar nucleus, the interpositus nucleus, result in impairments in the acquisition and retention of classically conditioned eyeblink reflexes, without affecting reflexive eyeblinks (URs). Consistent with the role of gene expression and cellular changes that underlie learning (see Chapters 2 and 3), inhibition of protein synthesis in the interpositus nucleus prevents establishment of the conditioned reflex. The cerebellar cortex plays a more complicated role, revealed in disruption of the timing of conditioned eyeblink responses following cerebellar cortical lesions.

These and other observations have led Richard Thompson and his colleagues to propose a model of eyeblink conditioning that includes a central set of elements by which the CS input is sent via the brain stem pontine nuclei to the interpositus as well as to the cortex of the cerebellum (Fig. 10–6A). The US input is relayed by the trigeminal nucleus and inferior olive of the brain stem to the same cerebellar sites where the essential plasticity occurs. Outputs for the CR are then mediated by projections from the interpositus to the red nucleus, which projects to the accessory abducens motor nucleus, which also executes the UR via direct inputs from the trigeminal nucleus.

The evidence for involvement of these particular structures in different aspects of eyeblink conditioning is substantial. Studies by Joseph Steinmetz and colleagues using stimulation and recording techniques within the cerebellar circuit have shown that stimulation of the auditory pathway via the pontine nucleus can substitute for the tone CS in establishing the conditioned response. Similarly, the US pathway has been traced through the trigeminal nucleus to a circumscribed area in the dorsal accessory inferior olive, by showing that lesions of this area prevent the UR and stimulation of this area substitutes for the US.

Additional compelling data come from studies using reversible inactivations of particular areas during training. These studies showed that drug inactivation of the motor nuclei that are essential for production of the CR and UR prevented the elicitation of behavior during training. However, in trials immediately following removal of the inactivation, CRs appeared in full form, showing that the neural circuit that supports UR production is not critical for learning *per se*. A similar pattern of results was obtained with inactivation of the axons leaving the interpositus or their target in the red nucleus (Fig. 10–6B), showing that the final pathway for CR production is also not required to establish the memory trace.

By contrast, inactivation of the anterior interpositus nucleus and over-lying cortex by drugs (muscimol, lidocaine) or temporary cooling did not affect reflexive blinking, yet resulted in failure of CR development during inactivation and the absence of savings in learning after removal of the inactivation (Fig. 10–6B). These results point to a small area of the anterior interpositus nucleus and overlying cerebellar cortex as the essential locus of plasticity. It is in this area, of course, where the interactions occur between the mossy and climbing fibers resulting in LTD, and the connections with the relevant outputs exist. Consistent with a view that this plasticity is essential, mice with gene knockouts resulting in deficient cerebellar LTD were impaired in eyeblink conditioning.

Recording studies have also been helpful, and are beginning to shed light on the nature of the neural coding in the cerebellar cortex and interpositus nucleus that mediates the conditioning. During the course of training, neurons in both areas developed increased firing to the CS. During subsequent extinction trials, during which the US was withheld while the CS was presented repeatedly, the CR gradually disappeared while interpositus cells ceased firing. By contrast the neural code remained in the activity of the cerebellar cortex long after extinction. These data support the view that the cortical and subcortical components of the cerebellum play somewhat different roles in maintaining and modulating this form of motor learning.

The hippocampus and eyeblink conditioning

An interesting contrast with the complex but circumscribed circuitry that supports standard eyeblink conditioning involves the larger set of brain structures that become involved with elaborations on this kind of motor learning. One particularly intriguing story involves the role of the hippocampus in an unusual kind of eyeblink conditioning called *trace conditioning*. Notably, the hippocampus is not required for the standard *delay conditioning* paradigm described so far. However, the hippocampus is required for the trace conditioning variant of the paradigm. In this version of the task, the conditioning stimulus (CS) involves a brief 100 ms tone followed by a silent 500 ms "trace" interval punctuated by the unconditioned stimulus (US). Rabbits develop conditioned responses (CRs) in this form of eyeblink conditioning, and hippocampal neurons also are active associated with the CS and US. This variant of eyeblink conditioning is sensitive to damage to the hippocampus. Thus, even though this form of learning does not fit the typical definitions of declarative or hippocampal-dependent memory, it is an example where the hippocampus is part of a larger circuit including the cerebellum in producing a form of reflex adaptation.

The extent of cerebellar involvement in procedural memory

Does the role of the cerebellum extend to other learning situations? The emerging evidence is that the cerebellum is involved in a broad scope of procedural learning. One of the most striking examples involves a demonstration of cerebellar plasticity in studies by William Greenough and his colleagues. In these studies rats were given "acrobatic" training by challenging them to acquire complex motor skills necessary to traverse a series of obstacles, involving moving over barriers and balancing on teeter-totters and tightropes. Rats with such training developed an increased volume of the parallel fiber layer in the cerebellar cortex, and increased number of synapses onto Purkinje cells without an increase in synaptic density. Control rats exercised in a running wheel without acrobatic training, having extensive motor activity without the requirement to acquire new motor skills. The cerebellum of these animals did not develop these characteristics of synaptogenesis. Instead, the cerebellum of control animals demonstrated increased blood vessel density associated with motor activity.

Evidence for the involvement of the cerebellum in procedural memory in humans

Studies on humans have shown that the scope of the cerebellum's role in habit or motor skill learning extends to classical conditioning in that species, and further to several other forms of motor adaptation. Patients with cerebellar damage are impaired in the acquisition of classically conditioned eyeblink responses and show other abnormalities of conditioned responses. In addition, patients with cerebellar damage are impaired in adaptation to lateral displacement of vision produced by prism glasses. When normal subjects first wear the prism glasses, their pointing to targets is typically off in a systematic way, but they gradually adapt and begin pointing correctly. When the glasses are subsequently removed, normal subjects' pointing is offset in the opposite direction and readapts to the normal matching. By contrast, patients with cerebellar damage show impaired adaptation. Patients with cerebellar damage are also impaired in skill learning tasks and in the serial reaction time test described earlier. Such patients have also been shown to be impaired at planning a sequence of actions in a problem-solving task. Functional imaging studies have documented decreases in cerebellar activation in association with learning of finger movement sequences, with learning in the sequential reaction time task, and with learning in drawing or tracking tasks.

By one view, virtually all skill learning tasks require motor adaptations, in which case the cerebellum may play its role in the execution of skill learning, that is, in the production of the learned responses, rather than the learning of movement sequences. Alternatively, the same results have been employed to suggest that the cerebellum plays a critical role in temporal sequencing itself. This conclusion follows from work with the serial reaction time task, in which cerebellar patients showed a sequence learning impairment not only in their reaction time performance but also in their explicit remembering of repeating sequences.

Other work on the cerebellum in humans has explored its possible role beyond the motor domain. Cerebellar activation was seen in the deep nuclei during sensory discrimination, and in the cortex during an attention demanding task without movement and during verb generation. In the verb generation task, subjects are presented with nouns (e.g., *ball*) and are to generate an appropriate verb (e.g., *throw*) for each one. Compared to a control condition in which subjects are just to repeat the nouns aloud, generating verbs to the same nouns resulted in activation of cerebellar cortex along with activation of dorsal frontal cortex. There are now a number of reports of cerebellar activation associated with frontal cortex activation in various tasks requiring search or selection among multiple response options or representations. This participation of cerebellum in nonmotor tasks, while initially surprising, is consistent with anatomical findings of cerebellar outputs to higher cortical areas. Moreover, the participation of such noncerebellar structures as the hippocampus, in humans as well as animals, in the trace variant of the cerebellum-dependent eyeblink conditioning task, further implicates the interaction of higher systems with essential cerebellar function.

The role of the motor cortex in procedural memory

The motor and premotor cortical areas mentioned at the outset of this chapter are involved in all the circuits for procedural learning, so it is likely that these areas participate in some important ways in virtually all types of adaptation and skill acquisition. This has been confirmed in various ways in studies of humans and of animals. Functional imaging studies have shown activation of the motor (and somatosensory) cortical areas during various examples of skill learning, such as learning a sequence of finger taps on a keyboard (see Chapter 4). Several studies in animals have reported evidence of expansion of the motor cortex representation associated with procedural learning. An increased number of synapses per neuron in motor cortex was found in rats who have learned complex motor skills in the "acrobat" task, and training-induced physiological changes in the cortical representation of reaching movements were found in the motor cortex of monkeys. Other studies in animals have shown other learning-dependent effects on the physiology of cells in the motor cortex. Pioneering studies by Charles Woody showed that cells in primary motor cortex demonstrated conditioning-dependent changes in activity and threshold in the eyeblink conditioning task. Considerable attention has focused on the development of long-term potentiation (LTP) and other cellular changes underlying alterations in excitability and in functional mappings of motor cortical cells as a function of learning (see Chapter 3).

Finally, the premotor areas may play a special role in conditional motor learning. This type of learning involves the acquisition of different motor responses to distinct stimulus conditions. Lesions of the premotor cortex in monkeys result in severe impairments in conditional motor learning tasks, but do not affect discrimination learning that involves only a single go/no-go response. Importantly, the other region especially important for conditional motor learning is the relay through the thalamus that brings striatal input to the frontal cortex. Parallel findings from neurophysiological studies confirm an important role for the premotor area in conditional motor learning. These studies involve recordings from single neurons in the premotor cortex of monkeys performing reaching or visual saccade tasks where distinct visual cues are associated with arbitrary arm or eye movement responses. The principal result of these studies is the appearance of visually evoked neural activity at the time when the correct conditional behavioral responses occur. These neurons did not respond to familiar and overlearned stimuli that signaled identical arm or eye movements. Many of these cells that developed responses during initial learning disappeared shortly after. These data suggest that the premotor cortex may be involved in the initial correct selection of responses associated with novel stimulus contingencies.

Summing up

The observations considered here indicate that procedural learning is mediated by a complex circuitry involving the motor cortical areas and two main subcortical loops, one through the striatum and another through the cerebellum. While we are still at a relatively early stage of understanding the brain circuits that support even the simpler forms of procedural learning, some distinctions are beginning to emerge. The motor cortex and surrounding premotor and somatosensory areas are involved in several forms of procedural learning. The striatum plays a critical role in habit learning, particularly in tasks involving the learning of specific responses or response sequences to specific stimuli. The critical circuitry includes cortical sensory input and direct motor outputs to mediate the association of stimuli with specific behavioral outputs. The role of the striatum is especially important in the acquisition of skills that require resolution of competition among multiple input or response options, particularly in tasks involving the learning of response sequences. This role becomes even more important in more "cognitive" tasks where temporal sequencing of information is involved. The cerebellum is critical to a variety of reflex adaptations that are played out in simple, direct form in conditioning situations, and may be fundamental parts of more complicated sequencing tasks. The critical anatomical components of this system involve brain stem sensory inputs and direct and indirect motor outputs, although connections with the cerebral cortex may be very important in the contribution of the cerebellum to higher aspects of learning. Timing is a critical aspect of the involvement of the cerebellum, and the fundamental contribution of the cerebellum may lie in its role in adjusting the timing of skeletal muscle movements in the course of adapting to new stimulus-response contingencies.

Whether the functional roles of the striatum and cerebellum in temporal sequencing are fundamentally the same, or are really quite different, is unclear. It is obvious that these areas have substantially different circuitries, and some studies have suggested dissociations in the functional roles of these systems. However, it is also clear that these structures, the motor cortex, and yet other structures not considered here, all modify their circuitries in the service of procedural memory. It is likely that the contributions of the two main subsystems, and other elements of motor systems in the brain, overlap in contributing to complex forms of procedural memory.

READINGS

Bloedel, J.R., Ebner, T.J., and Wise, S.P. (Eds.). *The Acquisition of Motor Behavior in Vertebrates*, Cambridge: MIT Press, pp. 289–302.
Cook, D., and Kesner, R.P. 1988. Caudate nucleus and memory for egocentric localization. *Behav. Neural Biol.* 49:332–343.

Graybiel, A.M. 1995. Building action repertoires: Memory and learning functions of the basal ganglia. *Curr. Opin. Neurobiol.* 5:733–741.

Houk, J.C., Davis, J.L., and Beiser, D.G. (Eds.). 1995. *Models of Information Processing in the Basal Ganglia.* Cambridge: MIT Press.

Byrne, J.H. 1997. The Cerebellum. Special Issues of *Learning and Memory* 3(6) & 3(7), Cold Spring Harbor Laboratory Press: Cold Spring Harbor, NY.

McDonald, R.J., and White, N.M. 1994. Parallel information processing in the water maze: Evidence for independent memory systems involving dorsal striatum and hippocampus. *Behav. Neural Biol.* 61:260–270.

Mink, J.W. 1996. The basal ganglia: Focused selection and inhibition of competing motor programs. *Prog. Neurobiol.* 50: 381–425.

Packard, M.G., and McGaugh, J.L. 1992. Double dissociation of fornix and caudate nucleus lesions on acquistion of two water maze tasks: Further evidence for multiple memory systems. *Behav. Neurosci.* 106:439–446.

Swanson, G. 1998. The Cerebellum—Development, Physiology and Plasticity. Special Issue of *Trends Cogn. Sci.* 2(9).

White, N.M. Mnemonic Functions of the Basal Ganglia.

Wise, S.P. 1996. The role of the basal ganglia in procedural memory. *The Neurosciences* 8:39–46.

Woodruf-pak, D.S. 1997. Classical conditioning. *Int. Rev. Neurobiol.* 41: 341–366.

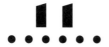

A Brain System for Emotional Memory

STUDY QUESTIONS

What is emotional memory?

What brain circuits mediate emotional expression and memory?

What circuitry in the amygdala makes it suited to play a central role in emotional perception, expression, and memory?

What is the range of emotional memories supported by this brain system?

One of my favorite memory experiences began when I entered an elevator in a busy downtown office building. I stepped in at the ground floor alone and pressed the button for the sixth floor where I had my upcoming appointment. At the second floor the elevator stopped for additional passengers. There were several, so I stepped to the back of the chamber to make room. The first passenger entering was a young woman who stopped just in front of me and turned around. I immediately noticed that she was wearing perfume, and it was a distantly familiar scent. As the next few seconds went by, I began to getting a great feeling of both familiarity and a sort of innocent sense of happiness. I found myself emotionally transported back to the "feeling" of high school. Within a few seconds, I began remembering girls I knew then, and then boys, too, classmates I hadn't thought of in many years. Finally, I fully recognized it—"Shalimar"—a perfume that was quite popular among teenagers in the early sixties. The latter specific recollections are run-of-the-mill declarative memories. But that initial "feeling of high school" was an example of emotional memory, an emotion evoked by a past association even before the conscious recollection of the experience that provoked it.

In this chapter our understanding of the brain pathways that mediate emotional experience and expression are reviewed. The early behavioral and anatomical studies identified specific brain areas, especially areas in the temporal lobe, that are involved in the appreciation of emotional cues and in the expression of emotional behaviors. Following this general review, I consider the current notion that some aspects of emotional memories involve a dedicated circuit of the brain that operates in parallel with other memory systems. In particular, it has been proposed that there is a specific memory system that mediates the learning and expression of emotional responses to stimuli of learned significance even in the absence of conscious memory for the events of the learning experience. Via this system, it is proposed, sometimes we can feel nervous or happy or scared at an image that evokes memory, even before, or independent of, our ability to declare the source of such feelings. This kind of learning is mediated by plasticity in components of the known pathways for emotional expression introduced earlier. Initially I consider the evidence for a specific system for the acquisition of learned fear, and then extend the review to consider whether the same brain system supports the acquisition and expression of a broad range of emotional associations.

The emergence of theories about brain pathways for emotional experience

The first theoretical proposal of a brain system for emotion was provided by James Papez in 1937. He postulated that sensory experiences took distinct pathways for "thought" and "feeling." The stream of thought, he proposed, involved channeling the sensory inputs from the thalamus to the wide expanse of the cerebral cortex on the lateral surface of the brain. The stream of feeling, he argued, followed a different path from the thalamus to the medial cortical areas known as the limbic lobe plus the neighboring hypothalamus. Based on gross anatomical evidence available at that time, Papez also speculated on the existence of a specific brain circuit for emotion (Fig. 11–1A). The system involves a *circular* sequence between several cortical and subcortical structures: The cingulate cortex, a major cortical division of the limbic lobe, connects to the hippocampal region. Then the hippocampus connects to an area of the hypothalamus called the mammilary bodies. Next the mammilary bodies connect to the anterior nuclei of the thalamus. These nuclei in turn project to the cingulate cortex, the beginning of the system, and so on around the circuit. Sensory in-

A. Papez circuit

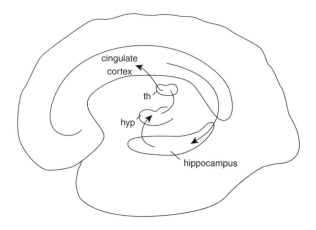

B. MacLean's limbic system

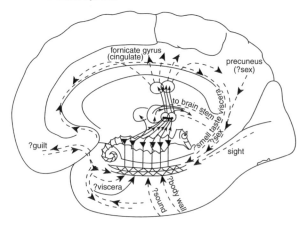

Figure 11–1. *A:* Pathway of the Papez circuit. *B:* Pathway of the limbic system as conceived by MacLean. In MacLean's illustration of the limbic system, the hippocampus is shown as a "seahorse" (hippocampus is Greek for seahorse). hyp = hypothalamus; th = thalamus.

puts from the posterior parts of the thalamus arrive into this circuit via either of two routes, either via inputs to the cingulate cortex from the lateral cortical areas that mediate the previously described "stream of thought" or from the posterior thalamus directly into the hypothalamus. Papez viewed the interactions between cortical and hypothalamic inputs as mediating the integration between cortical and subcortical processing of sensory inputs relevant to emotions. The outputs of this circuit course in two directions. One output is reflected by the cingulate cortex back to the stream of thought. The other output is via the hypothalamus to direct involuntary hormonal and autonomic nervous responses. The hormonal output route involves the release of stress hormones that activate the "fight or flight" response. The autonomic output route involves direct neural control over heart rate, blood pressure, and numerous other aspects of bodily regulation in the fight or flight response.

At around the same time, other evidence indicated a critical role for additional temporal lobe areas in emotion. In 1939 Kluver and Bucy described a syndrome of affective disorder following removal of the temporal lobe in monkeys. This disorder was characterized by "psychic blindness," which was observed mainly as a blunting of emotional reactions usually associated with fear of novel objects. Part of this disorder involved an impairment in object recognition known as agnosia. This part of the disorder is now associated with damage to the temporal cortex (see Chapter 7). Another part of the disorder, and the focus of this chapter, was the "taming" of these normally aggressive animals, as well as other abnormalities of social behavior. This part of the disorder has been attributed to the amygdala.

These distinct components of an emotional system in the brain were integrated into a more elaborate theoretical structure by Paul MacLean in 1949 (Fig. 11–1B). He combined the observations of Papez and Kluver and Bucy together with clinical observations on emotional disorders and electrophysiological evidence of internal organ sensory inputs to the hippocampus and other parts of the Papez circuit, arguing for the existence of a distinct "visceral brain," a system for regulation of internal organs. Using the full breadth of evidence from these various sources, MacLean expanded further on Papez's notion of distinct informational processing streams and on the anatomical components of the emotional system. He introduced the term "limbic system" as the anatomical designation of the emotional circuit and included within it Papez's circuit plus the amygdala, septum, and prefrontal cortex. MacLean proposed that the functional domain of this system encompassed all of emotional experience, from the role of lower brain stem structures in mediating instinctive and stereotyped behaviors, to that of the higher cortical areas in mediating real feelings.

Since then there have been numerous elaborations and modifications to the notion of the limbic system, and the boundaries of this system have become unclear. New anatomical evidence expanded the connections of the limbic system forward toward the frontal lobe and backward toward the midbrain. These interconnections are so strong that the anatomist

Walle Nauta proposed that we view this system as a continuum of structures throughout the entire brain. Interpretations about connections of the
classic limbic structures has today become so intertwined with those of
other brain systems such that today the term "limbic system" is somewhat
outmoded. This and other evidence brought into question whether the specific components of the limbic system were correctly identified, and indeed
whether one can circumscribe a complete and separate system for emotion. Nevertheless, more recent research has identified specific pathways
within the classic limbic system as critical elements in emotional output.
These are considered at some length next.

Pathways for emotional expression

Recent research has brought the focus on emotional memory specifically
to pathways through the amygdala. This is justly deserved because the
amygdala lies in a central position between cortical information processing, limbic circuitry, and hypothalamic outputs to the brain stem that mediate emotional responses. Thus, a brief summary of the organization of
the amygdala, including its main inputs, intrinsic connections, and outputs
is provided here (Fig. 11–2). The amygdala lies in the medial temporal

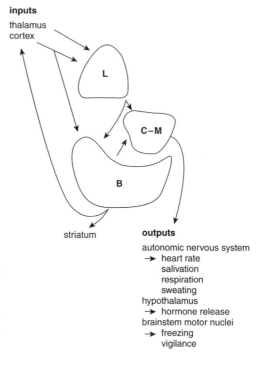

Figure 11–2. Schematic diagram of
some major inputs, outputs, and intrinsic circuitry of the amygdala. L =
lateral nucleus; C-M = centromedial
nucleus; B = basal (or basolateral)
nucleus.

lobe, just anterior to the hippocampus and surrounded by the parahip-pocampal cortical region. The amygdala involves a complex of many highly interconnected nuclei. The two most prominent major compartments are the group of nuclei that include the lateral nucleus and the basolateral complex, and the group of central and medial nuclei and their extensions. As it turns out, this division roughly corresponds to the major input and output sides of pathways of the amygdala. Thus, sensory inputs from the thalamus and cortex project mainly to the lateral and basolateral nuclei, whereas outputs of the amygdala to the cortex and subcortical areas orig-inate mainly in the central and medial nuclei.

Several studies have shown that the amygdala receives widespread sen-sory inputs from the thalamus and cerebral cortex. These are derived largely from gustatory, thoracic–abdominal (vagus nerve inputs), and au-ditory thalamic nuclei, but not the main somatosensory, or visual thala-mic nuclei. Cortical inputs are derived through the olfactory bulb and pir-iform (olfactory) cortex, plus higher-order sensory inputs from all sensory modalities via the entire cortex surrounding the rhinal sulcus (insular and perirhinal cortex). Joseph LeDoux and his colleagues have intensively stud-ied auditory inputs, and have shown that the main locus of input involves a convergence of thalamic and cortical projections to the lateral nucleus. In addition, the medial prefrontal cortex and hippocampal regions, specif-ically the subiculum and entorhinal cortex, send substantial inputs to the lateral nucleus. Some inputs, however, arrive in other amygdala nuclei. In particular, some of the olfactory inputs arrive mainly in the cortical nu-clei and the internal organ inputs arrive mainly in the central nuclei.

The intrinsic connectivity of amygdaloid nuclei is complex, and is char-acterized mainly by a distribution of connections from the lateral nucleus to the basal nuclear complex and central nucleus, which are also inter-connected. Thus, whatever segregation of inputs may have been preserved at the input stage is likely lost within the amygdala where all the inputs are mixed.

The amygdala has several output pathways that direct a widespread influence of emotional expression. Amygdala outputs to the cortex are largely derived indirectly from several nuclei to components of the thala-mus, in particular the mediodorsal nucleus. The basal nuclear complex sends direct outputs to several cortical areas, including the perirhinal, en-torhinal, and prefrontal areas. In addition, the amygdala projects heavily to multiple basal forebrain areas that secondarily influence widespread cor-tical areas. Also, the basal amygdaloid nuclei project to components of the substantia nigra and striatum, and to the subiculum (a part of the hip-pocampus). Other subcortical targets of amygdala output are directed mainly from the central and medial nuclei to the substantia nigra, lateral hypothalamus, and to several brain stem motor, autonomic (vagus nerve), and endocrine effector areas. This complicated scheme of outputs supports a correspondingly broad range of emotional responses that are generated by direct electrical stimulation of amygdala and are observed in the syndrome of behaviors associated with emotional experience. High emotional states induce increases in heart rate and respiration, decreased salivation, urination and defecation, and increased vigilance and freezing.

These pathways are complicated, but the bottom line is that these anatomical facts tell us the amygdala is the recipient of multimodal information about both lower-order visceral structures of the body as well as the crude sensory inputs from thalamus and higher-order sensory information originating in the cortex. The internal connectivity within the amygdala combines these inputs. This conclusion about the inputs and synthesis of sensory information is supported by physiological studies showing that single neurons in the amygdala respond to complex multimodal, affectively significant stimuli. On the output side, the amygdala orchestrates an enormous range of influences on behavior. These include influences back to the thalamic and cortical areas that provided sensory input, plus direct influences onto other systems important for different forms of memory, specifically the striatum and hippocampal regions. In addition, there are direct outputs from the amygdala to the autonomic, endocrine, and motor systems that generate diverse aspects of emotional expression.

The amygdala and emotional expression

Following Kluver and Bucy's initial reports of the "blunting" of affect in monkeys with temporal lobe damage including the amygdala, several studies have shown that selective amygdala damage results in a syndrome characterized by decreases in responsivity to affective stimuli. After amygdalotomy, monkeys fail to respond differentially to a wide range of painful shock intensities, and are poor at temperature discrimination. These animals also fail to show classic "orienting responses" to unexpected salient noises or visual stimuli, which normally include changes in heart rate and respiration. These animals also have a diminished galvanic skin response, the change in skin resistance associated with sweating. Monkeys with amygdala damage also demonstrate diminished selectivity in feeding, diminished sensitivity to food deprivation, and depressed shifts in behavioral performance normally associated with changes to food reward magnitude or type of food reward. Parallel impairments in responsiveness to food reward alterations have been observed in rats with amygdala damage.

A study on the amnesic patient H.M., whose surgical damage to the medial temporal lobe included removal of the amygdala bilaterally, provides confirmation of the blunting of affective responsiveness in humans with amygdala damage, and offers some further insights into the nature of this disorder. In the clinical setting, H.M. was known not to complain about normally painful conditions including hemorrhoids, and did not produce a normal skin-resistance change to electrical stimulation. He also was noted to rarely mention being hungry even when his meals were delayed, but he otherwise ate in a normal manner when given a meal. These observations were followed up in a systematic study of H.M.'s responsiveness to pain and hunger. In this study H.M's responses to thermal stimulation were compared to those of control subjects and amnesic patients without amygdala damage. H.M. showed a diminished ability to discriminate painful stimulation. Most prominent was his failure to identify any of the thermal stimuli as "painful" no matter how intense they were. By comparison, other amnesic patients without amygdala damage did not show loss of pain discrimination and were as likely as normal subjects to label the stimuli as painful. So, it does not appear that H.M.'s impairment in pain perception was secondary to his memory deficit.

A further experiment to characterize H.M.'s appreciation of hunger involved an assessment of his reaction to eating multiple dinners. Initially H.M. was asked to rate his hunger on a scale of 0 to 100, with 0 identified as "famished" and 100 identified as "too full to eat another bite." Just before dinner, H.M. rated his hunger level as 50. He was served a full meal and again rated his hunger level as 50. After a short rest period filled with conversation, by prearrangement with a dietician, he was served another full dinner as if the first had not occurred. As expected, H.M. had forgotten eating dinner and began eating the second meal at his usual slow, steady pace. However, he stopped before completing the meal, leaving his salad and cake. When asked about his break, H.M. remarked that he couldn't decide which to eat, and upon prompting why, simply decided to eat the cake. Following this he also rated his hunger level at 50. When probed further why he had not fully completed the second meal, H.M. would only say he was "finished," but would not characterize himself as "full" or "stuffed." In a separate set of ratings taken before and after regular meals, both amnesic patients and normal controls consistently rated themselves as less hungry and thirsty after meals, but H.M. showed small and inconsistent changes in his hunger rating. These findings were interpreted as demonstrating that, while there is evidence of modest decrease in sensitivity, the major effect of his surgery was diminished ability to access information about his internal states. Because this impairment was not observed in other amnesic patients without involvement of the amygdala, H.M.'s deficit was attributed to amygdala damage per se.

More recent studies on the role of the human amygdala in the perception of affective stimuli have focused on responses to faces. Several studies have now shown that bilateral damage to the amygdala results in impaired recognition of emotional expressions in pictures of human faces. These studies assessed the recognition of various facial expressions by human subjects with unilateral or bilateral removal of the amygdala and by one subject (S.M.) with a rare disorder known as Urbach-Wiethe disease, which is associated with calcification of the amygdala sparing the neighboring cortex and hippocampus (this disorder is introduced in Chapter 8). S.M. showed a selective impairment in recognizing facial expressions of fear, surprise, and anger. Also, S.M. showed a deficit in the normal capacity for recognizing similarities among different emotions expressed by others. In contrast, S.M. showed no general deficits in language, memory, or perception. She was able to recognize familiar faces, even ones not seen in considerable time. Furthermore, S.M. did perceive fearful faces as expressing emotion, but refused to characterize the expression as fearful, leading the investigators to conclude she could perceive the facial expression but that it did not activate responses associated with fear. The observation of inability to appreciate emotional expression is remarkably similar to H.M.'s emotional perception deficit, but without the accompanying memory impairment.

These findings are consistent with electrophysiological data showing that neurons in the amygdala respond to faces in both monkeys and humans. In addition, a recent brain imaging study using fMRI showed that the amygdala is preferentially active in response to viewing fearful versus neutral faces, although some response to other facial expressions over that of neutral expressions was also observed. These data bring into focus the importance of the amygdala as a critical part of a specialized system for the analysis of affective information and for the expression of emotional output.

Evidence for a dedicated emotional memory system

How is memory for emotions different from declarative memory? Certainly we do consciously recall emotional experiences, so these clearly can be a part of our declarative memories. However, there is also substantial emerging evidence that some aspects or types of emotional memory are accomplished by a distinct brain system, parallel to the system for declarative memory—this is the subject of the remainder of this chapter.

In a classic case study of amnesia performed in 1911, a neurologist named Cleparede pricked the hand of an unsuspecting patient with

Korsakoff disease. Subsequently, she refused to shake Cleparede's hand, although she could not recall the painful incident. Later, Antonio Damasio and colleagues described intact affective learning in their amnesic patient Boswell. Even though he could not learn to recognize the hospital staff, he consistently claimed he liked those with whom he had repeated positive encounters over those with whom he had negative encounters. In another study, amnesic patients were presented with pictures and biographical descriptions of two individuals, one characterized positively and the other negatively. Normal subjects preferred the positively described individual, and based this on their recall of the biographical information. Amnesic patients could not recall the individual or descriptions, but showed a strong preference for the "good guy." These and other case studies show that memory for emotional aspects of experiences can indeed be dissociated from declarative memory for the same experiences in amnesic patients.

Other findings from studies on normal human subjects provide an additional line of evidence that affective memory can occur independently of declarative memory. Perhaps most prominent among examples of unconscious affective memory is the "mere exposure" effect described by Robert Zajonc and his colleagues. They found that exposure to words, faces, and other stimuli produced a preference for the familiar items, even if the stimuli were not explicitly remembered. In some of these studies, the stimuli were even presented subliminally, so that their presentation did not reach consciousness. Nevertheless, subjects subsequently showed a preference for the stimuli that they had briefly experienced. These findings reflect the operation of an emotional system in the brain that can perceive and store information that is not adequately salient to reach attention and engage the declarative memory system. Furthermore, the mere exposure effect may reflect the operation of the emotional memory system in normal subjects in the same way it does in amnesic subjects who have a compromised declarative memory system. The identification and analysis of the critical elements of the emotional memory system have now proceeded to an extent that a preliminary understanding of its operation is available.

A brain system for emotional memory

Many laboratories have studied a variety of forms of emotional memory, and have focused on somewhat different brain areas and circuits, as well as different aspects of motivation and emotion that affect learning mechanisms. This section reviews a few prominent examples of circuit analyses of the brain system for emotional expression.

Perhaps the best studied example of emotional memory involves the brain system that mediates Pavlovian fear conditioning as studied by Joseph

LeDoux and by Michael Davis and their colleagues. This research has focused on the specific elements of the pathways through the amygdala that
support the learning of fearful responses to a simple auditory stimulus.
The critical elements of the relevant amygdala pathways include auditory
sensory inputs via the brain stem to circuits through the thalamus (Fig.
11–3A). Some of these auditory thalamic areas then project directly to the

A. pathway for fear conditioning

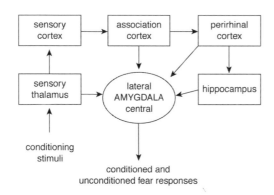

B. protocol

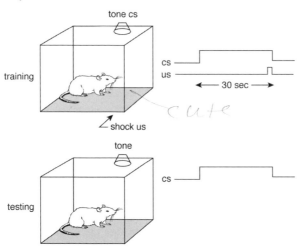

Figure 11–3. A: LeDoux's schematic diagram of a brain system for fear conditioning.
Signals from the conditioned stimulus can reach the lateral amygdala at several stages
of information processing. They converge in the lateral amygdala, which controls the
output of conditioned responses. *B:* The procedure for fear conditioning. During training, rats are placed in a chamber where a tone is presented for several seconds punctuated by a brief foot shock. During testing the tone is presented again, and the amount
of freezing, or other aspects of fear, are measured.

lateral amygdaloid nucleus. The other circuit involves auditory inputs to another part of the thalamus which projects to the primary auditory area of temporal cortex. This cortical area in turn projects to secondary temporal areas and the perirhinal cortex. These secondary auditory cortical areas are the source of cortical inputs to the amygdala, particularly the lateral and basolateral nuclei of this structure. Those areas of the amygdala project into the central nucleus, which is the source of outputs to subcortical areas controlling a broad range of fear-related behaviors, including autonomic and motor responses.

Learning to fear

LeDoux and colleagues have focused on the input side of these circuits. Their studies have examined the neuropsychology and neurophysiology of these structures in animals during the course of a simple tone-cued fear conditioning task (Fig. 11–3B). Rats are initially habituated to an operant chamber, then presented with multiple pairings of a prolonged pure tone terminating with a brief electric shock delivered through the floor of the cage. Subsequently, conditioned fear was assessed by measuring responses to the tone, including autonomic responses, such as changes in arterial pressure, and stereotypic behaviors, such as crouching or freezing. Unconditioned responses to the tone were evaluated by presenting other animals with unpaired tones and shocks. Under these conditions, the shocks produce the same set of autonomic and behavioral responses, but the tones do not acquire the capacity to evoke the responses.

Their initial experiments were aimed at identifying the critical input pathway to the amygdala. Animals with selective lesions in the lateral amygdala show dramatically reduced conditioned responses to the tone, both in the measures of autonomic and motor responses. Unconditioned responses consequent to unpaired presentations were not affected by this damage. Also, animals with damage to the adjacent striatum performed normally, showing anatomical specificity and confirming that the striatal system is not involved in emotional learning.

Subsequent efforts focused on identifying which of the two prominent auditory input pathways to the lateral amygdala was critical. Broad destruction of all auditory areas of the thalamus eliminated conditioned responses. However, selective ablation of either of the two prominent direct inputs to the lateral amygdala were individually ineffective. Lesions of the medial division of the medial geniculate, including all three nuclei that project directly to the lateral amygdala, *or* of the entire auditory cortex that projects to the amygdala did not reduce either the autonomic or freezing response. However, elimination of *both* of these inputs produced the full effect seen after lateral amygdala lesions. Thus, for this simple type of conditioning, either the direct thalamic input, which offers a crude identification of a sound, or the thalamocortical input pathway, which provides a sophisticated identification of auditory signal, is sufficient to mediate conditioning.

Additional experiments were aimed at another component of fear conditioning observed in these studies. After conditioning, when rats are replaced in the conditioning chamber, they begin to freeze even before the tone is presented. Thus, rats appear to condition both to the tone and to the environmental context in which tones and shock have previously been paired. This "contextual" fear conditioning is selective to the environment in which conditioning occurs. Furthermore, contextual fear conditioning can be dissociated from conditioning to the tone by presenting the conditioned tones in a different environment. Trained animals do not freeze prior to tone presentation in the unfamiliar environment, but do freeze when the tone is presented.

Moreover, contextual fear conditioning is mediated by a different pathway than tone-cued fear conditioning. To demonstrate this, the animals were trained on the standard version of the task, then their expression of memory was assessed both immediately after the rats were placed in the conditioning chamber and then subsequently in response to the tone. Amygdala lesions blocked conditioned freezing to both the context and the tone. By contrast, damage to the hippocampus selectively blocked contextual fear conditioning, sparing the conditioned response to the tone.

These data combined with the known anatomy of these brain structures demonstrate that the full set of circuits mediating fear conditioning in this task involves a set of parallel and serial pathways to the amygdala (see Fig. 11–3A). The most direct pathway is from areas within the auditory thalamus. A secondary path through the auditory thalamocortical circuit can also mediate tone-cued conditioning. Contextual fear conditioning involves a yet more indirect pathway by which multimodal information arrives in the hippocampus and is sent to the amygdala via the subiculum.

Additional studies by LeDoux and colleagues have elucidated the physiology of the neurons in the direct thalamic and thalamocortical auditory pathways to the amygdala. Cells in both the medial geniculate nuclei that project directly to the amygdala and in the thalamic nucleus that projects to the cortex demonstrate a variety of auditory responses. Finer auditory tuning was observed in the ventral medial geniculate than in areas that project directly to the amygdala. However, cells in the ventral nucleus responded only to auditory stimuli, whereas neurons in the medial geniculate nuclei that project to the amygdala also responded to foot shock stim-

rsency affect

ulation. Furthermore, some amygdala-projecting cells that responded to somatosensory stimulation but not auditory stimulation showed potentiated responses to simultaneous presentation of both stimuli.

In the amygdala, cells in the lateral nucleus that receives thalamic input were responsive to auditory stimuli at both short (12–25 msec) and long (60–150 msec) latencies. Some cells had clear tuning curves, whereas others responded to a broad spectrum of sounds. Cells in the lateral amygdala could also be driven by electrical stimulation of the medial geniculate, and their responses were typically shorter than those in the basolateral amygdala. In addition, LeDoux and colleagues have provided several lines of evidence suggesting that direct medial geniculate–lateral amygdala inputs exhibit learning related plasticity, including evidence for alterations in synaptic efficacy (see Chapter 3). At the level of neuronal firing patterns, fear conditioning selectively enhances the short latency auditory responses of lateral amygdala neurons. Furthermore, some cells that were not responsive to tones prior to training showed postconditioning short latency responses.

The potentiation of startle by learned fear

Michael Davis and his colleagues have investigated a different form of fear conditioning, and have provided an extensive line of evidence that runs in parallel with LeDoux and colleagues' findings, and involves much of the same brain circuit (Fig. 11–4A). Davis's research focuses on a simple behavioral response known as startle, the jump or other sudden movement performed by animals and people in response to an unexpected salient stimulus such as a loud sound. Their examination of fear learning in this situation is derived from the observation that when animals or people are in a fearful state, the startle response is magnified, and so their fear conditioning paradigm is known as *fear-potentiated startle*. All of us have experienced this phenomenon, for example, when we jump at a sudden noise that occurs while listening to a scary story.

In the formal laboratory version of this task, animals are initially exposed to pairings of a light or a tone with foot shock. Subsequently, their startle reflex to a loud noise is evaluated in the presence or absence of the conditioned stimulus. When the conditioned light or tone is present, the startle reflex is considerably augmented (Fig. 11–4B). Potentiated acoustic startle does not occur if the animal is pre-exposed to *un*paired presentations of the light or tone and shock, and is thus as valid a measure of fear conditioned to the tone or light. The brain pathway for fear-potentiated startle contains many of the same elements of the amygdala circuit studied by LeDoux and colleagues (Fig. 11–4A). An important advantage of

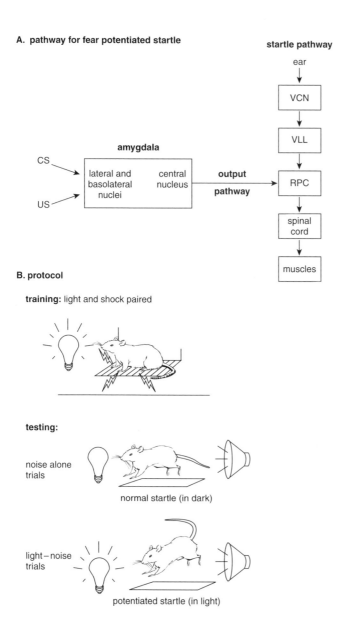

A. pathway for fear potentiated startle

startle pathway

ear

VCN

VLL

amygdala

CS

| lateral and basolateral nuclei | central nucleus |

US

output

pathway

RPC

spinal cord

muscles

B. protocol

training: light and shock paired

testing:

noise alone trials

normal startle (in dark)

light–noise trials

potentiated startle (in light)

Figure 11–4. A: Davis's schematic diagram of a brain pathway that mediates the potentiation of the acoustic startle response. CS = conditioned stimulus; RPC = caudal nucleus of the pontine reticular area; VCN = ventral cochlear nucleus; VLL = ventral nucleus of the lateral leminiscus; US = unconditioned stimulus. B: The protocol for training and testing in fear potentiation of startle.

• 275

the fear-potentiated startle paradigm is that the startle response can be measured independently of the influence of conditioned fear, allowing a rigorous analysis of the effects of manipulations on the fear component of the task as distinct from the behavioral response (startle) per se.

Davis and colleagues have independently demonstrated the importance of the amygdala in fear conditioning, showing that lesions of the lateral or basal amygdala or the central amygdala nucleus prevent conditioning and abolish expression of previously learned acoustic startle responses. Correspondingly, they found that electrical stimulation of the amygdala enhances acoustic startle.

Furthermore, Davis and his colleagues have shown that N-methyl-D-aspartate (NMDA)-dependent plasticity (see Chapter 3) in the amygdala is critical for the development of fear conditioning, but not for the expression of already learned fear responses. Thus, application of the NMDA receptor blocker AP5 prior to training prevents conditioning, but similar treatment after conditioning or prior to testing has no effect on later expression of potentiated acoustic startle. To further address the possibility that NMDA receptors are directly involved in the expression of conditioned fear, rats were initially conditioned to fear a "primary" conditioned stimulus (CS) and then subsequently trained to fear a second stimulus paired with the primary CS. AP5 infused into the amygdala during the final "second-order" conditioning stage actually enhanced the fear expression to the previously conditioned primary CS while at the same time preventing the second-order conditioning. This finding strongly supports the conclusion that NMDA receptors are differentially involved in plasticity of startle but not in the performance of potentiated startle.

Davis and colleagues have also extended our understanding of the specific input and output pathways of fear conditioning. They found that ablation of the auditory thalamus blocks tone-cued fear-potentiated startle, sparing visually cued potentiated startle. However, ablation of the perirhinal cortex eliminates previous conditioning in either modality, suggesting that the cortical pathway through this area is normally predominant. Like LeDoux and colleagues, Davis has shown that tone-cued conditioning can be supported by the direct thalamic pathway as well.

Other studies of Davis and colleagues have focused on identifying the critical output circuitry for fear-potentiated startle. These studies have shown that interruption of the pathway from the amygdala via the ventral output pathway to caudal brain stem regions to the nucleus reticularis pontis oralis constitutes the critical circuit for expression of potentiated startle.

Is the amygdala part of a general system
for emotional memory?

The notion that the amygdala is central to associating rewards, as well as fear, with stimuli has been traced to Lawrence Weiskrantz's observations in the 1950s on monkeys with amygdala lesions: ". . . the effect of amygdalectomy, it is suggested, is to make it difficult for reinforcing stimuli, whether positive or negative, to become established and recognized as such" (p. 390). Many amygdala neurons respond differentially to rewarded stimuli. Neurophysiological data showing strongly held reward-related responses, and their relation to unlearned reinforcing stimuli, have supported the view that the amygdala maintains neural representations of stimulus–reward associations. Thus, the notion that the amygdala plays a critical role in mediating stimulus–reward associations is widely held.

Yet, in studies on learning after damage to the amygdala, this notion has proven difficult to establish unambiguously in experimental analyses. Thus, the findings across a broad variety of learning tasks have indicated that amygdala lesions sometimes result in impairments in simple stimulus–reward learning tasks and sometimes do not. In addition, some studies have specifically contrasted the importance of the amygdala in appetitive and aversive learning. However, based on their experiment described in Chapter 9, McDonald and White suggested that the mixture of results may be explained by distinguishing cases where learning can be mediated by the establishment of stimulus–response associations even in the absence of normal stimulus–reward associations. Thus, in most simple conditioning and discrimination tasks, animals are rewarded for producing a specific behavior, for example, a choice and approach toward a particular stimulus. In such cases, they argue, two kinds of learning occur in parallel. In one type of learning, the positive reinforcer increases the likelihood of the behavioral response that preceded it—this is accomplished by brain systems that do not involve the amygdala. In particular, in McDonald and White's study of different forms of radial maze learning, animals with amygdala lesions normally acquired consistent approach responses to illuminated maze arms when specifically rewarded for such approach behaviors. In the other type of learning, the positive reinforcer enhances the attractive value of stimuli with which it is associated. In their study McDonald and White avoided the conditioning of habitual response by using a different training protocol (conditioned place preference) that involved simply feeding animals in an illuminated maze arm, with no requirement for an approach behavior. In this situation, amygdala lesions blocked the subsequent conditioned place preference. The distinction between stimulus–response and stimulus–reinforcer associations was made particularly compelling by the demonstration that striatal lesions had the opposite pattern of effects, blocking the learning of approach responses but not affecting the conditioned place preference.

Another behavioral paradigm that distinguished stimulus–reward from stimulus–response associations is "second-order conditioning," a procedure in which animals are first trained to associate a stimulus with reward, and then that stimulus is used as a reinforcer for subsequent conditioning. In an experiment by Barry Everitt and Trevor Robbins, thirsty rats were trained to associate a visual stimulus with their approach to a dispenser where they received water. Subsequently, they were trained to discriminate between two levers, one followed by the visual stimulus and an empty water dispenser, as a second-order reinforcer, and the other lever inactive. Normal animals pressed both levers somewhat, and much more on the lever associated with the second-order reinforcer. Amygdala lesions reduced responding on the lever associated with the second-order reinforcer to the same low level as that associated with the alternate lever. These findings are consistent with McDonald and White's proposal that simple stimulus–response learning is intact in animals with amygdala lesions, but they cannot differentially associate a specific lever with its acquired reinforcing properties. Similar results were obtained using second-order conditioning to a sexual reinforcer. Initially, male rats were allowed to interact sexually with a female in the presence of a visual stimulus (a light). Subsequently, the male rats were trained to bar press in the presence of the light. Normal animals bar press at high rates for this second-order reinforcer, and amygdala lesions reduced responding in that situation.

The same pattern of results has been obtained in experiments on monkeys. Amygdala lesions have no effect on traditional forms of simple discrimination learning. However, impairments have been observed in the acquisition of preferences to novel foods and when the animals must change responses to shifting reward contingencies. In addition, amygdala lesions interfere with the acquisition of a visual discrimination associated with a secondary auditory reinforcer. In an experiment performed by David Gaffan and his colleagues, intact monkeys were initially trained on visual discriminations in which the food reward was given along with an auditory stimulus. Following damage to the amygdala they were trained on new discrimination problems in which responses to one stimulus were followed by the second-order auditory reinforcer, and food reward was given only upon completion of the task. Amygdala damage severely retarded learning. In addition, disconnection of the amygdala from auditory input had the same effect, but disconnection of the amygdala from visual association cortex had no effect on this type of learning. These results confirm the findings on second-order conditioning in rats, and support the view that the effect of amygdala damage is to block the association between the primary reinforcer (food) and secondary reinforcer (auditory cue), but not the associations between the visual stimuli and the secondary reinforcer.

Additional evidence of the notion that the amygdala mediates stimulus–reward associations comes from an experiment performed by Raymond Kesner in which rats were presented with either one or seven pieces of food on different arms of a radial maze. After a delay period they could obtain an additional reward by choosing the arm with the larger reward. In this task, lesions of the basolateral nucleus had no effect, but lesions of the central nucleus produced a severe, delay-dependent deficit in memory for reward magnitude. This result confirms the role of the amygdala in affective discrimination and suggests a specific role for the central nucleus in this aspect of emotional learning.

Other experiments have also explored whether there are distinct pathways within or through the amygdala that support different types of stimulus-reinforcer learning. On the one hand, anatomical evidence indicates that the main sensory inputs to the amygdala arrive via the lateral, and to some extent the basolateral, nuclei, and that the main outputs are from the central nucleus. This suggests that damage to either set of nuclei would necessarily have similar effects on learning. However, there have been several reports that lesions within these amygdala nuclei have dissociable effects on performance in different tasks, making it tempting to speculate on the possibility that the minor inputs to all the amygdala nuclei, combined with the divergent output pathways, might support different forms of affective learning and memory.

The learning versus performance distinction

One final issue of importance to the analysis of the emotional memory system (as well as to the procedural memory system) is the extent to which one can distinguish the role of the amygdala and other structures in memory per se, as opposed to its role in emotional expression. This issue has most recently been brought to the forefront in comments by Larry Cahill and colleagues (1999), who have questioned the findings on the emotional memory system. In particular, they challenged the conclusion that lesions of the amygdala block conditioned fear responses, citing considerable evidence that indicates that amygdala lesions interfere with the expression of unconditioned as well as conditioned fear responses (see section on The amygdala and emotional expression). This suggests that the lesions affect performance functions of the amygdala but have no special role in blocking emotional memory. This alternative interpretation highlights the difficulty of identifying critical plasticity mechanisms within brain structures that are essential to performance functions involved in memory expression. However, two studies have addressed this criticism, with compelling results. One study, introduced previously, used the second-order conditioning test to show a sparing of a simple conditioned emotional response (fear-potentiated startle), in contrast to a total blocking of a second-order conditioned response. In a more recent study, Wallace and Rosen assessed freezing behavior of rats in contextual fear conditioning as well as unconditioned fear responses to a predator odor. Damage to the lateral amygdala using a toxin that selectively destroys cells in that region did not affect unconditioned freezing to the foot shocks, nor did this type of selective damage diminish unconditioned freezing to the predator odor. However, these lesions did produce an impairment in conditioned freezing. The combination of these studies, each involving the application of sophisticated behavioral and anatomical techniques, provides strong evidence favoring the view that a critical component of the emotional memory trace is formed in the amygdala.

Summing up

There is a distinct brain system that mediates the perception and appreciation of emotional stimuli as well as emotional expression. The system involves a complex set of cortical and subcortical areas in widespread areas of the brain. Recently, several studies have focused on the amygdala as a critical element of emotional perception and expression. The lateral and basolateral components of the amygdala receive both subcortical and cortical sensory inputs from both visceral and external stimuli. The central and basal nuclei send a broad range of outputs back to cortical areas, to subcortical areas involved in other memory systems and behavior, and to autonomic system and brain stem outputs for the expression of emotion through a variety of systems. Damage to the amygdala results in selective impairments in emotional perception and appreciation, as well as emotional expression in humans and animals.

There is substantial evidence that plasticity within this same brain system supports emotional memory in the absence of conscious recollection. The critical brain system involves pathways through the amygdala that are enhanced during emotional learning, leading to the appearance of emotional expression to previously neutral stimuli. This system mediates fear conditioning and the modulation of other behaviors by conditioned fear (e.g., fear-potentiated startle). The same system supports learned attractions, and there may be multiple distinct pathways through the system that support different aspects of learned emotional expression.

READINGS

Adolphs, R., Tranel, D., Damasio, H., and Damasio, A. 1994. Impaired recognition of emotion in facial expressions following bilateral damage to the human amygdala. *Nature*. 372:669–672.

Aggleton, J.P. (Ed.). 1992. *The Amygdala: Neurobiological Aspects of Emotion, Memory and Mental Dysfunction*. New York: Wiley-Liss.

Cahill, L., Weinberger, N., Roozendaal, B., and McGaugh, J.L. 1999. Is the amygdala a locus of conditioned fear? Some questions and caveats. *Neuron* 23: 227–228.

Damasio, A.R., Tranel, D., and Damasio, H. 1989. Amnesia caused by herpes simplex encephalitis, infarctions in basal forebrain, Alzheimer's disease and anoxia/ischemia. In *Handbook of Neuropsychology*, Vol. 3. F. Boller, and J. Grafman, (Eds.). Amsterdam: Elsevier.

Davis, M., Walker, D.L., and Lee Y. 1999. Neurophysiology and neuropharmacology of startle and its affective modulation. In *Startle Modification: Implications for Neuroscience, Cognitive Science, and Clinical Science*. M.E. Dawson, A.M. Schell, and A.H. Bohmelt, (Eds.). Cambridge University Press, pp. 95–113.

Gerwitz, J.C., and Davis, M. 1997. Second-order fear conditioning prevented by blocking NMDA receptors in the amygdala. *Nature* 388: 471–474.

Hebben, N., Corkin, S., Eichenbaum, H., and Shedlack, K. 1985. Diminished ability to interpret and report internal states after bilateral medial temporal resection: Case H.M. *Behav. Neurosci.* 99:1031–1039.

Kesner, R.P. 1992. Learning and memory in rats with an emphasis on the role of the amygdala. In *The Amygdala: Neurobiological Aspects of Emotion, Memory, and Mental Dysfunction*. J.P. Aggleton, (Ed.). New York: Wiley-Liss, pp. 379–399.

LeDoux, J. 1996. *The Emotional Brain*. New York: Simon & Schuster.

Wallace, K.J., and Rosen, J.B. 2001. Neurotoxic lesions of the lateral nucleus of the amygdala decrease conditioned fear but not unconditioned fear of a predator odor: Comparison with electrolytic lesions. *J. Neurosci.* 21:3619–3627.

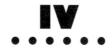

IV

CONSOLIDATION:
THE FIXATION AND
REORGANIZATION OF MEMORIES

Memory consolidation is the name given to the hypothetical process or set of processes by which new memories make a transition from an initially labile state to become permanently fixed for the long term. As introduced in Chapter 1, the notion of consolidation was first proposed formally in 1900 by Muller and Pilzecker, to account for the decrement in human memory performance caused by the presentation of other material shortly after exposure to the to-be-remembered items. They suggested that this memory phenomenon reflected the disruption, by the intervening material, of physiological activity that fixes associations established during learning. Until those associations were fixed, or *consolidated*, memory would be susceptible to disruption. The connection between these experiments and the observation of retrograde amnesia following brain trauma—impairment of memories acquired prior to the trauma—was made shortly thereafter. Burnham proposed that consolidation involves a time-consuming "process of organization" of newly obtained memories through some combination of physical reorganization and psychological processes of repetition and association. Accordingly, he proposed that retrograde amnesia was a consequence of interrupted organizational processing, which must normally occur for a considerable period of time after learning. Other, more physiologically based conceptions followed. In particular, the notion that the physical reorganization involved networks of neurons interacting for long periods was captured prominently in Hebb's concept of reverberating activity by cell assemblies.

Reverberation may well contribute to consolidation processes that last several seconds or even minutes, and might mediate or facilitate cellular and molecular processes that are initiated by brain activity (see Chapters

2 and 3). But it is difficult to conceive that a substantial level of meaningful neural activity can be sustained independent of other brain activities for days or months-long consolidation processes indicated by the findings on retrograde amnesia described in Chapter 1. So, instead, it is commonly accepted that another kind of processing must support prolonged processes in consolidation. The following chapter considers the evidence that there are indeed two major stages or forms of consolidation.

12

Two Distinct Stages of Memory Consolidation

STUDY QUESTIONS

What is memory consolidation? Are there different kinds of consolidation?

What are the steps in memory fixation? How is fixation modulated?

What memory system accomplishes the prolonged reorganization of memory following new experiences? What is the nature of that reorganization?

The term consolidation has been used in two ways in the memory literature. These two conceptions differ both in the presumed mechanisms that mediate consolidation and in the time scale of the relevant events. This difference has led to the view that there are two aspects of, or two kinds of consolidation, one that involves a *fixation* of memory within synapses over a period of minutes or hours, and another that involves a *reorganization* of memories that occurs over weeks to years.

Cellular events that mediate memory fixation

One approach to consolidation treats the phenomenon as a cascade of molecular and microstructural events by which short-term synaptic modifications lead to permanent changes in connectivity between neurons. These events are intended to capture the transition of memories from a short-term store to long-term memory, on a time scale of seconds and minutes. In principle these events can occur in any brain structure that participates in memory. Molecular events that mediate the formation of permanent structural changes associated with memory have been studied in a broad variety of invertebrate and mammalian brain structures that participate in memory.

The details of this work were described in Chapters 2 and 3. However, a few general points are reiterated and extended here. Studies on this conceptualization of consolidation focus on local network neural activity, that is, on highly integrated "cell assemblies," and on intracellular events that initiate nuclear transcription mechanisms for protein synthesis. The consolidation hypothesis received little attention in the twentieth century until the later 1940s, when studies showed that electrical currents applied to the head sufficient to produce overt convulsions (electroconvulsive shock; used successfully to treat psychiatric disorders such as major depression) produced a retrograde amnesia.

This finding led to many experiments that were aimed at determining the time course and features of memory lost following this treatment or various pharmacological treatments. For example, several studies showed that blockade of gene expression at the level of mRNA or protein synthesis did not affect learning but prevented later retention if the treatment was given shortly after learning but not if treatment was delayed by several minutes or hours. That is, these manipulations produce a temporally graded retrograde amnesia, similar in form if not time course to the observations of retrograde amnesia following head injury, brain damage, or disease. More recent studies on the molecular mechanisms of long-term potentiation have renewed the focus on protein synthesis as required for permanent physiological and microstructural alterations consequent both to long-term potentiation (LTP) or to learning. These studies have identified specific proteins, for example, CREB, the increased synthesis of which are seen as candidates for critical events in the formation of LTP and of permanent memory. Such cellular events begin immediately with the learning experience, but continue to unfold during the minutes and hours after learning. Treatments that disrupt the activity of cell assemblies and the molecular cascade leading to new protein synthesis are effective only within this relatively brief period, suggesting the time scale that characterizes this sense or this conception of memory consolidation.

The effort to identify specific molecules and the full cascade of molecular and cellular events that underlie memory fixation continues to be an area of considerable current research. One potentially important recent observation suggests that memory fixation processes may be labile for a period extending beyond several hours. Nader and colleagues trained rats in the fear conditioning protocol and then confirmed their memory as long as 14 days after. Then they infused a protein synthesis inhibitor into the amygdala either immediately or delayed following the retention test. If the infusion occurred shortly after the first retention test, subsequent memory in a second retention test was impaired. Delayed infusions had no effect on subsequent retention. The authors concluded that the first retention test "reactivated" the fear memory and that this reactivation was followed by a "reconsolidation" phase that requires protein synthesis. Currently, the generality and mechanism of the reconsolidation effect are under intense scrutiny.

Another major area of progress in understanding the short-term phase of consolidation has been in characterizing neural mechanisms that modulate the cellular processes of fixation. These discoveries are described next.

Modulation of memory fixation

James McGaugh and his colleagues observed that stimulant drugs could enhance the short-term process of memory consolidation. For example, they reported that the central stimulant picrotoxin given shortly after learning would facilitate later retention performance, but treatment several minutes after learning had no effect. This result, and many like it, showed that the neural information processing or molecular mechanisms of memory fixation could be influenced during a fixation period that extended for at least several minutes.

This situation provides an opportunity for events surrounding or following a learning experience to have some effect on the fixation or organization of memories. One of these modulatory influences that has been most studied is generated by the arousing nature of emotional experiences. Such experiences increase our attention toward particularly salient events, and can consequently increase the processing of memories for events as they occur during the emotional experiences, and indeed this has been shown to be the case. Another modulatory influence involves increments in memory processing that occur *even after the learning experience itself is completed,* and therefore can have their effects on subsequent retention, suggesting they operate on aspects of memory consolidation *per se.* This later influence of emotional arousal on the memory fixation is the main topic of this chapter.

Influencing memory by hormonal activation associated with emotional arousal

Stressful events that activate the sympathetic nervous system and pituitary–adrenal axis result in the release of epinephrine and glucocorticoids by the adrenal glands. These hormones have a variety of effects associated with the "flight or fight" response, including increased heart rate and blood pressure, diversion of blood flow to the brain and muscles, and mobilization of energy stores. There is now a wealth of evidence that another effect of this activation is to improve memory storage for experiences surrounding stress activation, and that the amygdala is critical to this influence on memory.

Investigations on the facilitation of memory by adrenal hormone activation in animals have largely focused on a step-through inhibitory avoidance task and post-training injections of drugs. In this task rats are initially placed in a small well-illuminated chamber that is attached to a larger, dimly lit area. When a door separating these chambers opens, the rat typically steps through to the larger compartment, where the floor is subsequently electrified. After a brief period of foot shocks the animal is allowed to escape back to the small chamber. In later tests of memory for this aversive experience, the animal is again placed into the small chamber and its latency to step through measured. Thus, the effect of training is to inhibit subsequent entry into the aversive compartment.

Many of the studies of memory modulation involve the systemic injection or brain infusion of drugs after the initial learning, with the common result that subsequent memory performance is altered. These effects typically depend on post-training drug administration within minutes after training, and have no effect if postponed for an hour or more. The post-training administration procedure eliminates the possibility that the drugs are altering perception, arousal, or motor performance during the learning experience. Conversely, this methodology, combined with the time-dependency of efficacy of the drug administration, provides strong evidence that neurochemical events strongly influence the consolidation of memories for several minutes after new learning.

There is now extensive evidence that administration of epinephrine (also called adrenaline) or adrenal glucocorticoids improves memory for inhibitory avoidance, and that these effects are mediated by the amygdala. In an elegant systematic series of studies, McGaugh, Larry Cahill, and their colleagues have provided a framework for the pathway by which these effects are exerted (Fig. 12–1). They have provided substantial and compelling evidence accumulated through a combination of behavioral analyses, selective lesions of parts of this system, and drugs that facilitate (agonists) or retard (antagonists) neurotransmitter receptors that are involved in the cascade of modulatory events that is generated by glucocorticoid release.

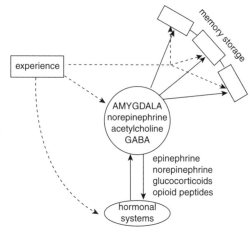

Figure 12–1. Schematic diagram of relationships between the amygdala and other systems, showing how the amygdala is influenced by hormonal systems and experience and can modulate memory storage in several memory systems.

According to their scheme, glucocorticoids released during stressful events, or administered by injection, can enter the blood brain barrier and influence receptors for this steroid in the brain directly. Epinephrine does not enter the blood brain barrier easily, however, and so it is likely that its effects are exerted via peripheral stimulation. This conclusion is supported by experiments showing that a β-adrenergic antagonist, a drug that blocks the β-subtype of epinephrine receptors, that does not pass the blood brain barrier blocks the memory-enhancing effects of epinephrine administration. The suspected target of peripheral epinephrine is β-adrenergic receptors on vagus nerve afferents that project to a brain stem area known as the nucleus of the solitary tract. This nucleus in turn projects into the amygdala where its afferents release norepinephrine (NE). This proposal is supported by studies showing that inactivation of the nucleus of the solitary tract by a local anesthetic blocks the effect of peripheral administration of epinephrine. In addition, other evidence shows that foot shock results in the release of NE within the amygdala. Furthermore, NE infused directly into the amygdala post-training enhances memory storage, and amygdala lesions or an NE antagonist infused into the amygdala block memory enhancement by peripheral epinephrine administration.

The effects of glucocorticoids on memory are remarkably similar to those of epinephrine. Peripheral treatment with glucocorticoids enhances memory, and this effect is blocked by lesions of outputs of the amygdala. The effect of glucocorticoids appears to be mediated selectively by the basolateral nucleus of the amygdala—a glucocorticoid receptor agonist infused into that nucleus, but not the central amygdala nucleus, enhances memory, and lesions of the basolateral nucleus, but not the central nucleus, block the memory-enhancing effects of glucocorticoids. Basolateral amygdala activation by glucocorticoids involves NE release, as shown by blockade of the effects of glucocorticoids by local infusion of a β-adrenergic antagonist. These responses of the amygdala are modulated by multiple other neurochemical systems. In particular, local infusions of agonists and antagonists of GABA (another neurotransmitter) and opioids (a type of neuromodulator) have demonstrated that these substances inhibit the release of NE in the amygdala and influence memory performance accordingly. In addition, other findings implicate a mechanism involving acetylcholine at a later synapse within the amygdala, providing yet another modulatory influence over this system.

Although most of the research on memory modulation involves the inhibitory avoidance task, consistent effects are observed on discrimination learning and maze learning tasks. In particular, one study has shown that these influences extend specifically to the types of memory mediated by the hippocampus and striatum. In this study, rats were trained on two different versions of the Morris water maze task, one in which learning was cued by a visible marker at the escape site, and the other where the platform was hidden (Fig. 12–2). In previous studies the same team had shown that learning the cued platform task depends on the striatum and learning the hidden platform task depends on the hippocampus. Animals were implanted bilaterally with cannuli in the striatum, hippocampus, or amygdala, then after recovery trained in a single session on one of the tasks. Post-training intrahippocampal infusions of d-amphetamine, which is an NE agonist, enhanced later retention on the spatial task, whereas intrastriatum infusions had no effect (Fig. 12–2A). Conversely, post-training intrastriatum infusions of d-amphetamine enhanced later retention on the cued task, whereas intrahippocampal infusions had no effect (Fig. 12–2B). Post-training intra-amygdala infusions of d-amphetamine enhanced retention on both tasks.

A follow-up study was conducted to examine whether the effect of amygdala infusions involved an influence on hippocampal and striatal mechanisms or whether the enhancement involved a direct involvement of the amygdala in performance. Animals were trained on the two versions of the task then given post-training injections of d-amphetamine into the amygdala, as in the first study. Then, prior to the retention testing, the amygdala was inactivated to eliminate the possibility that it was exerting a direct effect on retention performance. These inactivations did not block the enhancement effect, consistent with the view that the intra-amygdala infusions had exerted their effects via projections to the hippocampus and striatum.

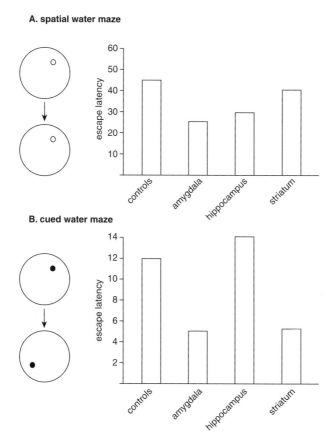

A. spatial water maze

B. cued water maze

Figure 12–2. The effects of d-amphetamine infused after training into the amygdala, hippocampus, or striatum on water maze retention. A: The spatial water maze task, where the position of a hidden platform is constant. B: The cued water maze task, trials where the position of a visible platform is varied across trials (data from Packard et al., 1994).

The amygdala also plays a role in enhancing memory in humans

Studies on human subjects have provided additional evidence that emotional arousal can affect different forms of memory and that this effect is mediated by the amygdala. In a series of experiments, Larry Cahill and his colleagues have examined the influence of emotional content on declarative memory. Their test involves presentation of a series of slides and a narrative that tell a story about a mother and son involved in a traumatic accident, or a control story with neutral emotional content (Fig. 12–3A). The story had three parts. In the beginning and end parts the emotional and neutral stories are similar and are low in emotional content. In

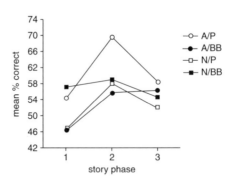

Narratives accompanying the slide presentation

	Neutral version	Arousal version
1.	A mother and her son are leaving home in the morning.	A mother and her son are leaving home in the morning.
2.	She is taking him to visit his father's workplace.	She is taking him to visit his father's workplace.
3.	The father is a laboratory technician at Victory Memorial hospital.	The father is a laboratory technician at Victory Memorial hospital.
4.	they check before crossing a busy road.	they check before crossing a busy road.
5.	While walking along, the boy sees some wrecked cars in a junkyard, which he finds interesting.	While crossing the road, the boy is caught in a terrible accident, which critically injures him.
6.	At the hospital, the staff are preparing for a practice disaster drill, which the boy will watch.	At the hospital, the staff prepares the emergency room, to which the boy is rushed.
7.	An image from a brain scan machine used in the drill attracts the boy's interest.	An image from a brain scan machine used in a trauma situation shows severe bleeding in the boy's brain.
8.	All morning long, a surgical team practiced the disaster drill procedures.	All morning long, a surgical team struggled to save the boy's life.
9.	Make-up artists were able to create realistic-looking injuries on actors for the drill.	Specialized surgeons were able to reattach the boy's severed feet.
10.	After the drill, while the father watched the boy, the mother left to phone her other child's preschool.	After the surgery, while the father stayed with the boy, the mother left to phone her other child's preschool.
11.	Running a little late, she phones the preschool to tell them she will soon pick up her child.	Feeling distraught, she phones the preschool to tell them she will soon pick up her child.
12.	Heading to pick up her child, she hails a taxi at the number 9 bus stop.	Heading to pick up her child, she hails a taxi at the number 9 bus stop.

Figure 12–3. The effects of arousal and a beta-blocker on story memory. *A:* Two versions of a story accompanied by slides. *B:* Performance on consistently neutral (phases 1 and 3; white background) and variable (phase 2; shaded background) components of the story. A/P = arousal story/ placebo treatment; A/BB = arousal story/ beta-blocker; N/P = neutral story/ placebo treatment; N/BB = neutral story/ beta-blocker (data from Cahill et al., 1994).

the middle section of the emotional story, the boy is critically injured and the events are depicted graphically; in the neutral story no accident occurs. In subsequent delayed memory testing, normal subjects show enhanced recall for the emotional component of the story, as compared to the parallel section of the neutral story (Fig. 12–3B). By contrast, subjects given a β-adrenergic antagonist (beta-blocker) showed no facilitation of declarative memory for the emotional component of the story, even though they rated that component of the story as strongly emotional and their memory performance on other parts of the story was fully normal. Performance on the neutral story was not affected by the beta-blocker, showing that there was no general effect of the drug on memory for the story. A subsequent study has now shown that an adrenergic agonist further enhances memory for the emotional component of the story.

The amygdala has been strongly implicated in the enhancement of memory for emotional events in humans. A patient with Urbach-Wiethe disease, the disorder that results in selective bilateral amygdala damage (see Chapter 8), was tested in the emotional story paradigm. Compared to control subjects this patient failed to show enhancement of memory for the emotional part of the story. The patient performed as well as controls on the initial neutral segment of the story, and rated the emotional material as affectively strong. In a complementary brain imaging study on normal human subjects, the amygdala was activated during the viewing of emotional material, and this activation was related to enhanced memory for that material. In different positron emission tomography (PET) scanning sessions, subjects viewed film clips that were strong or neutral in emotional content. The amount of PET activation in the amygdala was greater for the emotional than the neutral stories, and memory for this material was greater than for the neutral stories. Furthermore, the amount of amygdala activation was correlated with performance in a delayed test of memory for the material in the emotional films but not that in the neutral films.

Multiple emotional memory systems that involve the amygdala

Combining the findings across all the studies presented in this chapter, it is apparent that there are multiple influences of emotion on memory, and the nodal point in all these influences is the amygdala. It seems most likely that this confluence of emotional memory systems within the amygdala is a consequence of the convergent inputs and divergent outputs of this area of the brain. Thus, on the basis of the evidence presented here, it seems reasonable to suggest there are multiple emotional memory systems that involve the amygdala. One of these systems, or one set of systems, involves specific pathways for the attachment of perceptions to emotions, and to emotional output effectors. Another set of systems involves more general influences of emotional arousal on memory. One of these influences is mediated both by a neural pathway that increases memory processing during ongoing learning, whereas another influence involves a hormonal pathway for postlearning modulation of consolidation processes. These multiple aspects of emotional memory, and different types of emotional memory, are not incompatible. Instead, they could work largely in concert to acquire emotional responses and to mediate memory for associated information processed by other systems.

Brain systems that mediate prolonged processes in memory reorganization

The other conception of memory consolidation involves events above the level of cellular physiology; this kind of consolidation occurs at the brain systems level. The time scale of events involved in systems-level phenomena of consolidation are severalfold greater than that of the cellular fixation mechanisms. It appears that this kind of consolidation requires hours, days, months, or years, depending on the nature of the memory tested and the species tested. Indeed, it will be argued that this consolidation never ends completely, for reasons that are of considerable theoretical importance.

The notion of consolidation at the brain systems level, operating at this long time scale, is tied to the temporally graded retrograde amnesias discussed in Chapter 1, in which the susceptibility of recent memories to disruption extends over years. The neural processing that underlies this phenomenon is considered later in the chapter, addressing, along the way, various fundamental issues about consolidation. How long does this kind of consolidation go on? Precisely which brain structures are critical to mediate consolidation? Where are the memories stored after consolidation is complete? Are all kinds of memories subject to consolidation? How is the delay-dependent forgetting in anterograde amnesia related to this consolidation mechanism? Studies on both human amnesia and animal models of amnesia address different aspects of these issues, and provide an increasingly clear picture of the role of hippocampal involvement, and hippocampal–neocortical interaction, in consolidation.

Outlining the properties of this prolonged consolidation process is the focus of the remainder of this chapter. First, the literature on human retrograde amnesia is reviewed, including the methods used to test for retrograde amnesia in human subjects, the findings of temporally graded retrograde amnesia, and the identification of critical brain structures. Next, I review attempts to model retrograde amnesia in animals, again focusing on the testing methods, the findings of temporally graded memory loss, and on the critical brain structures. In addition, other relevant physiological findings are reviewed. Finally, conceptualizations of the information processing and circuitry critical to mechanisms of consolidation are considered, with the aim of combining the earlier discussed observations on the nature of memory representation in cortical and hippocampal areas with the phenomenology of consolidation.

The phenomenon of temporally graded retrograde amnesia

The main focus of studies on the long-term process of consolidation has been studies of amnesia following hippocampal system damage, and in particular the phenomenon of temporally graded retrograde amnesia. The conceptual linkage between the hippocampus and consolidation began with the earliest observations on the patient H.M. Scoville and Milner's report on H.M. focused on his disorder as a particularly good example of Ribot's law (see Chapter 1). They characterized his amnesia as a severe and selective impairment in "recent memory" in the face of spared remote memory capacities. Indeed, the dissociation in H.M. between impaired recent memories and intact remote memories was most striking. So far as could be ascertained by interviews with H.M. and his family, the retrograde memory loss dated back 2 years prior to the surgery, with remote memory seeming to be intact. More recent evaluations confirm that H.M.'s remote memory impairment is indeed temporally limited.

However, a large battery of tests of memory for public and personal events also extend the period of impairment back to 11 years prior to the surgery. These studies used several strategies to assess H.M.'s memory for material he was presumed to have acquired across the decades prior to his surgery. Some of these tests evaluated his memory for public events, including naming of tunes, verbal recognition of events, or identification of faces that became famous in a particular decade. For example, a test of recognition for famous events includes a series of questions about particularly important public events from the 1940s through the 1970s. H.M., whose surgery was performed in 1953, performed within the normal range of scores for questions about events that occurred in the 1940s, was borderline for events from the 1950s, and was clearly impaired on events from the 1960s onward.

A test for recognition of public scenes was included, in which pictures depicting important scenes from the 1940s to the 1980s were selected such that the famous event could not be deduced from the picture alone. Subjects were asked if they had seen the picture before and could identify the event, and then further questions were asked about details of the event depicted. H.M.'s content scores were deficient in all decades except the 1940s.

A method used to probe H.M.'s memory for personal events involved a test originally designed to access remote autobiographical memories. In this test, subjects were given concrete nouns and asked to relate them to some personally experienced event from any period in their life, and to describe when the event occurred. In addition, to assess the consistency of these memories, the test was readministered on another day. Normal subjects provided memories from throughout their life span, including especially the most recent time period. By contrast, the memories that H.M. retrieved to these cues all dated back to the age of 16 (i.e., 1942) or younger. Thus, he had no memories of the end of World War II or of his high school graduation (1947), or any other event onward. These data provided the strongest evidence that his retrograde amnesia extends back 11 years prior to his surgery. Note, however, that because this time frame corresponds with the onset of H.M.'s seizure disorder (that ultimately precipitated the surgery he received), there is the possibility that at least some of the loss of memories might be a result of compromised hippocampal function during the period prior to his surgery, that is, there might be a contribution here from a partial anterograde amnesia.

Subsequent studies on retrograde amnesia have provided confirmation of the phenomenon of temporally graded memory loss, in cases where the deficit is unambiguously a retrograde amnesia. For example, one line of studies with patients receiving electroconvulsive therapy for severe depression examined memory for television programs that were shown in a single viewing season. These patients were found to have a (temporary) retrograde amnesia extending back 1–3 years before the treatments. Other studies have shown temporally graded retrograde amnesia dating 10–20 years back from an anoxic or ischemic event.

In addition, in a recent study of temporally graded retrograde amnesia, Squire and his colleagues tied the severity of retrograde amnesia to the amount of damage to the medial temporal region. This study involved four patients who had become amnesic without other cognitive impairment following specific brain insult and who had, for unrelated reasons, subsequently died and come to autopsy involving histological analysis of the brain damage. Two patients developed moderately severe anterograde amnesia following a transient ischemic event. Both patients had a selective loss of cells in the CA1 field of the hippocampus, and had a very limited retrograde amnesia, extending only 1–2 years. Two other patients had more severe anterograde amnesia and more extensive retrograde amnesia extending back 15–25 years. The histopathological examination of these patients showed cell loss throughout the hippocampus and to some extent in entorhinal cortex as well. These studies further confirm that damage limited to the hippocampal region can result in temporally limited retrograde amnesia, and that the extent of the temporal gradient of retrograde amnesia might be associated with the anatomical extent of damage within the hippocampal region.

Recent studies by Squire and colleagues have also examined in detail whether the phenomenon of temporally graded retrograde amnesia extends to spatial memory. This study focused on a patient with extensive damage to the medial temporal lobe. The patient had lived in a neighborhood in California during the 1930s and 1940s, but had moved away and subsequently returned only occasionally. The patient's spatial memory for this period was evaluated by comparing his ability to construct routes between different locations in the community, as identified using archival maps of the areas from the relevant period. In addition, the patient's ability to plot alternative roundabout routes was examined, using tests where he was asked how to navigate among places when the major route between them was blocked. They also measured the patient's accuracy in pointing in the direction of major landmarks from an imagined position in the neighborhood. On all these tests, the patient scored as well as or better than a group of age-matched control subjects who had lived in the same area during the target period, and who had also subsequently moved away. By contrast, and unlike the control subjects, the patient failed completely in solving the same navigational problems based on knowledge about their current neighborhood. Thus, for this patient, the pattern of retrograde amnesia for spatial knowledge matched that of temporally graded nonspatial memory observed in previous studies in many amnesic patients.

Not all forms of retrograde amnesia are temporally graded, however. Thus, there are retrograde amnesias associated with a variety of etiologies in which gradients are flat, extending back to the earliest childhood memories. In addition, some researchers have argued that some retrograde amnesias show a pattern of memory loss characterized less by the age of the memories than by their nature. For example, in one study four patients with retrograde amnesia showed impairments in the ability to recall or recognize faces of people who had become famous in the news media dating back several decades. Some of these patients showed flat gradients of retrograde amnesia dating for all periods of their life span. A large number of cases of retrograde amnesia concluded that retrograde amnesia following medial temporal lobe damage affects memory for personal episodes more severely than semantic memory, and that this deficit in autobiographical memory extends back many years, and in many cases the entire life span.

It has been argued that flat gradients of retrograde amnesia, and particularly those involving autobiographical memory, occur only in cases where there is damage or suspected damage beyond the medial temporal lobe. Amnesia associated with Korsakoff syndrome, closed head injuries, seizure disorders, and certain other etiologies often include damage or cell loss in prefrontal cortex. This is important because damage to the prefrontal area is associated with disorders of "source memory," the ability to recall where and when information was acquired. Such an inability to identify the circumstances surrounding new learning might be expected to lead to a selective impairment in memory for personal experiences. In these cases, the content-selectivity of retrograde amnesia would *not* be related to hippocampal function.

Prospective studies of retrograde amnesia in animals

The relatively recent development of experimental protocols for studying retrograde amnesia in animals has been a major advance in understanding the role of brain structures in memory consolidation. The use of animals allows increased resolution of the anatomical structures under study. In addition, animal studies allow greater control over the learning experience prior to brain insult. Such prospective experiments can equalize the nature and extent of acquired information, and can precisely control when learning takes place before brain damage. There have now been several prospective studies of retrograde amnesia, using different species and different learning and memory protocols. The majority of these studies support the notion that damage to medial temporal structures results in a temporally graded retrograde amnesia. Nevertheless, this finding is not universal, and the severity and gradient of retrograde amnesia varies across studies with the species, types of tests, and locus of brain damage. The remainder of this section reviews a few of these studies that provide examples of the pattern of retrograde amnesia and the variety of memory tests employed.

Zola-Morgan and colleagues trained monkeys on a series of visual object discriminations at different times prior to ablation of the hippocampus and of some of the surrounding cortex. Animals were trained on 100 object discrimination problems, segregated into five 20-problem sets presented at 16, 12, 8, 4, or 2 weeks prior to the surgery. Each set of problems consisted of two problems per day, with each problem presented on 14 consecutive trials. Performance was typically very good in learning, averaging 88% correct on the last trial of all the problems. Two weeks after the surgery, memory was assessed for all 100 problems, with random order presentation of a single trial of each problem over 2 days of testing. Normal monkeys performed best at problems that had been learned in the 4 weeks just prior to the (sham) surgery, with significantly poorer performance on problems that had been learned earlier, thus showing the typical forgetting curve (Fig. 12–4A). Monkeys with hippocampal damage showed the opposite pattern, however. They were significantly impaired, and indeed performed poorest, for problems presented at the shortest interval prior to surgery. These monkeys were not impaired on problems presented 8–16 weeks before surgery. Accordingly, these findings document the existence of temporally graded retrograde amnesia, and hence the presumption of a consolidation deficit, in animals with damage limited to medial temporal lobe structures.

Several studies using rats and rabbits have also demonstrated temporally graded retrograde amnesia following damage to the hippocampal region. Winocur demonstrated temporally graded retrograde amnesia in rats using the social transmission of food preferences task described in Chapter 5. In this study, pairs of rats were housed together for 2 days, then one of the rats was fed rat chow mixed with either cinnamon or cocoa. Subsequent training involved reexposure of the fed rat to its cagemate for a 30-minute period. Then, either immediately, or after intervals varying between 2 and 10 days, rats were operated for lesions of the hippocampus, and were allowed to recover for 10 days. Thus, the retention interval varied between 10 and 20 days. Memory for the social learning of the food odor was tested by measuring the consumption of cinnamon-flavored versus cocoa-flavored chow in a preference test. Normal rats showed a striking preference for the trained odor that lasted at full strength for 15 days, with some subsequent forgetting on the 20-day test (Fig. 12–4B). Rats with hippocampal lesions were severely impaired when the interval between training and surgery was minimal, showing no significant preference for the odor trained soonest to the time of surgery. They showed some retention when the surgery was delayed to 2 days after training, and full recovery at longer training-to-surgery intervals. As in the experiment on monkeys described earlier, and as in human amnesia, the performance pattern after hippocampal damage was opposite to that seen in normal controls. Thus, whereas normal animals showed progressively poorer performance at progressively longer retention intervals, rats with hippocam-

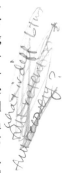

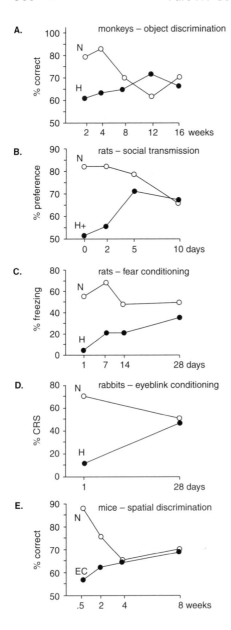

Figure 12–4. Several demonstrations of temporally graded retrograde memory impairments in animals following damage to the hippocampal region. *A:* Performance in normal (N) monkeys and that of monkeys with removal of the hippocampus plus some surrounding cortex (H+) on retention of 100 object discrimination problems learned at different times prior to surgery (data from Zola-Morgan and Squire, 1990). *B:* Performance of normal control rats (N) and rats with lesions of the hippocampus (H) on retention of the social transmission of food preference trained at different times prior to the surgery (data from Winocur, 1990). *C:* Performance of normal control rats (N) and rats with hippocampal lesions (H) on retention of contextual fear conditioning trained at different times prior to the surgery (data from Kim and Fanselow, 1992). *D:* Performance of normal control rabbits (N) and rabbits with hippocampal lesions (H) on retention of trace eyeblink conditioning performed at different times prior to the surgery (data from Kim et al., 1995). *E:* Performance of normal control mice (N) and mice with lesions of the entorhinal cortex (EC) on maze problems learned at different times prior to the surgery (data from Cho et al., 1993).

pal lesions performed better for learning that occurred at a more remote time.

Other evidence for temporally graded retrograde amnesia in rats comes from studies of contextual fear conditioning, a task described in Chapter 11. In a study by Fanselow and colleagues, like the one just described, animals were trained at different intervals prior to surgery. Then, all subjects were tested at a fixed interval postoperatively. Rats were placed in a conditioning chamber and presented a series of 15 tone-shock pairings in a single session. Hippocampal lesions were performed at 1–28 days after this training. Testing for conditioned fear associated with the shock was conducted separately for the context (the training chamber) and for the tone. To test for contextual fear, rats were placed back in the training chamber and freezing was measured for several minutes. To test for conditioned fear to the tone, animals were placed in a different chamber, and freezing during re-presentation of the tone was measured. As shown in Fig. 12–4C, normal rats exhibited substantial freezing across all retention intervals, indicating virtually no forgetting for the conditioned fear for both the context and the tone. By contrast, rats with hippocampal lesions showed impairment in contextual fear conditioning in a temporally graded way: They were severely impaired when the interval between training and surgery was 1 day, showing virtually no freezing in the familiar chamber; they showed some retention when the surgery occurred a week after training; and they demonstrated full retention when the surgery occurred a month after training. In addition, the retrograde amnesia was material specific in that rats with hippocampal damage showed fully normal retention of conditioned fear for the tone at all retention intervals.

A temporally graded retrograde amnesia has also been observed in rabbits trained on hippocampal-dependent trace (classical) conditioning, a task described in Chapter 10. Rabbits were trained using standard classical eyelid conditioning procedures for 100-trial-per-day sessions. On each trial, a 250 msec tone conditioning stimulus (CS) was followed by a 500 msec trace interval and then an airpuff unconditioned stimulus (US). Daily training continued until the rabbit elicited eyeblinks during the CS or trace interval on eight out of ten consecutive trials, requiring on average three to four training sessions. The rabbits then received hippocampal lesions, either 1 day or 1 month later. After a 7-day recovery period, all animals were tested for retention during retraining. As shown in Fig. 12–4D, normal rabbits showed complete savings of the conditioned eyeblink at both retention intervals. By contrast, rabbits given hippocampal lesions 1 day after training were severely impaired, exhibiting no retention of conditioning, and indeed were unable to acquire the task postoperatively. Nevertheless, when the surgery occurred 1 month after conditioning, rabbits were intact, showing as much savings as did control rabbits at both retention intervals.

Temporally graded retrograde amnesia has also been observed in mice and rats on spatial discrimination problems. In one study, mice were trained on a set of two-choice spatial discrimination problems using a radial maze. For each problem, the mouse was rewarded for selecting one of two adjacent maze arms, such that the same apparatus was used for multiple problems. Each problem was presented for 16 trials per day for 3–5 days, until the animals reached a performance criterion of 13 correct choices in a session. Training on successive problems was separated by 10 days. On the following day, animals were given ibotenic acid lesions of the entorhinal cortex, then allowed to recover for 10 days. Subsequent retention testing involved 16 trials on each problem presented concurrently on multiple problems. Control mice exhibited striking savings on problems presented 3 days prior to surgery, with significant forgetting at longer retention intervals (Fig. 12–5E). Mice with entorhinal lesions were severely impaired when the surgery had occurred 3 days after presentation of the problem, showing almost no retention at that interval, while some retention was observed when the surgery occurred 2 weeks after presentation of a problem, and normal retention was obtained for problems presented 4–8 weeks prior to surgery. Notably, as in the other studies presented, the patterns of performance across retention intervals for normal mice were the opposite of mice with damage to the entorhinal cortex.

A similar study using rats, run subsequently, replicated the main findings with entorhinal lesions, showing a severe retention deficit when the training-to-surgery interval was a few days, with better performance for more remotely acquired spatial discriminations and indeed normal performance for the longest interval. In addition, this study also examined the performance of animals given lesions of the parietal cortex at varying intervals after spatial discrimination training. In contrast to the pattern of findings on entorhinal lesions, rats with parietal lesions, though impaired, showed no sign of a temporal gradient. These data are consistent with the notion that the hippocampal region, but not parietal cortex, plays a role in the consolidation process.

There have also been failures to find retrograde amnesia following hippocampal damage, and reports of flat and not temporally graded deficits. These studies differ in the type of lesion and training, leaving open the critical parameters that determine the extent of the retrograde gradient in animals, as in humans. Notwithstanding the mixed results, the large number of successful demonstrations of temporally graded amnesia in animal models, using a compelling range of species and behavioral tests, adds to the conclusions from studies of human amnesia. At least some components of the hippocampal system play a critical role in consolidation of memory during the time after learning for at least some types of information.

Models of cortical–hippocampal
interactions in memory reorganization

There have been many theoretical proposals about the mechanisms of long-term consolidation. It is generally held that the final repository of long-term memories is the neocortex, and that hippocampal processing somehow facilitates, organizes, or otherwise mediates the creation of permanent memory representations in specific neocortical sites. The question to be addressed here is: What is the nature of the interaction of the hippocampal system with neocortical processors that permit memory storage and consolidation to occur?

Several models of hippocampal–cortical interactions have been proposed, including a number of computational models that implement various kinds of interactions that could occur. Two recent models that will be considered here focus on how the hippocampus could mediate a slow reorganization process.

Pablo Alvarez and Larry Squire offered a simple network model that highlighted several basic distinctions in the operating characteristics of the cerebral cortex and the hippocampus. They argued that the cerebral cortex was capable of storing an immense amount of information, but that cortical representations change slowly and incrementally. By contrast, the hippocampus had a limited storage capacity but recorded information rapidly through changing of synaptic weights using rapid LTP mechanisms. Their focus was to show how these properties instantiated within a simple neural network simulation could demonstrate key properties of consolidation.

The schematic diagram shown in Fig. 12–5A illustrates their model. The simulation contained two distinct cortical areas and a medial temporal lobe region (MTL). Each neural unit in these areas was connected to every other unit in other areas, and the connection strengths could be modified by a use-dependent competitive learning rule. The rate of change in connections between the MTL and cortex was designed to be rapid, but short-lasting, whereas the changes in connections between the two cortical areas was slow, but long-lasting. When new information was presented to the network that set up activations in each of the cortical areas, the MTL connections changed substantially and rapidly to represent the conjointly active units in the cortical areas, although very little permanent change had occurred in the cortical representations or their connection between them. Subsequently, when the MTL area was randomly activated, to simulate a subsequent consolidation event, the originally activated cortical input areas were reactivated, incrementally enhancing their connections.

A.

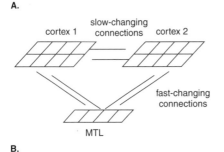

cortex 1   slow-changing connections   cortex 2

fast-changing connections

MTL

B.

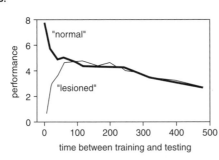

Figure 12–5. Alvarez and Squire's (1994) model of cortical–hippocampal interactions in consolidation. *A:* Conceptualization of the model. Eight units in two cortical areas and four in the medial temporal lobe (MTL) have different rates of change in connectivity. *B:* Performance of the intact model and the model with an MTL lesion on the capacity to excite units in one cortical area from the other in retention of associations acquired at different times prior to the surgery.

Memory performance of the model was assessed in terms of how well activation of one of the cortical representations could reinstate the associated representation in the other cortical area (Fig. 12–5B). The intact network showed strong performance in activating the associated representation shortly after learning, and showed some forgetting over time. By contrast, if the MTL was removed shortly after learning, memory performance was very poor, and the longer the period the MTL was left intact after learning, the stronger was the consequent memory performances. Accordingly, the model seemed to simulate the essential characteristics of memory consolidation.

Jay McClelland and his colleagues developed a more elaborate and larger-scale model, taking these ideas somewhat farther. In their model, cortical representations involved systematic organizations of related items in parallel, multidimensional hierarchies. They envisioned the operation of the cortex as identifying stimulus characteristics and sorting items into categories and subcategories within the large-scale organization. As an example, they considered the semantic network illustrated in Fig. 12–6A. In this network, birds and fish are characterized by a set of propositional properties, for example, a robin is an animal that has feathers and wings, is red, and can fly. They noted that elaborate parallel distributed networks can readily be trained on such sorting operations for a large set of ani-

A. propositional network

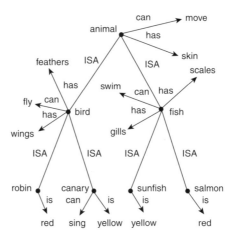

B. performance in new learning

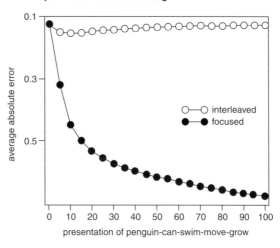

Figure 12–6. A semantic network used to train network models of the organization of propositional knowledge about living things. *A:* The propositional network which the model initially learned for the categorization of characteristics of fish and birds. ISA = is a. *B:* Overall categorization performance following either focused or interleaved training on a new item with characteristics of both birds and fish (penguins) (from McClelland et al., 1995).

mals according to these and similar characteristics. However, once a set of hierarchical organizations is established and stabilized, it is difficult to add new items smoothly, not because a network cannot be altered to include the new item by repetitive training—it will do so quite well. Rather, the problem is that such novel training causes changes in an already established network resulting, in turn, in catastrophic interference among the already existing items. New training alters a network to identify the new item, but such learning results in network modifications that interfere with the previously developed ability to correctly identify the old information. In the example network, catastrophic interference was illustrated by focused training on identification of a penguin, a bird that has some characteristics of other birds (e.g., wings) but also other characteristics of fish (can swim). The outcome of focused training was that network performance on overall categorization fell precipitously (Fig. 12–6B).

McClelland's solution to the problem of catastrophic interference was to add a new small network—a "hippocampus"—that could very rapidly acquire a representation of a new item, and then have this small network slowly and gradually "train" the large network. As a result, as in the Alvarez and Squire simulation, the synaptic weights in the hippocampal network changed rapidly, and that network sent its representation repetitively to the large—"cortical"—network. The cortical network modifications were slow and incremental. Also, in addition to the occasional input from the hippocampus, the cortical model was also repetitively exposed to the old materials it was built to represent, thereby resulting in an "interleaved learning" regimen that intermixed repetitions of old and new representations. This was key to the ability of the overall cortical network to be modified so as to incorporate new information without suffering from catastrophic interference. In the example, by contrast to focused training, such interleaved training led to successful preserved performance on all the categorizations (Fig. 12–6B).

Eventually, this process of interleaving produced an asymptotic state of the overall cortical representation, at which point it no longer benefited from hippocampal activations, and thus no longer depended upon the hippocampus. In this fashion, the model exhibited the critical features of consolidation. The duration of consolidation required would be expected to be indeterminate, depending on the nature and extent of new information to be obtained, as well as on any other new learning that must be incorporated during the course of consolidation of already stored information. Thus, consolidation should be conceived as a life-long evolution of cortical networks, one that only asymptotically approaches a state where more interleaving does not alter the network substantially. In this way, we can come to understand at least some of the mixed results regarding the duration and nature of temporal gradients in retrograde amnesia.

The nature of hippocampal representation and consolidation

How might information processing by the hippocampus support the reorganization of cortical information during a prolonged consolidation period? A further consideration of the nature of hippocampal representations discussed in Chapters 4–6, combined with our knowledge about cortical–hippocampal circuitry (Chapter 9), offers potential insights about the cortical–hippocampal interplay proposed to underlie memory consolidation. In the model of the hippocampal "memory space" developed in Chapters 5 and 6, the hippocampus was envisioned to represent learning episodes as a series of discrete events, each encoded within the activity of a single cell. Within the hippocampal memory space, some cells were characterized as encoding highly specific conjunctions or sequences of stimuli and actions that compose unique events that occurred in only one or a few learning episodes. Yet other cells were envisioned to encode "nodal" events, features of experience that are common across different episodes; these might mediate our capacity to link an ongoing event to previous episodes that share the nodal event.

In an extension of this model, Eichenbaum and colleagues suggested that the nodal codings could subserve the linking and interleaving processes of consolidation proposed by Alvarez and Squire and McClelland and his colleagues. According to this scheme, representations of discrete events and sequences of events within the hippocampus are conceived to occur within one or a few learning trials. Furthermore, "nodal" representations are conceived as developing in parallel with the variations in experience that occur across related learning episodes. Because of the very high level of interconnectivity of hippocampal pyramidal cells relative to that in all the cortical areas, the initial development of these nodal representations is envisioned as primarily within the hippocampus shortly after learning. Subsequent prolonged cortical memory consolidation involves the creation of the nodal properties within cortical cells, mediated through connections with the hippocampus and parahippocampal region.

Within this framework, memory reorganization may operate in two stages. The first stage involves interactions between the hippocampus and the parahippocampal region. Parahippocampal neurons receive direct inputs from many cortical areas, and so they would be expected to encode the configurations of stimuli to compose event representations and sequences based on simultaneity of these inputs alone. However, for some period immediately after learning, associations among the complex event representations within the parahippocampal region may depend upon the connections to and from the hippocampal cells that have encoded particular nodal events. At the same time, the feedback from the hippocampus to the parahippocampal cortex is envisioned to mediate the development of nodal representations within the parahippocampal region. This may occur by the hippocampus providing an indirect pathway that drives the coactivation of parahippocampal neurons, enhancing the connections within their intracortical network and producing nodal cell properties in parahippocampal neurons. Because parahippocampal neurons have an unusual capacity for prolonged firings following discrete events (see Chapter 9), cells in this region may rapidly support the coding of long event sequences through the interactions with the hippocampus. When long sequence and nodal properties have been acquired by parahippocampal cells, the memory can be considered to have consolidated there, in the sense that the memory abilities conferred by these cells would no longer require hippocampal feedback.

The second stage involves a similar interplay between the cortical association areas and the parahippocampal region. Initially, cortical associations are viewed to depend on the parahippocampal region to supply linkages between their representations. In addition, by simultaneously driving cells in cortical areas and activating their intracortical connections, these linkages would be expected to mediate the ultimate development of context and nodal properties in the cortical association areas. When this is accomplished the entire hippocampal circuit would no longer be necessary for the existence of event, long sequence, and nodal representations. Consistent with the proposal that the prolonged consolidation process occurs in stages involving first a reorganization within the parahippocampal region and then later in the cortex, human amnesics with damage extending into the parahippocampal region have a more extended retrograde amnesia than those with selective hippocampal damage.

The key aspects of this model involve the unusual associational structure of hippocampal anatomy that makes it the earliest site for arbitrary associations that underlie event, sequence, and nodal properties. At earliest stages of parahippocampal or neocortical processing, the range of associations and the speed of their formation may be much more limited. But they can mediate substantial development and reorganization of a memory space through the connections within the hippocampus initially. In this way the repeated invocation of hippocampal representations onto the cortex serves to reorganize cortical representations accommodating new information and new associations within the overall knowledge structure encoded there.

Summing up

There are two aspects of memory consolidation, one that involves molecular and cellular processes that support the *fixation* of memory within synapses over a period of minutes or hours, and another that involves interactions within the declarative memory system to support a *reorganization* of memories that occurs over weeks to years.

There is a cascade of molecular and microstructural events by which short-term synaptic modifications lead to permanent changes in connectivity between neurons, and this cascade is conserved across brain structures that participate in memory and across species in the phylogenetic scale. The fixation of memory can be halted or facilitated by postlearning treatments that interfere with the molecular/cellular cascade. There are also natural modulatory mechanisms that can facilitate fixation in the various memory systems of the mammalian brain. An important modulatory system involves the release of glucocorticoids and adrenergic mechanisms via the amygdala that can influence memory fixation in the declarative and habit systems in both animals and humans.

In addition, the declarative memory system mediates the prolonged reorganization of memories. This process has been identified in graded retrograde amnesia for declarative memories in both humans and animals. The nature of mechanisms within the declarative system is poorly understood. But current models propose that the role of the hippocampus is to rapidly store indices of cortical representations, and to slowly facilitate the interconnection of cortical representations by repeated two-way interactions between the cortex and hippocampus. Over a protracted period, these interactions ultimately result in an asymptotic level of reorganization and connections among cortical representations to incorporate new material into semantic knowledge.

READINGS

Alvarez, P., and Squire, L.R. 1994. Memory consolidation and the medial temporal lobe: A simple network model. *Proc. Natl. Acad. Sci. U.S.A.* 91: 7041–7045.

Cahill, L., and McGaugh, J.L. 1998. Mechanisms of emotional arousal and lasting declarative memory. *Trends Neurosci.* 21: 273–313.

McClelland, J.L., McNaughton, B.L., and O'Reilly, R.C. 1995. Why there are complementary learning systems in the hippocampus and neocortex: Insights from the successes and failures of connectionist models of learning and memory. *Psychol. Rev.* 102: 419–457.

McGaugh, J.L. 2000. Memory—a century of consolidation. *Science* 287: 248–251.

Nader, K., Schafe, G.E., and LeDoux, J.E. 2000. Fear memories require protein synthesis in the amygdala for reconsolidation after retrieval. *Nature* 406: 722–726.

13

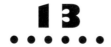

Working with Memory

STUDY QUESTIONS

What is working memory?

How does it differ from the mechanisms of declarative memory discussed so far?

What brain structures and systems support working memory?

What do we know about the anatomy and evolution of the prefrontal cortex?

What are the consequences of prefrontal damage in humans, in animals?

Do different parts of the prefrontal cortex have different functions?

What aspects of cognition and memory are encoded by prefrontal neurons?

The story of memory does not end with consolidation. Indeed, even after consolidation is completed, there is the issue of how we search for
information during retrieval, as well as how new information becomes incorporated into the established organization during additional learning experiences. I think of cognitive processing that guides encoding and retrieval
as "working-with-memory," the manipulation of information that is not
memory per se, but handles our memory processing. While the entire cerebral cortex is involved in memory processing, the chief brain area that mediates these processes is the prefrontal cortex, the area in the frontal lobe
whose functions are not fully understood but clearly involve strategic mechanisms of the sort that work with memory as a major part of its function.

The role of the prefrontal cortex is generally viewed as mediating
"working memory," a concept akin to my notion of working with memory. Working memory involves a combination of storing new incoming

information, plus some type of cognitive manipulation, during a brief period in consciousness. Consider a task in current common usage in memory research, called the "two-back" task. In this protocol, human subjects are presented with a string of stimuli (letters, words, or numbers). Their job is to say yes when the current item is the same as the one presented two back, that is, on the second trial previous to the current one. To succeed at this task one must create a buffer in memory that holds the last two items seen. Then when a new item is presented, one can match it to the first item in the buffer (the two-back item) and make a correct response. Then one must update the buffer by deleting that two-back item and adding in the current item, and so on.

We perform tasks that demand working memory in almost all of the activities of our conscious lives, from checking off the jobs accomplished in our morning routine, to keeping track of the flow of information in reading a text chapter, to solving the many complex problems we encounter during our work. Working memory is considered a form of declarative memory because this sort of processing goes on in consciousness and involves relational organization and inferential judgments, and is accessible to explicit forms of expression. However, our consideration of the short-term mechanisms of working memory here is also distinctly different from the mechanisms of long-term memory that have been the focus of this book so far (see also a discussion of short-term memory mechanisms of other cortical areas in Chapter 7).

Alan Baddeley and his colleagues first realized the importance of distinguishing the cognitive and storage processes in short-term memory, and replaced the concept of a unitary short-term memory with a multiple component conception of working memory. The multiple component model was inspired by findings from experiments in which they found an unexpected low degree of interference in the capacity for storing lists of visual patterns or word items when people performed cognitive tasks simultaneously. So, in their model of working memory they proposed the existence of a set of specialized subsystems that mediates the storage process, and a distinct "central executive" that controls the subsystems and performs the mental "work" of controlling the slave subsystems and forming strategies. Corresponding to the materials involved in Baddeley's studies, the model involved two distinct subsystems, a "visuospatial sketch pad" that could maintain nonverbal images and a "phonological loop" that mediated speech perception and subvocal rehearsal of verbal materials. These should be considered just examples of the full range of specialized subsystems available to the central executive.

Because this kind of conceptual model of working memory involves multiple types of cognitive processing combined with a range of stored material, it will come as no surprise that working memory relies on a widespread network of brain structures. Indeed, there is considerable evidence that the brain network for working memory is large and can be subdivided into a central executive with multiple subsystems. Considerable evidence points to the prefrontal cortex as the locus of the central executive, and to a variety of other cortical areas as the mediators of subsystem processes.

In this chapter, first, the anatomy of the prefrontal cortex is summarized. A review follows of the functional role of the prefrontal cortex, including a consideration of whether the prefrontal area is involved in memory *per se*, or other cognitive processes related to memory, and whether the expansive prefrontal area has specialized subdivisions between or within the hemispheres. Then the story is broadened to consider parcellation of functions and cooperation between the prefrontal cortex and other higher-order cortical areas. Finally, some of the main points made in earlier chapters are reviewed, with the aim of considering how the entire brain participates in ordinary learning and memory processing.

The anatomy of the prefrontal cortex

The assignment of the central executive function to the prefrontal cortex is supported by substantial anatomical data. The phenomenal expansion of the prefrontal area in primates and especially humans is impressively associated with the evolution of cognitive capacities (Fig. 13–1). The prefrontal cortex in humans is a diverse area, composed of several distinct subdivisions. There is considerable consensus on correspondences in monkeys with identified areas in the human prefrontal cortex. Although several anatomical areas have been characterized based on morphological appearance, most of the functional evidence has been related to four general regions. These include the medial, dorsolateral, ventrolateral, and orbital areas. Most of the attention with regard to working memory functions in monkeys and humans has focused on the dorsolateral and ventrolateral areas, and these areas are partially distinct in their connections with more posterior parts of the cerebral cortex. Each of the subdivisions receives input from a diverse set of rostral and causal cortical areas, and each has a distinctive input pattern.

In addition, prefrontal areas are characterized by considerable associative connections with other prefrontal areas. Nevertheless, despite this diversity and associativity with the prefrontal cortex, a few generalities

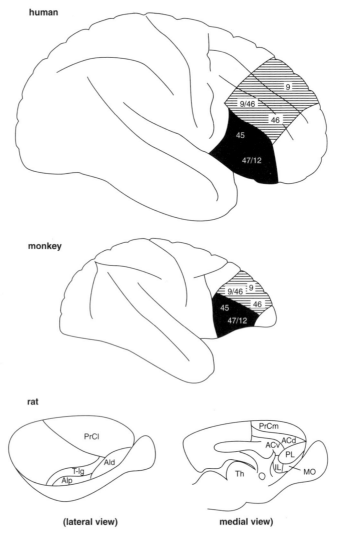

Figure 13–1. Designations of prefrontal areas in the human (top), monkey (middle), and rat (bottom; lateral and medial views). In the human and monkey, the designations are Brodman's areas. In the rat the designations are: AI = agranular insular; PrC = premotor; AC = anterior cingulate; PL = prelimbic; IL = infralimbic; MO = medial orbital; T-Ig = taste/granular insular; Th = thalamus; d = dorsal; l = lateral; m = medial; p = posterior; v = ventral.

have emerged about distinctions among prefrontal areas with regard to their inputs from posterior cortical areas. Thus, in general, the dorsolateral prefrontal area receives inputs mainly from medially and dorsolaterally located cortical areas that preferentially represent somatosensory and visuospatial information. Conversely, in general, the lateral prefrontal areas receive inputs mainly from ventrolateral and ventromedial cortical areas that represent auditory and visual pattern information. In particular, the differentiation of visuospatial input to the dorsolateral prefrontal area, and visual pattern input to the lateral prefrontal area has received considerable attention in studies on distinct working memory systems.

In rats there is also clear anatomical evidence for correspondences with some prefrontal regions in primates. However, the number of these areas is limited. And in particular, there is little evidence for the existence of rodent homologies for the dorsal and lateral convexity subdivisions of the prefrontal cortex prominent in views on working memory in primates and humans. Nevertheless, there is evidence that the medial and orbital areas in the rodent prefrontal cortex serve some of the general functions of working memory observed in primates.

The role of the prefrontal cortex in human memory function

Deficits in short-term or working memory can arise from a variety of disorders, including some associated with damage to multiple brain areas. Nevertheless, the greatest attention in behavioral studies has been accorded the prefrontal cortex, befitting its role as the putative "central executive" of working memory systems. However, prefrontal cortex function is a large issue, not limited to or even considered by some researchers as primarily an issue of memory processing, as suggested earlier. Rather, the role of the prefrontal cortex in human memory is differently viewed as only a part of its role in multiple higher cognitive functions including personality, affect, motor control, language, and problem solving.

Consistent with this view, in general, neuropsychological studies suggest that deficits in memory are secondary to an impairment in attention and problem-solving deficits. For example, one of the best studied and most profound impairments following prefrontal damage in humans is a deficit in the Wisconsin Card Sorting task. In this test, subjects are initially presented with four target items, playing cards each with a repeating pattern design that involves a unique combination of pattern color, shape, and number. Subsequently, the subjects are given a deck of similar cards and must sort the cards onto the target cards according to a criterion (color, shape, or number) the subject selects. The subject is given feedback with every choice, and must search for the correct sorting criterion. When the subject is sorting correctly, the experimenter shifts to a new criterion without warning and the subject must discover the new criterion.

This task contains an obvious working memory component, in that subjects must keep in mind the currently judged sorting criterion, and dispense with it and then select and maintain a new one. Patients with frontal lobe lesions are severely impaired on this task. However, the observed impairment in these patients is not that they forget the current sorting criterion. On the contrary, prefrontal patients have no difficulty learning the initial sorting criterion. Moreover, their disorder is that they subsequently *perseverate*, that is, continue to use a sorting criterion that is no longer operative. This pattern of findings is not consistent with the notion that the prefrontal cortex is specifically involved in the memory aspect of the task.

On the other hand, this does not mean that patients with prefrontal damage perform perfectly well in standard memory tasks. They do well at some, but not others. They perform normally in recall of stories or non-verbal diagrams. And they learn verbal paired associates as well as normal control subjects. These findings stand in marked contrast to the typically poor performance of amnesic subjects on the same paired associate learning tasks. By contrast, frontal patients perform poorly on other variants of memory tasks. For example, by contrast to their success in initial verbal paired associate learning, they are inordinately sensitive to proactive interference in learning paired associates composed of different pairings of the same target works. Frontal patients also perform poorly in "meta-memory," self-assessments of whether they feel they could recognize verbal memory items they cannot recall. Yet they perform just as well as normal subjects in the accuracy of recall of the same word items. Similarly, frontal patients do poorly in recalling the situation in which they learned correctly recalled materials. This deficit in "source memory" has been viewed as reflecting a deficit in memory for the context of learned items.

Another potentially related area of memory impairment in patients with prefrontal damage is a difficulty in remembering temporal order of recent events. In one study, patients were presented with a long series of cards in rapid succession, each card bearing two line drawings. Some cards also contained question marks, requiring the subject to indicate which of the two items had appeared more recently. In some cases both items had appeared earlier, but at different times in the sequence. In other cases one item has appeared before and the other item was new. Frontal patients could recognize the earlier-appearing items but could not identify their order. By contrast, patients with temporal lobe damage could identify the ordering of old items but showed impairments in recognizing new items, consistent with the typical pattern in amnesia. In another study, subjects were presented with a list of 15 words and were subsequently asked to reconstruct the order in which they appeared. Frontal patients performed poorly in replicating the presented order, but performed relatively well in recall and recognition of presented words. This pattern of deficits has led to the view that the fundamental deficit in humans with prefrontal damage is an inability to inhibit irrelevant information. Such a deficit could account straightforwardly for their difficulties on the Wisconsin Card Sorting and other tasks that require switching one's attention, and could underlie the impairments in source and meta-memory, as well as problem solving and temporal ordering, to the extent that performance on such tasks requires inhibiting irrelevant cognitive strategies.

The role of the prefrontal cortex in problem solving and memory in monkeys

Deficits in short-term memory following damage to the prefrontal cortex have been highlighted since the pioneering studies of Jacobsen and his colleagues in the 1930s. These studies focused on the delayed response task, a variant of the "shell game" in which the monkey views a reward being hidden under one of two plaques, then after a memory delay, must choose the location of the reward (see Fig. 5–1D). The specific demand for short-term memory was emphasized in an experiment where poor performance after prefrontal lesions was observed in delayed response, but not in a visual pattern discrimination task using the same stimuli.

Patricia Goldman-Rakic has shown that the deficit following damage to the dorsolateral prefrontal cortex is observed only when there is both a spatial and a memory component of the task. Other deficits in short-term memory, and sometimes in other types of learning, are observed after damage to different areas of the prefrontal cortex in monkeys. Most prominent among these are selective deficits associated with damage to three of the key areas of prefrontal cortex. Damage to the dorsolateral area produces a severe deficit in spatial delayed response and in the related spatial delayed alternation task where the food is hidden in the left and right locations on alternate trials. No deficits are observed on object alternation (choosing one of two objects on alternate trials), discrimination, or delayed nonmatch to sample, or a variety of other tasks with no spatial memory requirement. By contrast, damage to the lateral prefrontal cortex does not result in severe deficits in spatial delayed response or delayed alternation, but does produce severe impairments in object alternation and delayed nonmatch to sample. Damage to the orbital prefrontal area produces deficits in olfactory, taste, visual, and auditory discriminations and especially in discrimination reversal learning; orbital lesions also result in emotional disorders. These data are consistent with the heterogeneity of prefrontal connections, and with the proposal that areas of the prefrontal cortex may be distinct in the modality of information they process in memory.

More recent studies on the neuropsychology of prefrontal function in monkeys have expanded on these early findings, suggesting a broader role for the prefrontal cortex in cognition as observed in humans. For example, in one recent study by Angela Roberts and her colleagues, monkeys with lateral or orbital prefrontal lesions were trained on a variant of the attention switching tasks described before. In this experiment animals learned to discriminate compound visual stimuli each composed of a polygon and a curved line (Fig. 13–2). In the preliminary discrimination they

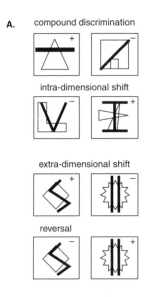

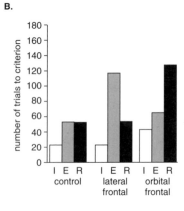

Figure 13–2. Attentional shift protocol. *A:* Examples of stimuli used in testing in each stage of training. The large polygon is the relevant dimension in all but the extradimensional shift and reversal conditions. *B:* Performance of monkeys with lateral or orbital prefrontal lesions on intradimensional shift (I), extradimensional shift (E), and reversal (R) conditions (data from Dias et al., 1996).

had to attend to one dimension (e.g., the polygon) and ignore the other (the line). Then they learned other discrimination problems: first, one involving an *intradimensional shift* (discrimination between new polygons, ignoring new lines); then one involving an *extradimensional shift* (discrimination between new lines, ignoring the new polygons; and, finally, a *reversal* of the last problem (where the reward assignments were switched for the same stimuli). Neither lesion affected performance on the intradimensional shift problem. Monkeys with lateral lesions were impaired on the extradimensional shift problem, but not on its reversal. Monkeys with orbital prefrontal lesions showed the opposite pattern—they were unimpaired on the extradimensional shift, but impaired on its reversal. These results indicate selective impairments after different prefrontal lesions not within the same visual modality, but associated with different cognitive demands. The lateral prefrontal region seems to be essential for switching the relevant visual perceptual dimension, whereas the orbital prefrontal area seems to be critical for reversing the affective association for the same stimuli.

Another recent study by Michael Petrides and his colleagues examined the capacity of monkeys with dorsolateral prefrontal lesions in working memory for temporal order. The key test for self-ordering involved presentations of three distinct objects on three successive trials each day. On the first trial all the objects were baited, and any could be selected to obtain a reward. After a 10-second delay the same objects were again presented with their positions randomized, and the initially selected item was not rebaited, so the subject was required to choose one of the remaining objects to obtain a second reward. On the third trial, the objects were again randomly rearranged, and the monkey had to select the remaining object. Monkeys with dorsolateral prefrontal lesions were impaired on this self-ordering task. They do no better when the same stimuli are presented one at a time during the first two trials, that is, when the stimuli are externally ordered. However, the same monkeys perform well on delayed object alternation (as observed following dorsolateral lesions in the above described studies), and a variant of the task showed that the central difference involved in the ordering task and delayed alternation is the number of stimuli that had to be remembered. In one more test, Petrides showed that the same monkeys could readily learn to appropriately select objects presented repeatedly in the same order, that is, in a task not requiring the monitoring of order in working memory. These findings demonstrate a strong parallel with the studies showing temporal ordering deficits in human patients with prefrontal damage, and suggest a common mechanism in strategic processing functions of the prefrontal area in humans and monkeys.

A similar role for the prefrontal cortex in rodents?

Other neuropsychological studies have provided parallel evidence of functionally heterogeneous areas in the prefrontal cortex of rats, suggesting these mechanisms of prefrontal function are common in mammalian evolution. Bryan Kolb reviewed the anatomical and behavioral evidence on rodent prefrontal areas, and concluded there are substantial similarities between rats and monkeys in the connections between the medial prefrontal area and spatial cortical areas, and between the orbital prefrontal area and subcortical limbic structures. The findings from neuropsychological investigations also suggest substantial similarities across species in the functions of these areas. Damage to the medial prefrontal area in rats results in deficits in spatial alternation, spatial working memory on the radial maze task, and impairments in the Morris water maze. These data indicate the rodent medial prefrontal area is involved in spatial memory performance similar to dorsolateral prefrontal involvement in spatial functions in monkeys. Notably, the poor performance in the water maze has been attributed to poor navigational strategies rather than memory *per se*, consistent with the findings from studies on human spatial working memory. A recent study showed that rats with medial prefrontal lesions normally acquired the water maze when trained from a single starting point, and accommodated successfully to finding the escape platform from a second location. However, they were impaired when the number of starting positions exceeded two, a finding reminiscent of Petrides's findings on object working memory in monkeys.

Also consistent with the findings on monkeys and humans, damage to the prefrontal cortex results in impairments in attention switching and temporal ordering. David Olton and colleagues trained rats to time each of two stimuli either independently or simultaneously by varying the rate at which they press a bar in anticipation of rewards delivered at different fixed intervals after each stimulus. Lesions of the prefrontal cortex severely disrupted performance on this task, consistent with an impairment in dividing or switching attention between two processing events. Hippocampal lesions do not impair performance on this divided attention task. In contrast, hippocampal lesions produce amnesia in a variant of the timing task where a gap is inserted in the timing procedure, whereas prefrontal lesions did not affect memory in the gap procedure. Thus, as in the previously described studies in monkeys, prefrontal damage results in a deficit in "executive" function, not memory, and hippocampal lesions result in the opposite pattern.

In addition, Raymond Kesner and colleagues have performed a series of experiments demonstrating that medial prefrontal lesions result in deficits in temporal ordering in rats. In experiments similar in design to those used with monkeys, rats were trained to enter arms on a radial maze to obtain rewards. On each trial, they were first allowed to visit each of four arms in a predetermined sequence for that day. Then they were give one of two types of memory tests. In the test for order they were presented with a choice of the first and second, or second and third, or third and fourth presented arms, with the contingency that another reward could be obtained in the arm that was presented earlier that day. Alternatively, they were presented with one of the arms that had been visited that day and another arm that was not presented in that trial. Animals were trained on the task preoperatively and retested after medial prefrontal lesions. They performed well on both tests preoperatively, but very poorly on the order test after surgery. They performed well when tested on recognition of the first arm presented on each day, but were impaired on subsequently presented arms. Thus, like monkeys with dorsolateral lesions, rats with medial prefrontal lesions are more severely impaired on order memory than on recognition. Unlike the monkeys in Petrides's study, the rats with medial prefrontal lesions remained impaired on order memory even when the same ordering was presented each day. However, the dissociation between order and recognition memory was more striking—these animals were completely unimpaired in recognizing repeatedly presented arms. In addition, Kolb documented several reports of medial prefrontal damage resulting in disruption of species-specific behavioral patterns including food hoarding, nest building, and maternal and sexual behavior. Kolb interpreted these findings as reflecting a general deficit in the temporal organization of behavioral sequences.

Several studies have demonstrated behavioral abnormalities in emotion and response inhibition after orbital prefrontal lesions in rats similar to those observed in monkeys. Furthermore, some studies have uncovered specific dissociations of function in medial and orbital lesions in rats similar to those seen in monkeys. Perhaps the most striking example comes from a double dissociation of the effects of selective prefrontal lesions on performance in spatial delayed alternation and olfactory discrimination. Preoperatively, all animals were trained on spatial delayed alternation in a standard Y-maze, and on a two-odor discrimination problem that involved a go/no-go response contingency (where the animal executed a response to one stimulus and inhibited that response to the other stimulus). Postoperatively, all animals were retrained on those tasks plus one more odor discrimination problem. Rats with medial prefrontal lesions were severely impaired on spatial delayed alternation, similar to the findings from several earlier studies, and were not impaired in retention or acquisition of odor discriminations (Fig. 13–3A). Rats with orbital prefrontal lesions showed the opposite pattern of effects, no deficit in reacquisition of the spatial delayed alternation, but severe impairment in both retention and acquisition of odor discriminations (Fig. 13–3B).

Subsequent analyses focused on the nature of the impairments and the perseverative tendencies in both tasks. In the spatial alternation task perseverative errors were measured as repetitive responses made during correction trials given following selection of the incorrect arm. This analysis showed that rats with medial prefrontal lesions made substantially more perseverative errors in the spatial alternation task than controls or rats with orbital prefrontal lesions. The analysis of perseveration in the odor discrimination task involved a replication of the previously described experiment, but with the addition of a symmetrical reward contingency by which animals were rewarded for correct go and no-go responses. Under these conditions intact rats showed relatively little overall bias toward go

A. spatial alteration

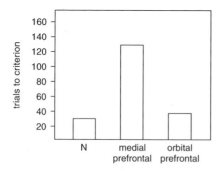

B. olfactory discrimination

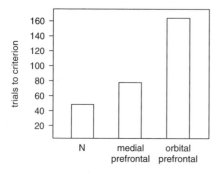

Figure 13–3. Double dissociation of areas of the rat prefrontal cortex. *A:* Performance of normal control rats (N) and rats with lesions of the medial prefrontal cortex or orbital prefrontal cortex on spatial delayed alternation. *B:* Performance of the same animals on a set of odor discrimination problems (data from Eichenbaum et al., 1983).

or no-go responses. Rats with orbital prefrontal lesions were again severely impaired, but the deficit was not attributable to a shift in their response bias. In addition, rats with orbital lesions showed an increased level of repetitive responses for both the go and no-go response types, showing that their impairment was associated with a general tendency to perseverate the last rewarded response. This pattern of findings shows that the different deficits associated with medial and orbital lesions can be characterized as modality-specific perseveration.

The scope of the deficit in olfactory guided learning following damage to the orbital prefrontal cortex in rodents has recently been extended by demonstrations of impairments in acquisition and performance of delayed nonmatch to sample, and conditional discrimination learning. In the odor-guided delayed nonmatch to sample task described in detail in Chapter 7, unlike hippocampal and parahippocampal cortical lesions, damage to the orbital prefrontal cortex results in a deficit in acquisition of the task even with brief memory delays. Conversely, unlike parahippocampal lesions, orbital prefrontal lesions resulted in no subsequent deficit in forgetting at extended delays. Rats with orbital prefrontal lesions were impaired, however, when the pool of repeating odor cues was reduced, that is, under conditions of increased inter-item interference. This pattern of results indicates once more that the effects of prefrontal and hippocampal lesions on performance in working memory tasks are quite different, and that the effects of prefrontal lesions are less attributable to a memory deficit *per se*, than to an impairment in strategic functions subject to interference.

Gordon Winocur reached a similar conclusion based on his studies that compared the effects of medial prefrontal and hippocampal lesions. Animals were tested on a delayed matching to sample task that required them to respond differentially to sample and choice lights that were of the same or different brightness. Normal rats performed the task very well and their accuracy declined only slightly as the memory delay was increased. Rats with prefrontal lesions were impaired at the matching judgment even with the shortest delay, but their accuracy declined over delays at the same rate as that of controls. By contrast, rats with hippocampal lesions performed normally at the shortest memory delay, whereas their performance across delays declined abnormally rapidly. These results suggested that the prefrontal cortex was essential to the working memory requirement for briefly remembering and matching the stimuli, whereas the hippocampus was essential to the maintenance of the stimulus representation.

Finally, Ian Whishaw and colleagues reported a severe impairment in conditional odor–tactile discrimination following orbital prefrontal lesions in rats. In this study rats were trained on a set of four discrimination problems between compound stimuli. The correct choice for each problem was a particular combination of two stimulus elements, although each element was individually equally often rewarded. The findings in this study parallel the findings from studies on humans and monkeys, showing that under conditions of high interference, the prefrontal cortex plays a critical role in learning stimulus–stimulus associations.

How information for working memory is encoded within the prefrontal cortex

In the early 1970s neurophysiologists began to study the activity of neurons in monkeys performing the delayed-response task. A large network of neurons was activated as animals performed each of the relevant task events. Some cells fired associated with presentation of the left or right cue in both the sample and choice periods, and subsequent work has shown that prefrontal neurons show considerable selectivity for visual and spatial properties of memory cues across a variety of working memory tasks. Moreover, many prefrontal neurons begin to fire upon presentation of the sample item or when it disappears, and many of these cells continued to fire throughout the ensuing delay period. These "delay cells" number half the recorded neurons in the prefrontal cortex and have received the most attention because they provided the first evidence of neuronal activity specifically involved in storing a short-term memory.

Recent studies have focused on the delay cells, using an oculomotor version of the delayed-response task developed by Goldman-Rakic and her colleagues (Fig. 13–4A). In this paradigm monkeys are trained to fixate a central spot on a display, and to maintain fixation while a target at one of eight locations is briefly illuminated. Following a delay period when the target must be remembered, the monkey then moved its eyes very rapidly (making what is called a "saccade") to the location of the former target to obtain a reward. In this variation of the delayed-response task, the prefrontal cortex is critical to memory, and this paradigm allowed a dissection of the topography of spatial memory in this cortical area. In a key experiment monkeys were trained to perform the task and then given small unilateral lesions of the dorsolateral prefrontal cortex. Subsequently, their performance was measured for each of the eight target locations, both in the memory task and in a simple task where the target stimulus was on at the time of the saccadic eye movement, eliminating the need for spatial memory. The lesions had no effect on eye movements in the nonmemory task, but resulted in poor delay-dependent performance within a spatially restricted region during the memory task. Furthermore, the deficit was re-

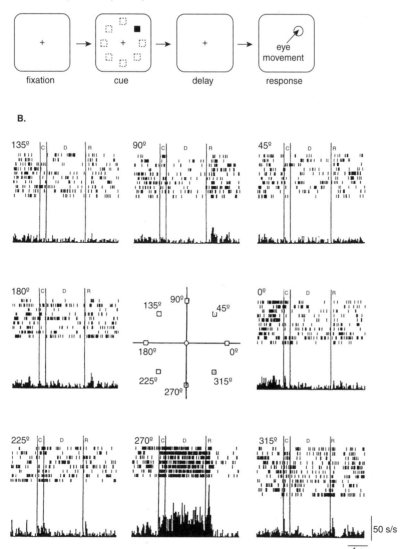

A. occular spatial delayed response

fixation → cue → delay → response

eye movement

B.

135° C D R

90° C D R

45° C D R

180° C D R

135° 90°
45°
180°   0°
225° 315°
270°

0° C D R

225° C D R

270° C D R

315° C D R

50 s/s

1 s

Figure 13–4. The oculomotor delayed-response task. *A:* The task protocol. Initially the animal fixates its eyes on a central cross-hair. Then a light flashes at one of eight positions, followed by a blank delay period when the animal must maintain fixated. Then, when the fixation cross-hairs turn off, the animal saccades to the locus where the cue was flashed. *B:* Responses of a prefrontal neuron during the cue (C), delay (D), and response (R) periods of the task when the cue was presented at different loci. Note selective response when the cue was at 270 degrees, and signs of inhibited activity when the cue was presented at 90 degrees (from Funahashi et al., 1989).

• 325

stricted to a portion of the contralateral visual field, and the magnitude of error in eye movements was minimal at short delays and greater at longer delays. These data provided the first evidence of a "mnemonic scotoma," a "blindness" in memory for a specific region of visual space.

Correspondingly, recordings made from prefrontal neurons in intact monkeys performing this task revealed that the majority of delay cells fired selectively while the animal was remembering a stimulus presented in a particular part of visual space (Fig. 13–4B). The average area of space where excitatory activity was observed was about 45 degrees, and most cells preferred the contralateral part of space, consistent with the findings in the lesion study. In addition, some cells showed distinct inhibitory activity for the direction opposite the preferred direction, suggesting a network mechanism for sharpening the spatial memory signal. Delay cells fired only on trials when a correct saccade was produced, indicating their activity reflected the maintenance of the spatial memory. Subsequent analyses showed that most of these cells maintained the memory of the target location, rather than firing in anticipation of the incipient response. To test this question directly, monkeys were trained in both the standard version of the task and an "antisaccade" version of the task where the monkey was required to move its eyes to the opposite location from where the spatial target had been illuminated. About 80% of the delay cells with directional activity fired during memory for a particular target stimulus location regardless of the direction of the subsequent response. The remaining 20% of the directional delay cells fired associated with the incipient direction of the saccade, indicating the prefrontal cortex also contains information about the intended response.

Reinforcing the view that the prefrontal cortex contains a specialized temporary store, Earl Miller and colleagues compared the capacity of prefrontal and temporal neurons in maintaining selective visual codings during the delay in monkeys performing a matching to sample task. A greater fraction of temporal cells showed selective responses to visual features, but the delay-related activity of these cells ceased abruptly when intervening stimuli were presented. Prefrontal cells that encoded specific visual features were not as prevalent, but these cells maintained elevated stimulus-specific activity throughout a delay filled with intervening stimuli.

A central current question about delay activity in the prefrontal cortex is whether there is regional parcellation of memory storage functions. Particularly striking evidence in favor of this view came from a study by Goldman-Rakic and colleagues in which monkeys were trained on two variants of the delayed-response task. One version was the standard oculomotor spatial delayed-response task, although only right and left target locations were employed. The other version was a visual pattern delayed-response task where one of two elaborate visual stimuli was presented at the central fixation point, and then after the delay the monkey was required to make a left or right saccade depending on which pattern was the sample cue. Neurons in the lateral prefrontal area were particularly responsive in the pattern delayed-response task, such that over three-quarters of the delay cells differentially fired associated with one visual cue. Some of these cells showed highly selective delay responses, such as cells that fired selectively associated with one of two faces, but did not differentiate two other visual patterns. The opposite result was obtained for cells in the dorsolateral prefrontal cortex, such that most delay cells fired selectively in the spatial task and not in the pattern task. The combination of these findings has been interpreted as strong support for the notion that there exist distinct working memory parcellations in the prefrontal cortex, one in the dorsolateral prefrontal area supporting spatial working memory and another in the lateral area supporting visual pattern working memory.

There are such considerable differences between working memory tasks used across species and in different laboratories that it is currently impossible to reach a conclusion about the nature of division of functions within the prefrontal cortex. Consistencies in the data across techniques and species implicate prefrontal processing as more "strategic" than "memory," even though there are also considerable data showing extensive intermixing of executive and storage functions in working memory. While a resolution of the functional mechanism of prefrontal cortex remains elusive, new studies on prefrontal neurons in monkeys performing novel working are providing insights that may supersede notions about division of function by modality or cognitive processing.

In one study Miller and his colleagues trained monkeys on a variant of the delayed matching to sample task in which subjects were shown a sample object stimulus at the central fixation point, then after a memory delay were shown that object plus another object choice at peripheral locations, then after another memory delay had to saccade to the location of the matching stimulus item (Fig. 13–5A). Thus, the monkeys had to remember two aspects of the sample object. During the initial delay they had to retain the visual content properties, or the "what" quality of the stimulus. Then in the second delay they had to retain the location where the object was again presented, that is, its "where" quality. Neurons in the lateral prefrontal area responded to the "what" and "where" qualities of objects. One example, shown in Fig. 13–5B (left), fired more to one particular object during the initial "what" delay. The example Fig. 13–5B

A. "what" then "where" task

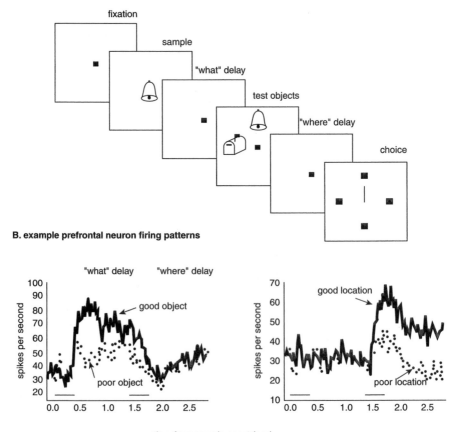

B. example prefrontal neuron firing patterns

time from sample onset (sec)

Figure 13–5. The "what" and "where" task. *A:* Sequence of trial stages in the protocol. After initial fixation, a sample stimulus is shown in the center. Then, after a delay, two choice stimuli are shown and the animal must saccade to the one that is the
same as the sample. Then, following another delay, the animal must saccade to the location where the sample was last shown. *B:* Examples of object-tuned (left) and loca-
tion-tuned (right) cells (from Rao et al., 1997).

(right) fired during the "where" delay more associated with location where
the sample reappeared, regardless of which object was remembered. Yet
other cells encoded both the "what" and "where" attributes, and fired either selectively both during the "what" and "where" delays, or fired maximally during the final delay associated with the combination of a particular object and a particular place it was presented. These data indicate

that cells in the same area of the prefrontal cortex can represent both visual and spatial information when demanded by the task requirements.

The prefrontal cortex may also be especially suited to retrieving and utilizing representations of associations in memory. In another study, neurons in the prefrontal cortex were recorded in monkeys who were initially presented with a sample visual stimulus and then, after a delay, had to identify an arbitrarily paired stimulus associate from multiple choices. During the sample stimulus presentation, and partially into the memory delay, the activity of prefrontal neurons was selective for the characteristics of the sample stimulus. However, toward the end of the delay, and prior to presentation of the choice stimuli, prefrontal neurons altered their activity associated with the characteristics of the appropriate stimulus associate. These findings suggest that prefrontal neurons may have access to long-term stored representations of visual as well as spatial associations, and employ them in sequence following the demands of the task.

The prefrontal cortex is activated in humans performing working memory tasks

The emergence of brain imaging techniques has allowed investigators to examine the areas of cortex activated during working memory performance in human subjects. Among the first of these studies, John Jonides, Edward Smith, and their colleagues characterized areas of the human brain activated during a variant of the spatial delayed response task. In this task subjects fixated a central point on a computer monitor and were presented with three dots as target sample stimuli. Following a 3-second delay period, a circle marked one location on the screen where one of the targets had appeared, or another location. Thus, subjects had to remember a set of target locations and later identify a choice item as one of the set. The control task was similar, except that the three dots were presented only during the end of the delay then during the choice period when one of them was circled, so that responses were guided by perception not memory. The brain areas prominently activated by positron emission tomography (PET) included all the components of the working memory circuit outlined in monkeys, but all on the right side of the human brain. These included the dorsolateral prefrontal cortex, the posterior parietal area, plus parts of the occipital and premotor areas. Confirming these findings, a neighboring area of dorsolateral prefrontal cortex was activated in a functional magnetic resonance imaging (fMRI) study when subjects were required to identify repetitions of stimuli among a series of items presented at various spatial locations.

In humans, of course, one can examine the very same verbal and visuospatial working memory processes that were the focus of the Baddeley model, and indeed there is evidence for the existence of distinct areas that mediate the visuospatial sketch pad and the phonological loop. Tasks that require subjects to rehearse verbal material activate a part of the parietal cortex, whereas different parietal areas are activated during visuo-spatial processing. All tasks that require working memory activate prefrontal areas. In addition, parts of the prefrontal cortex are especially strongly activated when subjects are required to update verbal information, consistent with the putative role of this area as the central executive.

There is considerable agreement that different posterior cortical areas are activated during modality-specific working memory processing. On the other hand, there is considerable controversy over whether different kinds of processing are parcellated within the prefrontal cortex, and about the nature of parcellation. One study by Smith and colleagues, directly modeled after the work on monkeys, examined this issue with the "three-back" task designed to test working memory for spatial or verbal material. In both versions of the task, on a series of trials subjects fixate a central location and are presented with a series of letters at a peripheral site, with one letter presented each trial with blank presentations intervening (Fig. 13–6). In the spatial memory condition, on each trial the subject must identify whether the target on the current trial matches in location the item presented three trials back, and must ignore the identity of the letters. In the verbal memory condition, the subject, conversely, must identify whether the current letter matches the identity of the letter presented three trials back, ignoring the location of presentations. Thus, the stimulus presentations in both tasks are identical, but the memory demands differ according to a spatial or verbal rule. The findings indicated a clear dissociation of brain regions involved in the two tasks. In the spatial task there was more activation on the right hemisphere, and included both a posterior parietal and a prefrontal site of most prominent activation. Conversely, the verbal task activated primarily parietal and prefrontal areas in the left hemisphere. This dissociation is consistent with clinical observations of selective spatial and verbal working memory deficits following damage to the right and left prefrontal cortex, respectively.

A separate set of PET studies by Petrides and colleagues modeled after experiments on self-ordering and conditional learning in monkeys, examined whether these cognitive operations could be dissociated in human brain activations. In one of these studies, subjects either performed the self-ordering task described earlier, or a conditional visual-motor response task in which subjects had to point to a different design assigned to each

A. spatial memory condition

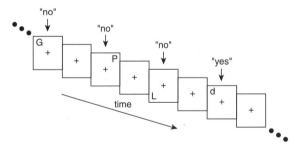

B. verbal memory condition

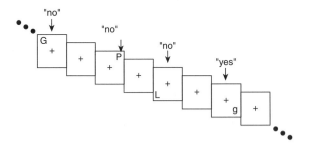

Figure 13–6. An example series of trials on each of two versions of the three-back task (from Jonides and Smith, 1997).

of a set of distinct color stimuli. Consistent with his studies on monkeys with selective prefrontal lesions, Petrides found that a middorsolateral part of the prefrontal cortex was selectively activated in the self-ordering task, whereas a premotor area was selectively activated in the conditional visual-motor task. In another study Petrides found that the same middorsolateral area is selectively activated in a verbal self-ordering task, showing the generality of function of this area over nonverbal and verbal stimulus materials. There was some degree of hemispheric lateralization consistent with the study described previously. In the nonverbal self-ordering task the right prefrontal area was differentially activated, whereas in the verbal task both hemispheres were equally activated.

In additional studies, Petrides and colleagues directly addressed potential distinctions between the dorsolateral and lateral areas of the human prefrontal cortex. These studies examined strategic retrieval from long-term memory for verbal and visuospatial materials. In the study on verbal strategic retrieval, Petrides scanned subjects performing different verbal recall tasks. In one task, subjects were required to recall a list of unrelated words, a task well acknowledged to depend on active retrieval mechanisms. To control specifically for strategic monitoring of the words that had been recalled, as opposed to the search in long-term memory *per se*, they compared the activation during word list retrieval with that during a control condition in which subjects produced correct responses in a previously well-learned verbal paired associate task. The latter task is much less demanding on active retrieval processes, but involves the same degree of self-monitoring. They found that indeed the left dorsolateral area was equally activated in both tasks, but the lateral prefrontal area was more activated in the list retrieval task. In the study on visuospatial strategic retrieval, subjects were trained to touch each of a set of displayed boxes on a screen, with each box touched as a nearby indicator light was illuminated. The sequence of indicated boxes was the same on each trial, so subjects reduced their reaction times over the course of training. This initially involved implicit learning, because the subjects could not generate the sequence explicitly. However, explicit training was then given by requiring subjects to touch each box in anticipation of the indicator.

Following training on this condition the subjects were scanned in both conditions of the task. Activity in the right lateral prefrontal area was greater in the explicit condition than in the implicit condition, consistent with the interpretation that only the explicit sequencing required active retrieval of the stored sequence. The combination of all these findings led Petrides to propose that the prefrontal cortex is parcellated, not according to different stimulus materials as Goldman-Rakic has argued, but rather according to the cognitive processing demands. Petrides argues that both verbal and nonverbal strategic ordering processes are reflected in selective activation of the dorsolateral prefrontal cortex, whereas strategic retrieval from long-term memory for both verbal and nonverbal materials selectively activates the lateral prefrontal cortical area. Notably, however, there are clear hemispheric differences in Petrides's findings on verbal and visuospatial materials, consistent with the proposal of Smith and colleagues. On the other hand, there are also considerable data showing hemispheric differences in the prefrontal cortex based on cognitive demands associated with long-term memory encoding and retrieval processes, such that encoding in episodic memory for various materials is associated with enhanced activity in the left prefrontal cortex, whereas retrieval of various materials is associated with enhanced activity on the right side.

A recent meta-analysis of a large number of studies using brain imaging techniques to characterize prefrontal activation in working memory has generally sided with Petrides's view of parcellation by cognitive functions. In his analysis Adrian Owen found that spatial working memory tasks can activate either the dorsolateral or lateral prefrontal region, such that the lateral region was activated when the task demanded retention of one or a few items, whereas the dorsolateral region was activated when the subject was required to constantly monitor and manipulate a series of ongoing spatial locations. A generally similar pattern was found across studies on visual working memory. Tasks that required subjects only to retain visual pattern information over a delay did not activate the dorsolateral area, whereas tasks that required constant monitoring and updating did. Overall, Owen concluded that the dorsolateral region is activated when the demand for continuous monitoring is high regardless of the materials to be remembered.

The orchestration of memory: Parcellation of functions among cortical areas

While the prefrontal cortex plays a critical and central role in working with memory, a role akin to that of an orchestra conductor, there are also other players in the orchestra distributed in other areas of the cerebral cortex. Two recent studies have promoted the view that different cognitive demands contribute to a distribution of functional activations among cortical areas during working memory performance in humans.

Jonathan Cohen and colleagues used variants of the "*n*-back" task combined with rapid fMRI scans to compare regional activations as a function of differing demands for executive control in managing memory load versus maintenance over time. They trained subjects to match verbal stimuli to items presented previously under four different conditions. These included comparisons to items either one, two, or three items back, and a zero-back condition where a particular stimulus was identified whenever it was presented. Scans were made during and just after the stimulus presentation, and repeatedly during the 10-second delay between trials. Areas in both the left prefrontal cortex and posterior visual areas were activated, but the extent of activation differed under the controlled conditions (Fig. 13–7). Prefrontal cortex activation was maximal under high memory load conditions, that is in the two- and three-back tasks, and less so in the zero- and one-back tasks, and the level of activation was constant throughout the memory delay. Conversely, the visual areas were more activated late in the delay when the memory demand was highest, regardless of load. In addition the amount of activation in Broca's area was affected by both factors, with the greatest activation for the highest load at the longest memory delay. These data are consistent with the notion that working memory circuits are widespread in the cortex, and with the findings from earlier described neuropsychological studies across species showing that the pre-

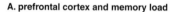

A. prefrontal cortex and memory load

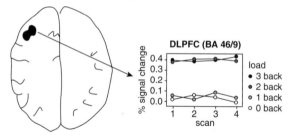

B. visual cortex and time

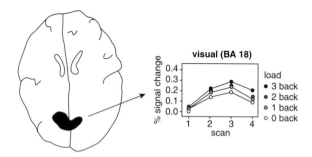

C. Broca's area and interaction of load and time

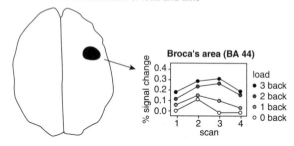

Figure 13–7. Activation of multiple brain areas during working memory. In each panel, the most activated brain area is shown, and the amount of activation is plotted over time during the memory delay and separately for the memory load zero, one, two, or three items. A: An area in the prefrontal cortex is activated more for higher memory load regardless of the delay. B: A visual area that is activated as the delay increased regardless of load. C: Broca's area is activated differentially associated with both the load and delay (data from Cohen et al., 1997).

frontal cortex is more involved in strategic processing associated with the number of items in memory, as opposed to storage of those items *per se.*

Another recent study by Courtney, Ungerleider, and their colleagues compared posterior and prefrontal cortical activations in humans performing a working task that required subjects to remember a face over a delay. They compared fMRI activations during presentations of face or visual "noise" stimulation, and during the memory delay between stimulus presentations. Responses of posterior and prefrontal cortical areas were characterized using complex statistical analyses aimed at three components of the task, transient nonselective visual responses, transient selective responses to faces, and sustained responses over the memory delay. They found that posterior visual cortical areas showed primarily transient nonselective or selective visual responses, whereas prefrontal areas exhibited strong delay responses plus face selectivity. Furthermore, the extent to which these factors activated areas throughout the cortex was graded, with the most posterior area responsive only nonselectively and without delay, and the most rostral prefrontal areas most responsive to delay with face selectivity. These findings again are consistent with the notion of widespread networks for working memory, with graded contributions of processing functions throughout the network.

In addition, recent studies of the firing patterns of single neurons in monkeys and rats have contributed to the view of a parcellation of functions in the prefrontal and posterior cortical areas during working memory. Miller and colleagues' studies on monkeys performing the visually cued working memory task described in Chapter 8 found that a greater proportion of cells in the lateral prefrontal region showed sustained responses during the delay, and conveyed more information about the match–nonmatch status of the test stimuli compared to perirhinal cortex. By contrast, more neurons in the perirhinal cortex and inferotemporal cortex show greater stimulus selectivity. Notably, in this task the memory delay was filled with interpolated material, which put a strong demand on working memory. By contrast, a study by Miyashita and Chang involved a visual recognition task where the memory delay was not filled with interpolated material, and they found that a large fraction of temporal neurons show sustained stimulus-specific delay activity. Similarly, in rats performing the continuous delayed nonmatch to sample task described in Chapter 7, it was found that more cells in the orbitofrontal area exhibited stimulus-selective match enhancement or suppression, whereas more cells in the parahippocampal region exhibited sustained stimulus-specific activity during the delay. This pattern of findings suggests that the posterior cortical areas play a strong role in encoding and maintaining sustained stimulus representations, and that the prefrontal cortex consistently plays a critical role in acquiring and employing the task rules as well as a variable role in maintaining stimulus representations depending on the demand for working memory.

Summing up

The prefrontal cortex performs a critical role in "working-with-memory" in rodents, monkeys, and humans. Most investigators regard its role as critical to working memory, the capacity to hold items and manipulate them in consciousness. The prefrontal cortex is parcellated into several distinct areas that have different inputs and whose functions can be dissociated according to different modalities of stimulus processing. However, they share common higher-order function in working memory and strategic processing, reflected in perseveration and other common strategic disorders following damage to any of the subdivisions.

Correspondingly, prefrontal neurons encode all events during working memory task performance, and large numbers of prefrontal cells are involved in maintaining item memories for brief periods and in encoding stimuli and events in accordance with acquired task rules. Prefrontal subdivisions are highly connected with one another and with posterior areas of the cortex to operate as a complex and widespread network for conscious control over memory and other intellectual functions.

READINGS

Baddeley, A. 1996. The fractionation of working memory. *Proc. Natl. Acad. Sci.* 93:13468–13472.

Cohen, J.D., Perlstein, W.M., Braver, T.S., Nystrom, L.E., Noll, D.C., Jonides, J., and Smith, E.E. 1997. Temporal dynamics of brain activation during a working memory task. *Nature* 386: 604–607.

Courtney, S.M., Ungerleider, L.G., Kell, K., and Haxby, J.V. 1997. Transient and sustained activity in a distributed neural system for human working memory. *Nature* 386: 608–611.

Eichenbaum, H. 2000. A cortical-hippocampal system for declarative memory. *Nat. Rev. Neurosci.* 1:41–50.

Goldman-Rakic, P.S. 1996. The prefrontal landscape: Implications of functional architecture for understanding human mentation and the central executive. *Phil. Trans. R. Soc. Lond. Ser. B*, 351: 1445–1453.

Jonides, J., Rugg, M.D. (Ed.) and Smith, E.E. 1997. The architecture of working memory. In *Cognitive Neuroscience*, Hove East Sussex: Psychology Press, pp. 243–276.

Kolb, B. 1990. Prefrontal cortex. In *The Cerebral Cortex of the Rat*, B. Kolb and R.C. Tees (Eds.). Cambridge: MIT Press, pp. 437–458.

Miller, E. The prefrontal cortex and cognitive control. *Nat. Rev. Neurosci* 1:59–65.

Owen, A.M. 1997. The functional organization of working memory processes within human lateral frontal cortex: The contribution of functional neuroimaging. *Eur. J. Neurosci.* 9:1329–1339.

Pandya, D.N., and Yeterian, E.H. 1996. Comparison of prefrontal architecture and connections. *Phil. Trans. R. Sec. Lond. B.* 351:1423–1432.

Roberts, A.C., Robbins, T.W., and Weiskrantz, L. (Eds.). 1996. Executive and cognitive functions of the prefrontal cortex. *Phil. Trans. Roy. Soc. Lond.* B351: 1387–1527.

Shimamura, A.P. 1995. Memory and frontal lobe function. In: *The Cognitive Neurosciences*, M.S. Gazzaniga (Ed.). Cambridge: MIT Press, pp. 803–813.

• • • • • •
Final Thoughts

Over a hundred years ago there was an amazing period of break-throughs in neuroscience, a Golden Era, in which major discoveries about the brain were made and during which the basic themes of memory research were generated. Recent decades have seen remarkable progress in clarifying questions raised in each of these themes, by elucidating the cellular bases for increased connectivity that underlies memory, by qualifying the nature of different forms of cognition in memory, by showing how the different forms of memory are compartmentalized into distinct memory systems in the brain, and by providing an understanding of the processes that underlie memory consolidation. It should also be clear from this book that progress in understanding each of these themes is inter-twined, such that the elements that support alterations in connectivity and consolidation reflect a continuum of mechanisms and processes among the memory systems. Furthermore, the seamless experience of memory suggests that the different memory systems share information and work to-gether to mediate our sense of "autobiography," that is, the individuality of a lifetime of memories.

• • • • • •
Glossary

Acetylcholine • One of the first discovered neurotransmitters, uses two major receptor subtypes, muscarinic and nicotinic.

Action potential • The active conduction of a depolarizing potential characteristic of axons. This potential is slower than electrotonic conduction but is faithful in magnitude over long distances. Its initiation and propagation involve an initial influx of sodium, then an outflow of potassium, and then a recovery period during which the cell is refractory to initiation of another action potential.

Adrenergic • Pertaining to the hormone adrenaline (also called epinephrine) or the neurotransmitter noradrenaline (norepinephrine). The two major subtypes of the neurotransmitter are α and β.

Agonist • A drug that facilitates or prolongs the action of a neurotransmitter, by enhancing its production, release, or persistence, or by triggering the receptors for that neurotransmitter.

Allocentric space • Position in the environment independent of the orientation or location of the subject.

Ammon's horn • A subdivision of the hippocampus that receives major inputs from the dentate gyrus and the parahippocampal region, and projects to the subiculum; composed of sequentially connected areas CA3 and CA1.

Amygdala • A complex set of nuclei located underneath the cortex and just anterior to the hippocampus in the temporal lobe. A critical component of the system for emotional learning and emotional expression, and for the modulation of memory consolidation by emotional state.

Antagonist • A drug that inhibits the action of a neurotransmitter, by retarding its production, release, or persistence, or by blocking the receptors for that neurotransmitter.

Anterior • Also called **rostral**. Toward the front of the brain.

Anterograde amnesia • Loss of the ability to acquire new information following head injury or brain damage.

AP5 • D-2-amino-5-phosphonovalerate. Selective and competitive antagonist of NMDA receptors.

Autonomic nervous system • Components of the peripheral nervous system that regulate various organs of the body including the heart, blood pressure, respiration, sweating, pupil dilation, digestion, and more.

Axon • The single long neuronal extension that conducts the action potential to the synapse.

Basal ganglia • Forebrain components of the extrapyramidal motor system that include the striatum.

Behavioral LTP • Changes in synaptic efficacy following and due to the formation of new memories.

Behaviorism • The view that all learned behaviors can be explained on the basis of elements of conditioned responses.

Bilateral • Pertaining to both sides of the brain.

Brain stem • Components of the brain that lie beneath the cortex and thalamus, typically in the midbrain or hindbrain.

Caudal • Towards thr rear of the brain.

Cell assembly • Hebb's notion of a local or diffuse circuit of connected neurons that develop to represent a specific percept and concepts.

Cerebellum • Major structure of the brain stem involved in motor control, a critical component of motor systems involved in conditioning of skeletal muscle responses. Major components include an outer cerebellar cortex composed of many folia and an inner complex of cerebellar nuclei.

Cerebral cortex • Structure on the outer surface of the brain, usually with six distinct layers, separated into major frontal, parietal, occipital, and temporal regions and many functionally distinct zones.

Classical conditioning (or conditioning) • The association of an arbitrary external stimulus (the conditioning stimulus, or CS) with another stimulus (the unconditioned stimulus, or US) that produces an unconditioned reflexive response (UR), resulting in the gradual acquisition of a conditioned response (CR) to the CS.

Cognitive map • A systematic representation of the topology of the physical environment.

Cognitivism • The view that the complexity of learned behavior requires consideration of capabilities for insight and planning, and cannot be explained by a combination of conditioned responses.

Conditioned reflex or conditioned response (CR) • Behavioral response arising from the association between an arbitrary external stimulus (the conditioned stimulus, or CS) and an unconditioned stimulus (US) that evokes a reflexive unconditioned response (UR).

Consolidation • The process by which initially labile memories become permanent and impervious to disruption. Separated into a molecular/celluar process of fixation of a memory trace that occurs for several minutes after learning, and a prolonged period of reorganization of memories mediated by interactions between structures of the declarative memory system.

Contralateral • Opposite side of the head or body. The alternative is ipsilateral, on the same side of the body.

Cortical column • Functional and anatomical organization in the cortex by which closely connected and functionally similar cells are arranged vertically across layers into parallel columns. For example, in the primary visual cortex of higher mammals, there are alternating columns for ocular dominance and orientation selectivity.

"Cued" learning • A term often used to describe learning guided by a single simple or complex stimulus, as contrasted with spatial learning that involves spatial relations among multiple cues. Synonymous with "nonspatial" learning.

Cytoarchitecture • The types and arrangement of cells that characterize each brain area, and each distinct area of the cerebral cortex.

Deafferentation • Disconnection of inputs.

Declarative memory • Everyday memory for facts and events that are subject to conscious recollection and can be explicitly expressed in many ways outside the conditions of original learning. The combination of episodic and semantic memory.

Delay conditioning • The standard version of classical conditioning where the conditioning stimulus (CS) is presented continuously until and through the presentation of the unconditioned stimulus (US).

Delayed alternation • A task in which the subject must alternate between two conditions or stimuli to obtain rewards. In delayed spatial alternation, the subject alternates between two spatial directions or locations.

Delayed nonmatch to sample (DNMS) • A task in which the subject must remember the identity of a stimulus across a delay period when no cues are present. Typically divided into three phases: a sample phase when the subject views the stimulus but cannot respond, a delay phase when the stimulus cannot be seen, and a choice phase when the subject must select an alternative stimulus to obtain a reward. Typical variants involve whether a small number of stimuli are used repeated across trials or unique stimuli are used on each trial, and the "delayed match to sample" version where during the choice phase the subject must select the sample stimulus and not the alternative to obtain the reward.

Delayed response • A task in which the subject must remember the position of a reward across a delay period when no cues are present. Typically divided into three phases: a sample phase when the subject views the location of the reward but cannot respond, a delay phase when no spatial cues are provided to identify the reward location, and a choice phase when the subject is allowed to select the location of the hidden reward.

Dendrite • One of several multiple fine processes that extend the neuron cell body that receives neural signals from other neurons.

Depolarization • Change in the polarity of the cell membrane such that the inside of the cell becomes more positive relative to the outside, as compared to the resting state.

Discrimination learning • Tasks in which the subject is presented with multiple (usually two) stimuli and must consistently select one of them and not the other to obtain a reward. Variants include simultaneous discrimination when all the stimuli are presented at the same time on each trial versus successive discrimination when only one stimulus is presented on each trial and the stimuli are presented in a random sequence.

Dorsal • Toward the top of the brain.

Double dissociation • The observation that damage to brain structure A, but not structure B, results in impairment on task X, but not task Y, while damage to brain structure B and not structure A results in impairment on task Y and not task X.

Effector • Brain structures that directly control muscle or hormonal responses.

Egocentric space • Position in the environment relative to the orientation and location of the body, e.g., left or right. Note the egocentric positions of fixed objects will change as the subject moves through space.

Electrotonic conduction • The passive conduction of a potential difference (depolarizing or hyperpolarizing) along any part of the neuron. It is fast but decremental, dissipating over a short distance.

Emotional memory • An unconsciously expressed, acquired aversion or attraction toward a previously arbitrary stimulus.

Entorhinal cortex • A subdivision of the parahippocampal region, the region closest to the hippocampus, which has the greatest connections with it.

Episodic memory • Representations of specific personal experiences that occur in a unique spatial and temporal context, typically involving the capacity to reexperience particular events in one's life by conscious recollection.

Excitatory postsynaptic potential (EPSP) • Depolarizing electrical potential created at the postsynaptic site of *excitatory synapses* as a result of neurotransmitter recognition, usually due to the influx of sodium.

Explicit memory • Memory expression based on conscious recollection involving direct efforts to access memories.

Exteroceptive • Reception of stimulus information from the external world.

Extramaze • Pertaining to the environment outside of a maze.

Fear conditioning • The acquired association between an arbitrary, conditioned, external stimulus and a natural, fear-producing, unconditioned stimulus. The most common example is the association between a tone and shock to the feet. Often categorized into "cued" fear conditioning, when the relevant conditioned stimulus is a punctate stimulus that has a close temporal association with the unconditioned stimulus (e.g., presentation of a tone just before the shock), and "contextual" fear conditioning, referring to acquired association between the static environmental context, typically the testing chamber, and the shock or other unconditioned stimulus.

Fear-potentiated startle • Magnification of the startle response when animals or people are in a fearful state.

Field EPSP • The summed excitatory postsynaptic potentials from many simultaneously activated synapses.

Fornix • A major axon bundle that connects the hippocampus with several subcortical areas including the hypothalamus, thalamus, septum, and brain stem. Likely carries nonspecific information that modulates the arousal and paces the processing rhythm of the hippocampus.

Gene expression • The cascade of molecular processes involving reading the DNA sequence, mediated via RNA, to direct new protein synthesis.

Go/no-go • A response modality in which subjects make an active movement (go) under one condition or to one stimulus, and make no response (no-go) under an alternative condition or to another stimulus.

Habit • An acquired and well-practiced response to a particular stimulus.

Habituation • The decrement in responsiveness to repeated sensory stimulation without reinforcement.

Hebb rule • Hebb proposed that increases in synaptic strength result from the combination of repeated activation of a presynaptic element and its participation in the success in firing the postsynaptic cell.

Hippocampus • Structure in the medial temporal lobe involved in declarative memory. Composed of distinct subdivisions, including Ammon's horn (CA1 and CA3), the dentate gyrus, and the subiculum.

H.M. • The patient who suffered a highly selective and severe global amnesia following bilateral removal of the medial temporal lobe region.

Hyperpolarization • Change in the polarity of the cell membrane such that the inside of the cell becomes more negative relative to the outside, as compared to the resting state.

Implicit memory • Unconscious changes in performance of a task as influenced by some previous experience, typically revealed by indirect measures such as changes in the speed of performance or in biases in choices made while reperforming a task.

Inferential memory expression • The capacity to deduce solutions to novel problems based on indirect relations among items retrieved from distinct memories.

Inferotemporal cortex • Cortical area of the lateral and inferior temporal lobe that is involved in higher-order visual pattern recognition.

Inhibitory postsynaptic potential (IPSP) • Hyperpolarizing electrical potential created at the postsynaptic site of *inhibitory synapses* as a result of neurotransmitter recognition, usually due to the influx of chloride.

Intermediate term memory • A period that follows short-term or working memory, but involves representations that are not yet permanently stored.

Intramaze • Pertaining to local stimuli available inside a maze.

Ionotropic receptor • Conventional neurotransmitter receptors found in postsynaptic elements that are transmitter-gated and allow charged molecules to flow briefly inducing the postsynaptic excitatory and inhibitory potentials.

Law of effect • Principle by which behaviors that lead to a positive reinforcement are more likely to reoccur under the same circumstances. Considered a formulation of the basis for strengthening stimulus–response connections.

Limbic system • The anatomical designation of the emotional circuit in the brain, including Papez's circuit (cingulate cortex, hippocampal region, mammillary bodies, thalamus) plus the amygdala, septum, and prefrontal cortex, and more recently the orbital frontal cortex and areas of the midbrain.

Localization • The view that specific psychological functions, or memories, can be identified with specific areas of the cortex or other parts of the brain.

Long-term depression (LTD) • Long-lasting decrease of synaptic transmission, that is, a permanent decrement in synaptic efficacy, resulting from lack of coincident presynaptic activation and generation of a postsynaptic action potential.

Long-term potentiation (LTP) • Long-lasting facilitation of synaptic transmission, that is, a permanent increase in synaptic efficacy, resulting from repeated activation of a presynaptic element and its participation in the success in firing the postsynaptic cell.

Medial temporal lobe • The area of the temporal lobe that lies nearest the midline, including the hippocampus, the amygdala, and the immediately surrounding cortex of the parahippocampal region.

Memory space • A large-scale neural network that organizes the codings for the sequences of events that compose episodic memories, and links these memories together by codings for common features among the episodic memories.

Metabotropic receptors • Receptors that are activated by transmitters or other molecules, but do not open channels and directly cause changes in the membrane potential, and instead produce other changes in the cell that can have lasting effects on its responsiveness.

Modulation of memory • Facilitation or retardation of memory fixation, mediated by hormones including a pathway through the amygdala.

Multiple memory systems • The notion that there are several at least partially distinct brain systems that mediate different forms of memory.

Neuromodulators • Molecules that influence the activity of synapses or the production of action potentials. These are often released at distant sites and act at metabotropic receptors.

Neuron doctrine • The hypothesis that the brain is composed of discrete nerve cells that communicate with one another via specialized connections (synapses).

Neuropsychological studies • Examinations that attempt to identify and characterize specific perceptual, cognitive, or behavioral effects of brain damage.

Neurotransmitter • Molecules that are released and recognized within a synapse to mediate changes in the potential of the postsynaptic cell.

Neurotrophins • Molecules that promote morphological change and increased connectivity.

NMDA • N-methyl-D-aspartate. A molecule that acts as a first messenger (neurotransmitter) that regulates the flow of Ca^{2+} into the cell membrane. Normally the NMDA receptor is blocked by magnesium (Mg^{2+}). However, NMDA receptors have the unusual property of being modulated by the voltage of the cell membrane such that when the membrane is depolarized the magnesium block is eliminated and Ca^{2+} can flow into the cell.

Nonsense syllable • A meaningless letter string composed of two consonants separated by a vowel (e.g., "ket," "poc," "baf").

Norepinephrine • An early discovered neurotransmitter. Uses two major subtypes of receptors, α and β. Also called noradrenaline.

Ocular dominance • Pertaining to the situation when a visual neuron is better stimulated by presentation of a stimulus from the ipsilateral or contralateral side of visual space.

Oculomotor • Pertaining to eye movement.

Orientation selectivity • Pertaining to the situation in primary visual neurons where cells are selectively responsive to the orientation (e.g., vertical, horizontal) of a contrast edge.

Paired associate learning • The acquisition of associations among arbitrarily paired stimuli. In humans, most commonly involves learning novel associations between unrelated works, (e.g., army-table, ball-elephant, etc). In animals, involves novel associations among perceptual stimuli that are not reinforcers.

Papez circuit • A set of structures proposed by James Papez to mediate emotion. The structures are connected in a circular arrangement and viewed to mediate the integration of external and visceral signals and expression.

Parahippocampal region • A set of cortical areas of the temporal lobe immediately surrounding the hippocampus. Includes the perirhinal cortex, the parahippocampal cortex (in monkeys, and called the postrhinal cortex in rats), and the entorhinal cortex. Connects the hippocampus with neocortical association areas.

Perirhinal cortex • A subdivision of the parahippocampal region in rats and monkeys.

Perseveration • Continuing or repetitive behavioral responses emitted when no longer appropriate or intruding from previous events into the current situation.

Place cell • A neuron, typically in the hippocampus, that is activated when the animal is in a particular location in its environment, most purely regardless of the direction of its orientation or the ongoing behavior.

Place learning • Acquisition of a maze or other spatial problem guided by the expectancy of reward at an absolute (allocentric) location.

Population spike • The summed waveform of action potentials from many simultaneously activated neurons.

Posterior • Also called *caudal*. Toward the back of the brain.

Postrhinal cortex • A subdivision of the parahippocampal region in rats, called the parahippocampal gyrus in monkeys.

Postsynaptic site • The specialization of the cell membrane of a dendrite, cell body, or presynaptic site for recognition of a neurotransmitter molecule. Contains neurotransmitter receptors specialized for one or more forms of a neurotransmitter and mechanisms for influx of specific ions as a result of recognition of the transmitter at the receptor.

Prefrontal cortex • A large region of the cerebral cortex that lies anterior to the primary motor cortex, composed of many subdivisions including premotor cortex, dorsolateral, medial, and orbital subdivisions.

Premotor cortex • A specific zone of the cerebral cortex that lies just anterior to the primary motor cortex and is involved in motor learning.

Presynaptic site • The specialization of the ending of the axon where the connection is made with another neuron, characteristically filled with synaptic vesicles that contain neurotransmitter molecules and molecular machinery for manufacture and packaging of neurotransmitter and special processes for release of vesicles and reuptake of the transmitter.

Procedural memory • A set of learning abilities that involves tuning and modifying the networks of many brain systems that support skilled performance.

Radial maze • A maze with a central platform and multiple (usually eight) arms radiating out in all directions, like spokes of a wheel. Typically the rat must traverse each arm to find rewards at the end of some or all arms.

Receptive field • The location of a stimulus for optimal activation of a neuronal response. For visual stimuli the receptive fields are locations in visual space. For auditory stimuli the receptive fields are frequencies of sounds. For touch the receptive fields are locations on the body surface.

Reference memory • Memory for items that have a constant significance across many episodes.

Reflex • Automatic, unconditioned behavioral or endocrine response to an external stimulus. Mediated by a reflex arc composed of sensory neurons that connect to motor neurons that connect to effectors (muscles or glands).

Refractory period • A brief time following the action potential when another cannot be initiated due to the imbalance of ionic concentrations.

Reinforcer • A stimulus of innate biological significance that can drive behavior. Common positive reinforcers include food, water, sex, and warmth. Common negative reinforcers include electrical shock or other forms of painful stimulation.

Relational representation • An organization of episodic memories according to common items among them, leading to the development and modification of semantic memory networks.

Representational flexibility • The capacity to compare and contrast memories in a relational representation, and to infer solutions to new problems as a result of such comparisons.

Response learning • Maze learning guided by the acquisition of specific stimulus–response (left and right turn) associations.

Resting potential • Normal potential of the cell membrane, usually negative on the inside relative to the outside.

Retrograde amnesia • Loss of information acquired prior to head injury or brain damage. Often *temporally graded*, such that information acquired remotely prior to the damage is preserved, whereas information acquired recently prior to the damage is lost.

Reverberatory activity • Regenerative activity in a neural circuit that could mediate the persistence of a representation.

Rostral • Also called *anterior*. Towards the front of the brain.

Savings • Retention of a memory measured as the decrease in amount of training on some occasion after learning required to reattain the originally successful level of learned performance.

Schema • An active organization of memories whose structure determines the framework in which new memories are added, and can be employed during remembering to reconstruct or infer the probable constituents of a memory and the order in which they occurred.

Second messenger • Intracellular signaling molecule that causes downstream effects in the molecular cascade of events that follows activation of membrane receptors by neurotransmitters (the "first" messenger).

Second-order conditioning • A procedure that begins with a trained association between an arbitrary stimulus, as a conditioned stimulus, and a primary reinforcer, such as food or shock, followed by training on the association between another arbitrary stimulus and the previous conditioned stimulus which now acts as a second-order reinforcer. For example, initially a tone and shock are associated, such that the tone now produces a fearful reaction. Then the tone can be used as a secondary reinforcer on second-order conditioning of a light–tone association.

Semantic memory • The body of one's world knowledge, the large-scale organization of memories not bound to any specific experience in which they were acquired.

Sensitization • The increment in responsiveness to sensory stimulation following other strong stimulation.

Septum • Subcortical structure of the forebrain that is interconnected with the hippocampus.

Somatosensory • Sensations of touch on the skin, including texture, pressure, heat, and pain.

Spatial learning • Learning guided by the use of spatial relations among external stimuli.

Spine • Protrusion of the postsynaptic element of dendrites.

Startle response • A jump or other sudden movement performed by animals and people in response to an unexpected salient stimulus such as a loud sound.

Stimulus–reinforcer (reward or punishment) association • The acquired attraction or aversion to a stimulus associated with a primary reinforcer, such as food reward or shock. The fundamental mechanism of emotional memory.

Stimulus–response (SR) association • The learned execution of a specific behavior following presentation of a particular stimulus, reinforced by positive or negative outcomes following the behavior.

Striatum • Subcortical structure of the forebrain, composed of the caudate and putamen, a component of the extrapyramidal motor system and critical to habit memory.

Subcortical • Brain structures that lie under the cerebral cortex, such as the thalamus, striatum, hippocampus, amygdala, and many other nuclei and axon tracts.

Subiculum • A subdivision of the hippocampus that receives major inputs from CA1 and the parahippocampal region, and projects to the parahippocampal region and through the fornix to subcortical areas.

Synapse • Specialization for communication between neurons composed of the end of an axon (called the presynaptic site) and its contact area (the postsynaptic site) on the dendrite, cell body, or presynaptic site of another neuron.

Topographic map • Continuous point-to-point correspondence of adjacent parameters of external stimuli (e.g., locations in visual space or on the body surface), and sensitivities of neurons in neighboring locations in a structure of the brain.

Trace conditioning • A nonstandard version of classical conditioning where the conditioning stimulus (CS) is brief and followed by a blank "trace" period prior to the presentation of the unconditioned stimulus (US).

Transitive inference • The capacity to deduce indirect relations among items that share a common feature and a set of logical rules. For example, if A>B and B>C, then A>C.

Trigger feature • The optimal quality of a stimulus for activation of a neuron. For example, for neurons in primary visual cortex, the trigger feature is a particular contrast orientation of an edge presented to one eye.

Trisynaptic circuit • The series of connections within the hippocampus from the entorhinal cortex to the dentate gyrus, then to field CA3, then to field CA1. Originally thought to be the main processing route through the hippocampus, but expanded by another stage in the circuit from CA1 to the subiculum and direct parahippocampal inputs to CA3 and CA1, and the subiculum.

Unilateral • Pertaining to one side of the brain.

Ventral • Toward the bottom of the brain.

Visual field • A part of the environment one can see, or in which a presented stimulus will cause a neuron to fire. The center and reference point of the visual fields is the fixation point, the locus in space where the eyes converge. All parts of the visual field are relative to the fixation point.

Visuospatial • Pertaining to the location in space of visual stimuli.

Water maze • Device developed by Richard Morris to test spatial memory. Made of a large (usually 2 meter) diameter swimming pool filled with tepid water made opaque with the addition of a milky powder. An escape platform is hidden at one location just beneath the surface of the water and cannot be seen. In the conventional version of the task the rat is released from one of four randomly selected starting points and must find its way to the escape platform guided by cues outside the maze.

Working memory • A combination of storing new incoming information, plus some type of cognitive manipulation, held over a brief period in consciousness. The same term was used by Olton to refer to memory for items that were useful on only a single trial; however, his definition confuses episodic memory and working memory as the contents of current consciousness.

References in Figure Captions

Alvarez, P., Zola-Morgan, S., and Squire, L.R. 1995 Damage limited to the hippocampal region produces long-lasting memory impairment in monkeys. *J. Neurosci.* 15:5 3796–3807.

Alvarez, P., and Squire, L.R. 1994. Memory consolidation and the medial temporal lobe: A simple network model. *Proc. Natl. Acad. Sci. U.S.A.* 91: 7041–7045.

Bear, M.F. 1996. A synaptic basis for memory storage in the cerebral cortex. *Proc. Natl. Acad. Sci. U.S.A.* 93: 13453–13459.

Bechera, A., Tranel, D., Hanna, D., Adolphs, R., Rockland, C., and Damasio, A.R. 1995. Double dissociation of conditioning and declarative knowledge relative to the amygdala and hippocampus in humans. *Science*, 269: 1115–1118.

Bliss, T.V.P., and Collingridge, G.L. 1993. A synaptic model of memory: Long-term potentiation in the hippocampus. *Nature* 361: 31–39.

Brodmann, K. 1909. *Vergleichen de Lokalisationslehre der Grosshirnrinde in irhen Prinzipien dargestellt auf Grund des Zellenbaues.* Leipzig: Barth.

Bunsey, M., and Eichenbaum, H. 1995. Selective damage to the hippocampal region blocks long term retention of a natural and nonspatial stimulus-stimulus association. *Hippocampus* 5: 546–556.

Bunsey, M., and Eichenbaum, H. 1996. Conservation of hippocampal memory function in rats and humans. *Nature* 379: 255–257.

Cahill, L., Prins, B., Weber, M., and McGaugh, J.L. 1994. β-adrenergic activation and memory for emotional events. *Nature* 371: 702–704.

Cho, Y.H., Beracochea, D., and Jaffard, R. 1993. Extended temporal gradient for the retrograde and anterograde amnesia produced by ibotenate entorhinal cortex lesions in mice. *J. Neurosci.* 13: 1759–1766.

Cohen, J.D., Perlstein, W.M., Braver, T.S., Nystrom, L.E., Noll, D.C., Jonides, J., and Smith, E.E. 1997. Temporal dynamics of brain activation during a working memory task. *Nature* 386: 604–607.

Constantine-Paton, M., and Law, M.I. 1982. The development of maps and stripes in the brain. *Sci. Am.* 247: 62–70.

Corkin, S., Amaral, D.G., Gonzalez, R.G., Johnson, K.A., and Hyman, B.T. 1997. H.M.'s medial temporal lobe lesion: Findings from magnetic resonance imaging. *J. Neurosci.* 17: 3964–3979.

Defelipe, J., and Jones, E.G. 1988. *Cajal on the Cerebral Cortex.* New York: Oxford University Press.

Dias, R., Robbins, T.W., and Roberts, A.C. 1996. Dissociation in prefrontal cortex of affective and attentional shifts. *Nature* 380: 69–72.

Dusek J.A., and Eichenbaum, H. 1997. The hippocampus and memory for orderly stimulus relations. *Proc. Natl. Acad. Sci. U.S.A.* 94: 7109–7114.

Eichenbaum, H, Clegg, R.A., Feeley, A. 1983. A re-examination of functional subdivisions of the rodent prefrontal cortex. *Exp. Neurol.* 79: 434–451.

Eichenbaum, H., Stewart, C., and Morris, R.G.M. 1990. Hippocampal representation in spatial learning. *J. Neurosci.* 10: 331–339.

Eichenbaum, H., Dudchenko, P., Wood, E., Shapiro, M., and Tanila, H. 1999. The hippocampus, memory, and place cells: Is it spatial memory or memory space? *Neuron* 23: 1–20.

Eichenbaum, H. 2000. A cortical-hippocampal system for declarative memory. *Nat. Rev. Neurosci.* 1: 41–50.

Funahashi, S., Bruce, C.J., and Goldman-Rakic, P.S. 1989. Mnemonic coding of visual space in the monkey's dorsolateral prefronatl cortex. *J. Neurophysiol.* 61: 331–349.

Gabrieli, J.D.E., Milberg, W., Keane, M., and Corkin, S. 1990. Intact priming of patterns despite impaired memory. *Neuropsychologia* 28: 417–427.

Jonides, J., Rugg, M.D., and Smith, E.E. (Ed.). 1997. The architecture of working memory. In *Cognitive Neuroscience*, Hove East Sussex: Psychology Press, pp. 243–276.

Kermadi I., and Joseph, J.P. 1995. Activity in the caudate nucleus of monkey during spatial sequencing. *J. Neurophysiol.* 74: 911–933.

Kim, J.J., and Fanselow, M.S. 1992. Modality-specific retrograde amnesia of fear. *Science,* 256: 675–677.

Kim, J.J., Clark, R.E., and Thompson, R.F. 1995. Hippocamectomy impairs the memory of recently, but not remotely, aquired trace eyeblink conditioned responses. *Behav. Neurosci.* 109: 195–203.

Knowlton, B.J., Ramus, S., and Squire, L.R. 1992. Intact artificial grammar learning in amnesia. *Psychol. Sci.* 3:3 172–179.

Krupa, D.J., Thompson, J.K., and Thompsom, R.F. 1993. Localization of a memory trace in the mammalian brain. *Nature.* 260: 989—991.

Lashley, K.S. 1929. *Brain Mechanisms and Intelligence: A Quantitative Study of Injuries to the Brain.* New York: Dover (1963 edition).

Maguire, E.A., and Mummery, C.J. 1999. Differential modulation of a common memory retrieval network revealed by positron emission tomography. *Hippocampus,* 9: 54–61.

Martin, A. 1999. Automatic activation of the medial temporal lobe during encoding: Lateralized influences of meaning and novelty. *Hippocampus* 9: 62–70.

McClelland, J.L., McNaughton, B.L., and O'Reilly, R.C. 1995. Why there are complementary learning systems in the hippocampus and neocortex: Insights from the successes and failures of connectionist models of learning and memory. *Psychol. Rev.* 102: 419–457.

McDonald, R.J., and White, N.M. 1993. A triple dissociation of memory systems: Hippocampus, amygdala, and dorsal striatum. *Behav. Neurosci.* 107: 3–22.

McDonald, R.J., and White, N.M. 1994. Parallel information processing in the water maze: Evidence for independent memory systems involving dorsal striatum and hippocampus. *Behav. Neural Biol.* 61: 260–270.

Milner, B., Corkin, S., and Teuber, H.L. 1968. Further analysis of the hippocampal amnesic syndrome: 14- year followup study of H.M. *Neuropsychologia* 6: 215–234.

Morris, R.G.M., and Frey, U. 1997. Hippocampal synaptic plasticity: role in spatial learning or the automatic recording of attended experience? *Phil. Trans. R. Soc. Lond.* 352: 1489–1503.

Morris, R.G.M., Garrud, P., Rawlins, J.P, and O'Keefe, J. 1982. Place navigation impaired in rats with hippocampal lesions. *Nature* 297: 681–683.

Murray, E.A., and Mishkin, M. 1998. Object recognition and location memory in monkeys with excitotoxic lesions of the amygdala and hippocampus *J. Neurosci.* 18: 6568–6582.

Nicoll, R.A., Kauer, J.A., and Malenka, R.C. 1988. The current excitement in long-term potentiation. *Neuron* 1: 87–103.

Otto, T., and Eichenbaum, H. 1992. Complementary roles of orbital prefrontal cortex and the perirhinal-entorhinal cortices in an odor-guided delayed non-matching to sample task. *Behav. Neurosci.* 106: 763–776.

Packard, M.G., and McGaugh, J.L. 1992. Double dissociation of fornix and caudate nucleus lesions on acquistion of two water maze tasks: Further evidence for multiple memory systems. *Behav. Neurosci.* 106: 439–446.

Packard, M.G., and McGaugh, J.L. 1996. Inactivation of hippocampus or caudate nucleus with lidocaine differentially affects expression of place and response learning. *Neurobiol. Learn. Mem.* 65: 65–72.

Packard, M.G., Cahill, L., and McGaugh, J.L. 1994. Amygdala modulation of hippocampal-dependent and caudate nucleus-dependent memory processes. *Proc. Natl. Acad. Sci.* 91: 8477–8481.

Rao, S., C., R., G., and Miller, E.K. 1997. Integration of what and where in the primate prefrontal cortex. *Science* 276: 821–824.

Recanzone, G.H., and Merzenich, M.M. 1991. Alterations of the functional organization of primary somatosensory cortex following intracortical microstimulation or behavioral training. In *Memory: Organization and Locus of Change*, L.R. Squire, N.M. Weinberger, G. Lynch, and J.L. McGaugh, (Eds.). New York: Oxford University Press, pp. 217–238.

Rioult-Pedotti, M.-S., Feriedman, D., Hess, G., and Donoghue, J. 1998. Strengthening of horizontal cortical connections following skill learning. *Nat. Neurosci.* 1: 230–234.

Rogan, M.T., and LeDoux, J.E. 1995. LTP is accompanied by commensurate enhancement of auditory-evoked responses in a fear conditioning circuit. *Neuron* 15: 127–136.

Rogan, M.T., Staubli, U.V., and LeDoux, J.E. 1997. Fear conditioning induces associative long-term potentiation in the amygdala. *Nature* 390: 604–607.

Sakai, K., Naya, Y., Miyashita, Y. 1994. Neuronal tuning and associative mechanisms in form representation. *Learn. Mem.* 1: 83–105.

Squire, L.R. 1987. *Memory and Brain*. New York: Oxford University Press.

Warrington, E.K., and Weiskrantz, L. 1968. New method for testing long-term retention with special reference to amnesic patients. *Nature* 217: 972–974.

Weinberger, N.M. 1993. Learning-induced changes of auditory receptive fields. *Curr. Opin. Neurobiol.* 3: 570–577.

Winocur, G. 1990. Anterograde and retrograde amnesia in rats with dorsal hippocampal or dorsomedial thalamic lesions. *Behav. Brain Res.*, 38: 145–154.

Wood, E.R., Dudchenko, P.A., and Eichenbaum, H. 1999. The global record of memory in hippocampal neuronal activity. *Nature*, 397: 613–616.

Wood, E., Dudchenko, P., Robitsek, J.R., and Eichenbaum, H. 2000. Hippocampal neurons encode information about different types of memory episodes occurring in the same location. *Neuron* 27: 623–633.

Young, B.J., Otto, T., Fox, G.D., and Eichenbaum, H. 1997. Memory representation within the parahippocampal region. *J. Neurosci.*, 17: 5183–5195.

Zola-Morgan, S.M., and Squire, L.R. 1990. The primate hippocampal formation : Evidence for a time-limited role in memory storage. *Science* 250: 288–290.

Zola-Morgan, S., Squire, L.R., and Amaral, D.G. 1989. Lesions of the amygdala that spare adjacent cortical regions do not impair memory or exacerbate the impairment following lesions of the hippocampal formation. *J. Neurosci.* 9: 1922–1936.

Index

Page numbers followed by "f" indicate figures.